Myeloproliferative Neoplasms

Editors

RONALD HOFFMAN
ROSS LEVINE
JOHN MASCARENHAS
RAAJIT K. RAMPAL

HEMATOLOGY/ONCOLOGY CLINICS OF NORTH AMERICA

www.hemonc.theclinics.com

Consulting Editors
GEORGE P. CANELLOS
EDWARD J. BENZ Jr

April 2021 • Volume 35 • Number 2

ELSEVIER

1600 John F. Kennedy Boulevard • Suite 1800 • Philadelphia, Pennsylvania, 19103-2899

http://www.theclinics.com

HEMATOLOGY/ONCOLOGY CLINICS OF NORTH AMERICA Volume 35, Number 2
April 2021 ISSN 0889-8588, ISBN 13: 978-0-323-79588-3

Editor: Stacy Eastman
Developmental Editor: Ann Gielou M. Posedio

Hematology/Oncology Clinics (ISSN 0889-8588) is published bimonthly by Elsevier Inc., 360 Park Avenue South, New York, NY 10010-1710. Months of issue are February, April, June, August, October, and December. Business and Editorial Offices: 1600 John F. Kennedy Blvd., Ste. 1800, Philadelphia, PA 19103–2899. Customer Service Office: 3251 Riverport Lane, Maryland Heights, MO 63043. Periodicals postage paid at New York, NY and at additional mailing offices. Subscription prices are $456.00 per year (domestic individuals), $1150.00 per year (domestic institutions), $100.00 per year (domestic students/residents), $480.00 per year (Canadian individuals), $100.00 per year (Canadian students/residents), $1213.00 per year (Canadian institutions) $547.00 per year (international individuals), $1213.00 per year (international institutions), and $255.00 per year (international students/residents). International air speed delivery is included in all *Clinics* subscription prices. All prices are subject to change without notice. **POSTMASTER:** Send address changes to *Hematology/Oncology Clinics of North America*, Elsevier Health Sciences Division, Subscription Customer Service, 3251 Riverport Lane, Maryland Heights, MO 63043. Customer Service (orders, claims, online, change of address): Elsevier Health Sciences Division, Subscription **Customer Service, 3251 Riverport Lane, Maryland Heights, MO 63043. Tel: 1-800-654-2452 (U.S. and Canada); 314-447-8871 (outside U.S. and Canada). Fax: 314-447-8029. E-mail: journalscustomerservice-usa@elsevier.com (for print support); journalsonlinesupport-usa@elsevier.com (for online support).**

Reprints. For copies of 100 or more, of articles in this publication, please contact the Commercial Reprints Department, Elsevier Inc., 360 Park Avenue South, New York, New York 10010-1710; Tel.: 212-633-3874, Fax: 212-633-3820, E-mail: reprints@elsevier.com.

Hematology/Oncology Clinics of North America is covered in *MEDLINE/PubMed (Index Medicus), EMBASE/ Excerpta Medica, and BIOSIS.*

Contributors

CONSULTING EDITORS

GEORGE P. CANELLOS, MD
William Rosenberg Professor of Medicine, Department of Medical Oncology, Dana-Farber Cancer Institute, Boston, Massachusetts, USA

EDWARD J. BENZ Jr, MD
Professor, Pediatrics, Richard and Susan Smith Professor, Medicine, Professor, Genetics, Harvard Medical School, President and CEO Emeritus, Office of the President, Dana-Farber Cancer Institute, Boston, Massachusetts, USA

EDITORS

RONALD HOFFMAN, MD
Albert A. and Vera G. List Professor of Medicine, Director, Myeloproliferative Disorders Research Program, Tisch Cancer Institute, Division of Hematology and Medical Oncology, Icahn School of Medicine at Mount Sinai, New York, New York, USA

ROSS LEVINE, MD
Laurence Joseph Dineen Chair in Leukemia Research, Chief, Molecular Cancer Medicine Service, Human Oncology and Pathogenesis Program, Leukemia Service, Department of Medicine, Center for Hematologic Malignancies, Center for Epigenetics Research, Memorial Sloan Kettering Cancer Center, New York, New York, USA

JOHN MASCARENHAS, MD
Director, Adult Leukemia Program, Leader, Myeloproliferative Disorders Clinical Research Program, Associate Professor of Medicine, Division of Hematology/Oncology, Tisch Cancer Institute, Icahn School of Medicine at Mount Sinai, New York, New York, USA

RAAJIT K. RAMPAL, MD, PhD
Assistant Member, Leukemia Service, Department of Medicine, Center for Hematologic Malignancies, Memorial Sloan Kettering Cancer Service, New York, New York, USA

AUTHORS

KARIE CHEN, MS
Department of Medicine, Division of Hematology/Oncology, Icahn School of Medicine at Mount Sinai, New York, New York, USA

NATALIE C. CHEN, MD, PhD
Resident, Department of Internal Medicine, The University of Texas School of Health Sciences at Houston, Houston, Texas, USA

JOHN D. CRISPINO, PhD
Chief, Division of Experimental Hematology, St. Jude Children's Research Hospital, Memphis, Tennessee, USA

MARTA B. DAVIDSON, PhD, MD, FRCPC
Clinical Research Fellow, Division of Medical Oncology and Hematology, University Health Network, Princess Margaret Cancer Centre, Toronto, Ontario, Canada

AMYLOU C. DUECK, PhD
Associate Professor of Biostatistics and Vice Chair, Department of Health Sciences Research, Division of Biomedical Statistics and Informatics, Scottsdale, Arizona, USA

ANDREW DUNBAR, MD
Department of Medicine, Leukemia Service, Center for Hematologic Malignancies, Memorial Sloan Kettering Cancer Center, New York, New York, USA

RYAN ECKERT, MS
Research Coordinator, Mays Cancer Center, UT Health San Antonio MD Anderson Cancer Center, San Antonio, Texas, USA; Research Affiliate, Arizona State University College of Health Solutions, Phoenix, Arizona, USA

ANGELA G. FLEISCHMAN, MD, PhD
Associate Professor, Division of Hematology/Oncology, Department of Medicine, Department of Biological Chemistry, Irvine Chao Family Comprehensive Cancer Center, University of California, Irvine, California, USA

AARON T. GERDS, MD, MS
Leukemia and Myeloid Disorders Program, Cleveland Clinic Taussig Cancer Institute, Cleveland, Ohio, USA

VIKAS GUPTA, MD, FRCP, FRCPath
Professor, Department of Medicine, Princess Margaret Cancer Centre, University of Toronto, Toronto, Ontario, Canada

RONALD HOFFMAN, MD
Albert A. and Vera G. List Professor of Medicine, Director, Myeloproliferative Disorders Research Program, Tisch Cancer Institute, Division of Hematology and Medical Oncology, Icahn School of Medicine at Mount Sinai, New York, New York, USA

JENNIFER HUBERTY, PhD
Associate Professor, Arizona State University College of Health Solutions, Phoenix, Arizona, USA; Adjunct Faculty, Mays Cancer Center, UT Health San Antonio MD Anderson Cancer Center, San Antonio, Texas, USA

TANIA JAIN, MBBS
Assistant Professor, Division of Hematological Malignancies and Stem Cell Transplantation, Department of Oncology, The Sidney Kimmel Comprehensive Cancer Center at Johns Hopkins University, Baltimore, Maryland, USA

ASHWIN KISHTAGARI, MD
Leukemia and Myeloid Disorders Program, Cleveland Clinic Taussig Cancer Institute, Cleveland, Ohio, USA

RAMI S. KOMROKJI, MD
Senior Member, Department of Malignant Hematology, Moffitt Cancer Center, Tampa, Florida, USA

HEIDI E. KOSIOREK, MS
Assistant Supervisor and Statistician, Department of Health Sciences Research, Division of Biomedical Statistics and Informatics, Mayo Clinic, Scottsdale, Arizona, USA

ANDREW T. KUYKENDALL, MD
Assistant Member, Department of Malignant Hematology, Moffitt Cancer Center, Tampa, Florida, USA

ROSS LEVINE, MD
Laurence Joseph Dineen Chair in Leukemia Research, Chief, Molecular Cancer Medicine Service, Human Oncology and Pathogenesis Program, Leukemia Service, Department of Medicine, Center for Hematologic Malignancies, Center for Epigenetics Research, Memorial Sloan Kettering Cancer Center, New York, New York, USA

JOHN MASCARENHAS, MD
Director, Adult Leukemia Program, Leader, Myeloproliferative Disorders Clinical Research Program, Associate Professor of Medicine, Division of Hematology/Oncology, Tisch Cancer Institute, Icahn School of Medicine at Mount Sinai, New York, New York, USA

ADAM J. MEAD, MA, BMBCh, FTCP, FRCPath, PhD
Medical Research Council (MRC) Molecular Haematology Unit, MRC Weatherall Institute of Molecular Medicine, NIHR Biomedical Research Centre, University of Oxford, Oxford, United Kingdom

JOHANNA MELO-CARDENAS, PhD
Postdoctoral Research Associate, Division of Experimental Hematology, St. Jude Children's Research Hospital, Memphis, Tennessee, USA

RUBEN MESA, MD
Director, Mays Cancer Center, UT Health San Antonio MD Anderson Cancer Center, San Antonio, Texas, USA

SARA C. MEYER, MD, PhD
Attending Physician and Research Group Leader, Division of Hematology and Department of Biomedicine, University Hospital Basel and University of Basel, Basel, Switzerland

ANNA RITA MIGLIACCIO, PhD
Professor, Department of Biomedical and Neuromotor Sciences, University of Bologna, Bologna, Italy

JEANNE PALMER, MD
Division of Hematology and Medical Oncology, Mayo Clinic, Phoenix, Arizona, USA

YOUNG PARK, MS
Center for Epigenetics Research, Memorial Sloan Kettering Cancer Center, New York, New York, USA

NAVEEN PEMMARAJU, MD
Associate Professor, Department of Leukemia, The University of Texas MD Anderson Cancer Center, Houston, Texas, USA

NIKOLAI A. PODOLTSEV, MD, PhD
Associate Professor, Section of Hematology, Department of Internal Medicine, Yale School of Medicine and Yale Cancer Center, New Haven, Connecticut, USA

BETHAN PSAILA, MA, MBBS, MRCP, FRCPath, PhD
Medical Research Council (MRC) Molecular Haematology Unit, MRC Weatherall Institute of Molecular Medicine, NIHR Biomedical Research Centre, University of Oxford, Oxford, United Kingdom

GAJALAKSHMI RAMANATHAN, PhD
Division of Hematology/Oncology, Department of Medicine, University of California, Irvine, California, USA

RAAJIT K. RAMPAL, MD, PhD
Assistant Member, Leukemia Service, Department of Medicine, Center for Hematologic Malignancies, Memorial Sloan Kettering Cancer Service, New York, New York, USA

DANIEL ROYSTON, MBChB, BMSc, DPhil, FRCPath
Nuffield Division of Clinical Laboratory Sciences, Radcliffe Department of Medicine and NIHR Biomedical Research Centre, University of Oxford, Oxford, United Kingdom

MOHAMED E. SALAMA, MD
Professor, Department of Laboratory Medicine and Pathology, Division of Hematopathology, Professor, Mayo Clinic School of Medicine, Mayo Clinic, Rochester, Minnesota, USA

ANDREW I. SCHAFER, MD
Professor of Medicine, Director, Richard T. Silver, M.D. Myeloproliferative Neoplasms Center, Emeritus Chairman, Department of Medicine, Weill Cornell Medical College, New York, New York, USA

RORY M. SHALLIS, MD
Assistant Professor, Section of Hematology, Department of Internal Medicine, Yale School of Medicine and Yale Cancer Center, New Haven, Connecticut, USA

ALAN H. SHIH, MD, PhD
Assistant Professor, Department of Medicine, Division of Hematology/Oncology, Icahn School of Medicine at Mount Sinai, New York, New York, USA

JAKUB SZYBINSKI, PhD
Department of Biomedicine, University Hospital Basel and University of Basel, Basel, Switzerland

FRANCO CASTILLO TOKUMORI, MD
Department of Internal Medicine, University of South Florida, Tampa, Florida, USA

DOUGLAS TREMBLAY, MD
Clinical Fellow, Division of Hematology and Medical Oncology, Tisch Cancer Institute, Icahn School of Medicine at Mount Sinai, New York, New York, USA

SANGEETHA VENUGOPAL, MD
Division of Hematology/Oncology, Tisch Cancer Institute, Icahn School of Medicine at Mount Sinai, New York, New York, USA; Fellow, Department of Leukemia, The University of Texas MD Anderson Cancer Center, Houston, New York, USA

SRDAN VERSTOVSEK, MD, PhD
Professor, Department of Leukemia, The University of Texas MD Anderson Cancer Center, Houston, Texas, USA

RONG WANG, PhD
Research Scientist, Department of Chronic Disease Epidemiology, Yale School of Public Health, Yale University, New Haven, Connecticut, USA

ABDULRAHEEM YACOUB, MD
Associate Professor, Division of Hematologic Malignancies and Cellular Therapeutics, Department of Internal Medicine, The University of Kansas Cancer Center, Westwood, Kansas, USA

AMER M. ZEIDAN, MBBS, MHS
Associate Professor, Section of Hematology, Department of Internal Medicine, Yale School of Medicine and Yale Cancer Center, New Haven, Connecticut, USA

Contents

Myeloproliferative disorders are a group of diseases morphologically linked by terminal myeloid cell expansion that frequently evolve from one clinical phenotype to another and eventually progress to acute myeloid leukemia. Diagnostic criteria for the Philadelphia chromosome–negative myeloproliferative neoplasms (MPNs) have been established by the World Health Organization and they are recognized as blood cancers. MPNs have a complex and incompletely understood pathogenesis that includes systemic inflammation, clonal hematopoiesis, and constitutive activation of the JAK-STAT pathway. Complications, such as thrombosis and progression to overt forms of myelofibrosis and acute leukemia, contribute significantly to morbidity and mortality of patients with MPN.

Polycythemia vera (PV), essential thrombocythemia (ET), and primary myelofibrosis (PMF) comprise the BCR-ABL-negative classical myeloproliferative neoplasms (MPNs). These clonal myeloid diseases are principally driven by well-described molecular events; however, factors leading to their acquisition are not well understood. Beyond increasing age, male sex, and race/ethnicity differences, few consistent risk factors for the MPNs are known. PV and ET have an incidence of 0.5 to 4.0 and 1.1 to 2.0 cases per 100,000 person-years, respectively, and predict similar survival. PMF, which has an incidence of about 0.3 to 2.0 cases per 100,000 person-years, is associated with the shortest survival of the MPNs.

Megakaryocytes give rise to platelets, which have a wide variety of functions in coagulation, immune response, inflammation, and tissue repair. Dysregulation of megakaryocytes is a key feature of in the myeloproliferative neoplasms, especially myelofibrosis. Megakaryocytes are among the main drivers of myelofibrosis by promoting myeloproliferation and bone marrow fibrosis. In vivo targeting of megakaryocytes by genetic and pharmacologic approaches ameliorates the disease, underscoring the important role of megakaryocytes in myeloproliferative neoplasms. Here we review the current knowledge of the function of megakaryocytes in the JAK2, CALR, and MPL-mutant myeloproliferative neoplasms

Gajalakshmi Ramanathan and Angela G. Fleischman

Chronic inflammation is a hallmark of myeloproliferative neoplasms (MPNs), with elevated levels of proinflammatory cytokines being commonly found in all 3 subtypes. Systemic inflammation is responsible for the constitutional symptoms, thrombosis risk, premature atherosclerosis, and disease evolution in MPN. Although the neoplastic clone and their differentiated progeny drive the inflammatory process, they also induce ancillary cytokine secretion from nonmalignant cells. Here, the authors describe the inflammatory milieu in MPN based on soluble factors and cellular mediators. They also discuss the prognostic value of cytokine measurements in patients with MPN and potential therapeutic strategies that target the cellular players in inflammation.

Jakub Szybinski and Sara C. Meyer

Myeloproliferative neoplasms are hematopoietic stem cell disorders based on somatic mutations in JAK2, calreticulin, or MPL activating JAK-STAT signaling. Modern sequencing efforts have revealed the genomic landscape of myeloproliferative neoplasms with additional genetic alterations mainly in epigenetic modifiers and splicing factors. High molecular risk mutations with adverse outcomes have been identified and clonal evolution may promote progression to fibrosis and acute myeloid leukemia. JAK2V617F is recurrently detected in clonal hematopoiesis of indeterminate potential with increased risk for vascular events. Insights into the genetics of myeloproliferative neoplasms has facilitated diagnosis and prognostication and poses novel candidates for targeted therapeutic intervention.

Andrew Dunbar, Young Park, and Ross Levine

This article reviews the genetic data on epigenetic modifying mutations in myeloproliferative neoplasms and their clinical implications, preclinical studies exploring our current understanding of how mutations in epigenetic modifying proteins cooperate with myeloproliferative neoplasms drivers to promote disease progression, and recent advances in novel therapeutics supporting the role of targeting epigenetic pathways to treat fibrotic progression.

Karie Chen and Alan H. Shih

Myeloproliferative neoplasms, such as polycythemia vera, essential thrombocythemia, and primary myelofibrosis, are bone marrow disorders that result in the overproduction of mature clonal myeloid elements. Identification of recurrent genetic mutations has been described and aid in diagnosis and prognostic determination. Mouse models of these mutations have confirmed the biologic significance of these mutations in myeloproliferative neoplasm disease biology and provided greater insights on the pathways that are dysregulated with each mutation. The models are useful tools that have led to preclinical testing and provided data as validation for future myeloproliferative neoplasm clinical trials.

Important Pathologic Considerations for Establishing the Diagnosis of Myelofibrosis

Mohamed E. Salama

Diagnostic criteria for primary myelofibrosis as defined by the 2017 revised World Health Organization (WHO) classification system incorporate clinical and laboratory findings, including driver mutational status (JAK2, MPL, CALR. and triple negative). The WHO emphasized the role of histopathology in making an accurate diagnosis of primary myelofibrosis and successfully incorporated a fibrosis scoring system and scoring schemas for collagen fibrosis and osteosclerosis. These steps represent a significant addition to the standardization of myelofibrosis evaluation and minimize the risk for misdiagnosis. This article reviews important pathologic considerations along with highlights of potentially relevant pitfalls relevant to histopathological diagnosis of myelofibrosis.

Application of Single-Cell Approaches to Study Myeloproliferative Neoplasm Biology

Daniel Royston, Adam J. Mead, and Bethan Psaila

Philadelphia-negative myeloproliferative neoplasms (MPNs) are an excellent tractable disease model of a number of aspects of human cancer biology, including genetic evolution, tissue-associated fibrosis, and cancer stem cells. In this review, we discuss recent insights into MPN biology gained from the application of a number of new single-cell technologies to study human disease, with a specific focus on single-cell genomics, single-cell transcriptomics, and digital pathology.

Unmet Need in Essential Thrombocythemia and Polycythemia Vera

Ashwin Kishtagari and Aaron T. Gerds

Consensus guidelines have helped to standardize the care of patients with essential thrombocythemia and polycythemia vera, focusing on reducing the risk of thrombosis, mitigating symptoms, and avoiding therapies that may accelerate disease progression. However, many unmet needs still exist ranging from the roll of antiplatelet therapy in ET to medications that reduce disease progression. Retrospective studies suggest an improvement in myelofibrosis-free survival for treatment with interferons; new agents are looking to also enact disease modification.

Thrombotic, Vascular, and Bleeding Complications of the Myeloproliferative Neoplasms

Andrew I. Schafer

Thrombotic, vascular, and bleeding complications are the most frequent causes of morbidity and mortality in myeloproliferative neoplasms

(MPNs). The interplay and reciprocal amplification between two factors are considered to lead to thrombosis in MPNs: (1) circulating blood cell–intrinsic abnormalities caused by an MPN driver mutation in their hematopoietic progenitor/stem cells, interacting with vascular endothelial cells, show prothrombotic and proadhesive phenotypes; and (2) a state of usually subclinical systemic inflammation that fuels the thrombotic tendency. Prevention and treatment require maintenance of hematocrit less than 45% and cytoreductive therapy in patients with a high risk for thrombotic and vascular complications.

Accelerated and blast phase myeloproliferative neoplasms are advanced stages of the disease with historically a poor prognosis and little improvement in outcomes thus far. The lack of responses to standard treatments likely results from the more aggressive biology reflected by the higher incidence of complex karyotype and high-risk somatic mutations, which are enriched at the time of transformation. Treatment options include induction chemotherapy (7 + 3) as that used on de novo acute myeloid leukemia or hypomethylating agent–based therapy, which has shown similar outcomes. Allogeneic stem cell transplantation remains the only potential for cure.

Myelodysplastic syndrome/Myeloproliferative neoplasms (MDS/MPNs) are molecularly complex, clinically heterogeneous diseases that exhibit proliferative and dysplastic features. Diagnostic criteria use clinical, pathologic, and genomic features to distinguish between disease entities, though considerable clinical and genetic overlap persists. MDS/MPNs are associated with a poor prognosis, save for MDS/MPN with ring sideroblasts and thrombocytosis, which can behave more indolently. The current treatment approach is risk-adapted and symptom-directed and largely extrapolated from experience in MDS or MPN. Gene sequencing has demonstrated frequent mutations involving signaling, epigenetic, and splicing pathways, which present numerous therapeutic opportunities for clinical investigation.

The US Food and Drug Administration (FDA) approval of Janus kinase 2 inhibitors, ruxolitinib and fedratinib for the treatment of intermediate-2 or high-risk primary or secondary myelofibrosis (MF) has revolutionized the management of MF. Nevertheless, these drugs do not reliably alter the natural history of disease. Burgeoning understanding of the molecular pathogenesis and the bone marrow microenvironment in MF has galvanized the development of targeted therapeutics. This review provides insight into the novel therapies under clinical evaluation.

Myeloproliferative neoplasms include essential thrombocythemia, polycythemia vera, and myelofibrosis. They are characterized by abnormal myeloid proliferation. Patients suffer from debilitating constitutional symptoms and splenomegaly. There have been advances in understanding the impact on quality of life in myeloproliferative neoplasms. Owing to the chronicity of these diseases, symptoms are considered in response criteria for clinical trials. This review wills cover how quality of life is measured in patients with myeloproliferative neoplasm. We review the impact of treatment options, including JAK inhibitors, allogeneic stem cell transplantation, and medications in development. We discuss non-pharmacologic methods of improving symptoms and quality of life.

Myelofibrosis (MF) belongs to a group of clonal stem cell disorders known as the *BCR-ABL*-negative myeloproliferative neoplasms. Allogeneic hematopoietic stem cell transplantation (HCT) is currently the only curative treatment option for MF. Because HCT can be associated with significant morbidity and mortality, patients need to be carefully selected based on disease-risk, fitness, and transplant factors. Furthermore, in the era of JAK inhibitors, the timing of transplantation has become a challenging question. Here the authors review recent developments in HCT for MF, focusing on risk stratification and optimal timing.

Myeloproliferative neoplasms are characterized by chronic inflammation. The discovery of constitutively active JAK-STAT signaling associated with driver mutations has led to clinical and translational breakthroughs. Insights into the other pathways and novel factors of potential importance are being actively investigated. Various classes of agents with immunomodulating or immunosuppressive properties have been used with varying degrees of success in treating myeloproliferative neoplasms. Early clinical trials are investigating the feasibility, effectiveness, and safety of immune checkpoint inhibitors, cell-based immunotherapies, and SMAC mimetics. The dynamic landscape of immunotherapy and immunomodulation in myeloproliferative neoplasms is the topic of the present review.

Design features of phase I, II, and III clinical trials of pharmaceutical interventions in myelofibrosis (MF) are discussed. Model-assisted and model-based designs for phase I trials are useful for maximizing therapeutic benefit and include novel approaches to dose escalation. Trials in MF have shifted to accommodate new challenges following approval of JAK inhibitor therapies. Standardized response criteria exist; however, alternative measures of response when evaluating newer agents may be needed. Noninferiority and other adaptive designs can be used to incorporate design changes over time. Patient-reported outcomes, including quality-of-life and symptom assessment, should be included as outcome measures.

HEMATOLOGY/ONCOLOGY CLINICS OF NORTH AMERICA

SERIES OF RELATED INTEREST

Surgical Oncology Clinics of North America
https://www.surgonc.theclinics.com/

THE CLINICS ARE AVAILABLE ONLINE!
Access your subscription at:
www.theclinics.com

Preface

The New Science and Concepts That Underlie Current and Future Treatments for Myeloproliferative Neoplasms

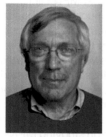
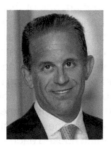
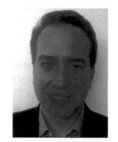

Ronald Hoffman, MD   Ross Levine, MD   John Mascarenhas, MD

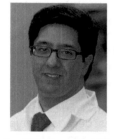

Raajit K. Rampal, MD,
PhD

Editors

The myeloproliferative neoplasms (MPNs) represent a group of chronic hematologic malignancies that have been recently the subject of more intense investigation since the discovery 15 years ago of driver mutations that underlie their biology and clinical manifestations. Previously, these disorders, which include polycythemia vera, essential thrombocythemia, and primary myelofibrosis, were thought to represent diseases that shared many clinical features and were unique in their ability to evolve from one clinical phenotype to another and to eventually evolve into an untreatable form of secondary leukemia. Each of the guest editors (Ronald Hoffman, Ross Levine, John Mascarenhas, and Raajit K. Rampal) represents one in a long line of distinguished hematologists and cancer biologists who have spent their careers studying these

Hematol Oncol Clin N Am 35 (2021) xvii–xix
https://doi.org/10.1016/j.hoc.2021.01.004
0889-8588/21/© 2021 Published by Elsevier Inc.

hemonc.theclinics.com

diseases and made innumerable contributions to this field. Our editorship of this issue might seem to exemplify hubris, but we must apologize in that we clearly recognize that the work presented here is the result of the whole community of past and present MPN researchers and their patients. These efforts of the hematology community have led to steady progress in the diagnosis and treatment of the MPNs, and fortunately, the pace of success has heightened over the last decade. The focus of these efforts has always been to improve the outcomes of patients with MPNs and to eventually cure patients with these debilitating disorders. Many have frequently asked why these relatively rare malignancies are the subject of so much interest. The answer to this question was obtained by one of the authors (R.H.) when he was a hematology fellow at the Mount Sinai Hospital in New York in the mid-1970s and his responsibilities included rounding daily with Dr Louis Wasserman, one of the leading MPN clinicians of that day. Although Wasserman was a connoisseur of art and much of the banter during these rounds dealt with the education of the then young hematology fellow in art, R.H. once asked Dr Wasserman why he was so interested in this group of diseases. Wasserman looked out in amazement and provided an answer that resonates with the content of this issue. The aging and often intimidating professor clearly stated that by studying the MPNs one had the opportunity to learn about every aspect of not only hematology but actually medicine and that lessons learned from studying MPNs could be applied to numerous other areas of medicine. Our editorial team continues to think about this response and its wisdom, which hooked each of us on studying MPNs. As you review the Table of Contents for this issue, you will quickly realize that the work dealing with MPNs summarized here involves diverse areas of not only hematology but also medicine and biology, including megakaryocyte and stem cell biology, epigenetics, genetics, epidemiology, stem cell transplantation, inflammation, thrombosis, bleeding, atherosclerosis, quality-of-life issues, murine modeling of hematologic malignancies, classifications of hematologic malignancies, new diagnostic and investigative laboratory techniques, and therapeutic options. The knowledge summarized here by our talented group of authors is useful for individuals working with not only MPNs but also many other disciplines. The science and medicine of the MPNs remain in their infancy, but if we can be judged by the progress made during the last decade summarized here, we remain optimistic that this multidisciplinary, scientific, and systematic approach will soon result in important therapeutic options that will be life-changing for the MPN patients, who remain our focus.

Ronald Hoffman, MD
Tisch Cancer Institute
Division of Hematology/Oncology
Icahn School of Medicine at Mount Sinai
One Gustave L. Levy Place, Box 1079
New York, NY 10029, USA

Ross Levine, MD
Molecular Cancer Medicine Service
Human Oncology and Pathogenesis Program
Leukemia Service, Department of Medicine
Center for Hematologic Malignancies
Center for Epigenetics Research
Memorial Sloan Kettering Cancer Center
1275 York Avenue, Box 20
New York, NY 10065, USA

John Mascarenhas, MD
Tisch Cancer Institute
Division of Hematology/Oncology
Icahn School of Medicine at Mount Sinai
One Gustave L. Levy Place, Box 1079
New York, NY 10029, USA

Raajit K. Rampal, MD, PhD
Leukemia Service, Department of Medicine
Center for Hematologic Malignancies
Memorial Sloan Kettering Cancer Service
530 East 74th Street
New York, NY 10021, USA

E-mail addresses:
ronald.hoffman@mssm.edu (R. Hoffman)
leviner@mskcc.org (R. Levine)
john.mascarenhas@mssm.edu (J. Mascarenhas)
rampalr@mskcc.org (R.K. Rampal)

Overview of Myeloproliferative Neoplasms
History, Pathogenesis, Diagnostic Criteria, and Complications

Douglas Tremblay, MD[a], Abdulraheem Yacoub, MD[b],
Ronald Hoffman, MD[a],*

KEYWORDS

- Myeloproliferative neoplasms • Myelofibrosis • Polycythemia vera
- Essential thrombocythemia • History • Diagnostic criteria

KEY POINTS

- Myeloproliferative neoplasms (MPNs) are clinically and biologically related but clinically and histopathologically distinct chronic hematopoietic disorders.
- Diagnostic criteria for each MPN have been established by the World Health Organization and often include a bone marrow biopsy.
- Pathobiologically, MPNs are progressive clonal diseases originating at the level of the hematopoietic stem cell, which are associated with three specific driver mutations resulting in constitutive activation of the JAK-STAT pathway, systemic inflammation, constitutional symptoms, and splenomegaly.
- Major complications include thrombosis and progression of disease, either to a fibrotic stage or blast phase.

INTRODUCTION

Myeloproliferative neoplasms (MPNs) are a group of clonal hematologic malignancies morphologically characterized by expansion of terminally differentiated myeloid cells (white blood cells erythrocytes and platelets).[1] There are three classical Philadelphia-negative MPNs (hereafter referred to as MPNs): (1) polycythemia vera (PV), (2) essential thrombocythemia (ET), and (3) primary myelofibrosis (PMF). In addition, a prefibrotic form of myelofibrosis (pre-PMF) is increasingly recognized

[a] Division of Hematology and Medical Oncology, Tisch Cancer Institute, Icahn School of Medicine at Mount Sinai, One Gustave L. Levy Place, New York, NY 10029, USA; [b] Division of Hematologic Malignancies and Cellular Therapeutics, Department of Internal Medicine, The University of Kansas Cancer Center, 2330 Shawnee Mission Parkway, Westwood, KS 66205, USA
* Corresponding author.
E-mail address: ronald.hoffman@mssm.edu

Hematol Oncol Clin N Am 35 (2021) 159–176
https://doi.org/10.1016/j.hoc.2020.12.001
0889-8588/21/© 2020 Elsevier Inc. All rights reserved.

hemonc.theclinics.com

as a distinct member of the MPNs. Moreover, there are a group of patients that share many features of an MPN that do not meet diagnostic criteria for PMF, ET, and PV and they fall into a grab bag group termed MPNs-unclassifiable. MPNs are often discussed together because they share similar pathobiologic and clinical features. In addition, patients with ET and PV can progress to myelofibrosis (MF), termed post-ET MF and post-PV MF, respectively.[2] Other rarer diseases classified as MPNs by the World Health Organization (WHO) include chronic neutrophilic leukemia, mastocytosis, and chronic eosinophilic leukemia but are not discussed here.[3]

Initially chronic myeloid leukemia (CML) was included as a classical MPN, in addition to paroxysmal nocturnal hemoglobinuria. However, CML was found to be associated with a specific cytogenetic abnormality, a translocation between chromosome 9 and 22 resulting in the generation of the BCR/ABL fusion gene, which possessed tyrosine kinase activity.[4] Patients with CML inevitably progressed to a universally fatal form of acute leukemia termed CML blast crisis, which was refractory to chemotherapy. This progression of CML to CML blast phase was associated with the progressive acquisition of new cytogenetic abnormalities, which provided evidence of the multistep pathogenesis of a hematologic malignancy.[5] During the 1970s, 1980s, and 1990s patients with CML could only be cured in the chronic phase of their disease by allogeneic stem cell transplantation, confirming that CML was a stem cell disease.[6] In fact, during this period CML was the most frequent indication for allogeneic stem cell transplantation.[7] However, this picture dramatically changed in the 1990s with the discovery of specific tyrosine kinase inhibitors that inhibited the BCR/ABL fusion protein and led to the depletion of CML progenitor and stem cells.[8] This first-in-class tyrosine kinase inhibitor, imatinib, was approved by the Food and Drug Administration in 2001 and changed the outcomes of virtually all patients with CML.[9] The discovery of imatinib was a result of synergistic interactions between academic scientists and clinicians with the pharmaceutical industry focusing on discovery science and translating these findings into the development of strategies to improve the lives of patients with cancer. The other Philadelphia chromosome–negative MPNs, including ET, PV, and PMF, share many clinical characteristics with CML. Although their clinical courses are frequently more indolent than CML, their origins have proven to be more complex, which has hampered success in developing therapeutic agents that share the clinical efficacy of imatinib.

Clinical manifestations across MPNs include panmyelosis (marrow hypercellularity with multilineage involvement), splenomegaly, constitutional symptoms, and a propensity toward thrombosis or bleeding. An overactive JAK-STAT pathway is a unifying pathobiologic feature of all the MPNs.[10] Thrombotic complications and disease progression are the most serious complications of MPNs and often the most common causes of death in patients with MPNs.[11] Current treatment approaches involve cytoreductive therapy; aspirin; and JAK1/2 inhibitors, such as ruxolitinib and fedratinib. Although these agents have demonstrated success in terms of symptom control and reduction in spleen volume, they do not necessarily halt disease progression.[12–14] At present, the only curative therapy for patients with MPNs is allogeneic stem cell transplantation, which is offered to a limited proportion of patients with MF with advanced-risk disease and without prohibitive comorbidities.[15] Thus, there is considerable interest in the development of novel agents for patients with MPNs, particularly MF.[16,17] These new therapeutic strategies are detailed in Sangeetha Venugopal and John Mascarenhas' article, "Current Clinical Investigations in Myelofibrosis," in this issue.

Epidemiologically, the MPNs are considered to be a rare disease. The incidence of PV and ET is around 1 to 2 per 100,000 in the United States, whereas the incidence of

PMF is 0.3 per 100,000.[18] Although typically thought of as a disease of older adults, with a median age of around 60 years, MPNs can also arise in young adults and children.[19,20] MPNs are generally more common in males as compared with females, with the notable exception of ET, which is more prevalent among females.[21] Amer Zeiden and Nikolai Podoltsev delve into more specifics of the epidemiology of MPNs in their article "Epidemiology of the Philadelphia Chromosome-Negative Classical Myeloproliferative Neoplasms," in this issue.

In this introductory article on the series, we first detail the history of MPNs including original observations and relevant scientific and clinical figures in the early conceptual development. To set the stage for the remainder of this series, we detail diagnostic criteria as defined by the WHO. We then briefly describe the pathophysiology, concentrating on unifying themes that run across each of the MPNs. Finally, we describe complications of MPNs including thrombosis and progression.

HISTORY

The dawn of hematology occurred in the mid-1650s. The refinement of the light microscope in the 1600s allowed Dutch biologist Jan Swammerdam to visualize the red blood cells of a frog in 1658.[22] Unaware of his work, Antonie van Leeuwenhoek also visualized the red blood cells (from blood pricked from his thumb) and estimated their size as "25,000 times smaller than a fine grain of sand."[23] White blood cells were first described in 1749 by Joseph Lieutaud, calling them *globuli albicantes*.[24] Platelets were the last blood cell lineage to be identified by Alfred François Donné in 1842.[25] The first MPN to be described was CML, which was detailed in a 1845 case report by the English pathologist John Hughes Bennett.[26] It was not until 1879 that cases of MF were reported by Gustav Heuck, a German surgeon, who detailed two young patients with massive splenomegaly, leukoerythroblastosis, and bone marrow fibrosis, differentiating it from CML.[27] The first description of PV came in 1882, when the French physician Louis Henri Vaquez described a 40-year-old man with chronic vascular congestion with marked erythrocytosis. On autopsy, no cardiac abnormalities were noted but he did observe splenomegaly and hepatomegaly. Vaquez concluded that this disease was caused by hematopoietic hyperactivity, a remarkable conclusion considering the time.[28] This description was further defined by William Osler 1903 when he described four cases of "chronic cyanosis, with polycythemia and enlarged spleen: a new clinical entity."[29] ET was the last MPN to be formally described. Two Austrian pathologists, Emil Epstein and Alfred Goedel, described a patient with extreme thrombocytosis ("more than three times normal values") associated with megakaryocytic hyperplasia. This patient had recurrent mucocutaneous bleeding.[30]

One of the most important figures responsible for developing the concept that the MPNs are an interrelated group of disorders was William Dameshek. In 1951, he hypothesized that trilineage myeloproliferation unified CML PMF, PV, and ET and coined this group of diseases as "myeloproliferative disorders." He considered these disease to be clinically and biologically related and "perhaps due to a hitherto undiscovered stimulus."[31] A major step in understanding the underlying cause of MPNs was made by Philip Fialkow, who studied polymorphisms in the X-linked glucose-6-phosphate dehydrogenase locus to confirm the clonal nature of PV,[32] ET,[33] and PMF.[34] Although many hematologists had debated whether these myeloproliferative disorders represented blood cancers, the seminal investigations of Fialkow and his talented group of collaborators indicated that these disorders were clonal in origin and involved all types of myeloid cells, supplying the first indications that they represented hematologic malignancies that originated at the level of the hematopoietic stem cell. Although the pathobiologic understanding of MPNs progressed, methodologic rigor was not applied to therapeutic efforts. Louis Wasserman, an American hematologist from Mount Sinai Hospital, formed the Polycythemia Vera Study Group in 1967. This group formalized clinical investigation of PV and included seminal multi-institutional, international studies establishing the leukemogenicity of chlorambucil and intravenous P-32,[35] providing early evidence of hydroxyurea efficacy in reducing thrombosis,[36] and describing the dangers of high-dose antiplatelet therapy.[37] The next paradigm shift in the MPN field occurred in 2005 when four independent laboratories identified the gain-of-function *JAK2V617F* mutation that is possessed by virtually all patients with PV and 50% of patients with ET and MF.[38–41] There have been numerous other important discoveries over the last 15 years. Subsequently, driver mutations in the thrombopoietin receptor (*MPL*) and chaperone protein calreticulin (*CALR*) were reported in patients with ET and MF and a mutation in exon 12 of *JAK2* rather than exon 14 as occurs in *JAK2V617F* was shown to be associated with a form of PV characterized by isolated erythrocytosis. As this issue outlines, the understanding of MPNs has deepened dramatically since the days of Dameshek. However, observations made by these pioneers in the field (**Fig. 1**) are still fundamental to the current understanding of the pathogenesis and treatment of MPNs.

DIAGNOSTIC CRITERIA

The WHO has proposed the most widely used diagnostic criteria for MPNs. The 2016 revision of these criteria for PV, ET, and PMF are listed in **Boxes 1–3**, respectively.[3] Megakaryocytic hyperplasia and atypia is one of the cardinal histopathologic features of each of the MPNs. The cause and consequences of this megakaryocytic hyperplasia in the MPNs is discussed by Johanna Melo-Cardenas and colleagues' article, "The Role of Megakaryocytes in Myelofibrosis," in this issue. The WHO criteria are far from perfect and numerous investigators debate their value. They have, however, proven useful in identifying patients with a particular MPN for entry in clinical trials but in everyday practice they should be used as guides to diagnosis rather than rigid criteria.

PV is suspected in a patient with an elevated hematocrit; however, a full evaluation is required. Polycythemia must be classified as relative or absolute. Relative polycythemia occurs in the setting of an absolute increase in hematocrit without an increase in red cell mass. This is typically a spurious finding caused by a contraction in plasma volume in the setting of protracted vomiting or diarrhea; plasma loss from an external burn; insensible fluid loss in the setting of fever; or Gaisböck syndrome, a benign condition classically found in middle-age, obese men who smoke.[42,43] Absolute polycythemia is characterized by an increase in red cell mass from primary or secondary causes. Causes of secondary erythrocytosis include hypoxemia as a result of pulmonary or cardiac disease; erythropoietin-secreting tumors (eg, renal cell carcinoma); and drug-induced, such as erythropoiesis stimulating agents, androgens, and corticosteroids.[44] There are congenital polycythemias that result from mutations in the hemoglobin genes that lead to an increase in oxygen affinity with resultant compensatory erythrocytosis.[45] Other causes of congenital polycythemias include 2,3-BPG deficiency; methemoglobinemia; or genetic disorders of oxygen sensing including Chuvash polycythemia (caused by a mutation in the Von Hippel Landau *VHL* gene), gain of function mutations in the *HIF*-2 gene, and prolyl hydroxylases mutations.[46–49] These mutations in the oxygen-sensing pathway each ultimately result in increased production of erythropoietin, which results in lifelong erythrocytosis. Chuvash polycythemia has been reported more frequently in Asia, Chuvashia, and the island of Ischia in Italy and is associated with an abbreviated life span.[50,51]

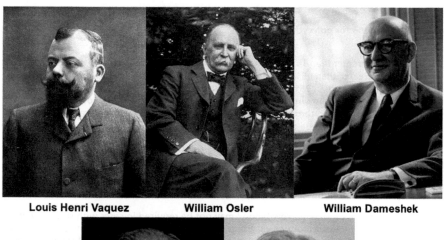

Louis Henri Vaquez   William Osler   William Dameshek

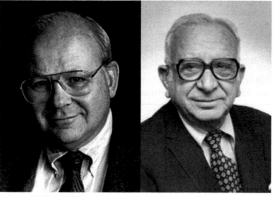

Philip Fialkow   Louis Wasserman

Fig. 1. Major clinical investigators responsible for early diagnostic and therapeutic advances in myeloproliferative neoplasms. Louis Henri Vaquez was the first to describe polycythemia vera, which was later expanded by William Osler. William Dameshek described pathologic links and coined the term "myeloproliferative disorders." Philip Fialkow identified myeloproliferative neoplasms as a stem cell disease and Louis Wasserman formed the Polycythemia Vera Study Group, the first dedicated organization to study therapies in myeloproliferative neoplasms.

PV encompasses most primary polycythemias; however, there are familial causes of erythrocytosis that result from activating gene mutations of the erythropoietin receptor.[45] The *JAK2V617F* mutation is the genetic sine qua non of the diagnosis of PV, being present in about 98% of patients.[52] In a patient with a subnormal EPO and absence of *JAK2V617F*, evaluation for *JAK2* exon 12 mutation identifies another variant of PV.[53] A bone marrow biopsy may not be necessary to make a diagnosis of PV in cases of extreme erythrocytosis (>18.5 g/dL in men or >16.5 g/dL in women) when a *JAK2* mutation is identified (see **Box 1**).[3] Many investigators, however, argue that red cell mass studies are necessary and hematocrit/hemoglobin values are at best imperfect parameters for documenting the presence of erythrocytosis.[54] Unfortunately, red cell mass measurements are rarely available at most institutions throughout the world.

Thrombocytosis is often secondary to an acute inflammatory condition and termed "reactive thrombocytosis," which is often transient and resolves after resolution of the precipitating process. Common causes of reactive thrombocytosis include infection,

Box 1
Diagnostic criteria for polycythemia vera

Major criteria
- Hemoglobin greater than 16.5 g/dL in men, hemoglobin greater than 16.0 g/dL in women; or hematocrit greater than 49% in men, hematocrit greater than 48% in women; or increased red cell mass, more than 25% higher than mean normal predicted value
- Bone marrow biopsy showing hypercellularity for age with trilineage growth (panmyelosis) including prominent erythroid, granulocytic, and megakaryocytic proliferation with pleomorphic, mature megakaryocytes (differences in size)
- Presence of *JAK2V617F* or *JAK2* exon 12 mutation

Minor criterion
- Subnormal serum erythropoietin level
  Diagnosis of PV requires meeting either all three major criteria, or the first two major criteria and the minor criterion†.

† Criterion number 2 (bone marrow biopsy) may not be required in cases with sustained absolute erythrocytosis: hemoglobin levels greater than 18.5 g/dL in men (hematocrit, 55.5%) or greater than 16.5 g/dL in women (hematocrit, 49.5%) if major criterion 3 and the minor criterion are present. However, initial myelofibrosis (present in up to 20% of patients) can only be detected by performing a bone marrow biopsy; this finding may predict a more rapid progression to overt myelofibrosis (post-PV MF).

From Arber DA, Orazi A, Hasserjian R, et al. The 2016 revision to the World Health Organization classification of myeloid neoplasms and acute leukemia. Blood 2016;127(20):2391-2405.

surgery, inflammatory conditions, and malignancy.[55] Even with high platelet counts, thrombosis is rare in patients with reactive forms of thrombocytosis.[56] There are also rare familial forms of thrombocytosis. Different mutant TPO alleles have been described in families with an autosomal-dominant form of thrombocytosis.[57] Each of these mutations act by augmenting the efficiency of translation of the TPO mRNA.[57,58] The rate of thrombotic and hemorrhagic complications in family members from two different kindreds has been reported to be comparable with that of patients with sporadic ET.[59] Most commonly, persistent thrombocytosis absent a prolonged

Box 2
Diagnostic criteria for essential thrombocythemia

Major criteria
- Platelet count $\geq$450 $\times$ 10^9/L.
- Bone marrow biopsy showing proliferation mainly of the megakaryocyte lineage with increased numbers of enlarged, mature megakaryocytes with hyperlobulated nuclei. No significant increase or left shift in neutrophil granulopoiesis or erythropoiesis and rarely minor (grade 1) increase in reticulin fibers.
- Not meeting WHO criteria for *BCR-ABL1*[+] CML, PV, PMF, myelodysplastic syndromes, or other myeloid neoplasms.
- Presence of *JAK2*, *CALR*, or *MPL* mutation.

Minor criterion
- Presence of a clonal marker or absence of evidence for reactive thrombocytosis.

Diagnosis of ET requires meeting all four major criteria or the first three major criteria and the minor criterion.

From Arber DA, Orazi A, Hasserjian R, et al. The 2016 revision to the World Health Organization classification of myeloid neoplasms and acute leukemia. Blood 2016;127(20):2391-2405.

Box 3
Diagnostic criteria for primary myelofibrosis

Major criteria
- Presence of megakaryocytic proliferation and atypia, accompanied by either reticulin and/or collagen fibrosis grades 2 or 3
- Not meeting WHO criteria for ET, PV, *BCR-ABL1*+ CML, myelodysplastic syndromes, or other myeloid neoplasms
- Presence of *JAK2*, *CALR*, or *MPL* mutation or in the absence of these mutations, presence of another clonal marker,[a] or absence of reactive myelofibrosis[b]

Minor criteria
Presence of at least one of the following, confirmed in two consecutive determinations:
- Anemia not attributed to a comorbid condition
- Leukocytosis $\geq 11 \times 10^9/L$
- Palpable splenomegaly
- LDH increased to greater than upper normal limit of institutional reference range
- Leukoerythroblastosis

Diagnosis of overt PMF requires meeting all three major criteria, and at least one minor criterion.[a] In the absence of any of the three major clonal mutations, the search for the most frequent accompanying mutations (eg, ASXL1, EZH2, TET2, IDH1/IDH2, SRSF2, SF3B1) is of help in determining the clonal nature of the disease.[b] Bone marrow fibrosis secondary to infection, autoimmune disorder or other chronic inflammatory conditions, hairy cell leukemia or other lymphoid neoplasm, metastatic malignancy, or toxic (chronic) myelopathies.

From Arber DA, Orazi A, Hasserjian R, et al. The 2016 revision to the World Health Organization classification of myeloid neoplasms and acute leukemia. Blood 2016;127(20):2391-2405. LDH, Lactate dehydrogenase

underlying condition identified previously raises the concern for an underlying MPN. CML must always be ruled out in patients with isolated thrombocytosis because this presentation is not unusual. Diagnostic evaluation of suspected ET includes evaluation of a driver mutation, specifically *JAK2*, *CALR*, and *MPL*, and a polymerase chain reaction testing for *BCR/ABL* (see **Box 2**). However, 10% to 15% of patients with ET may be negative for these three driver mutations and are classified as so-called "triple negative" ET.[60] A minority of these patients may have noncanonical mutations in *JAK2* or *MPL* detected with whole exome sequencing.[61] A bone marrow biopsy is essential for establishing a diagnosis of ET because it can distinguish ET from pre-PMF.[3]

The diagnosis of PMF requires exclusion of other MPNs, secondary forms of marrow fibrosis (eg, metastatic cancer to the marrow, tuberculosis and fungal diseases, hairy cell leukemia, autoimmune etiologies), myelodysplastic syndrome (MDS), and CML (see **Box 3**). A bone marrow biopsy is essential because grade 2 to 3 fibrosis is a requisite for the diagnosis, which is accompanied by megakaryocytic atypia and proliferation. Similar to ET, mutational assessment for a driver mutation is also important; however, 8% to 10% of patients have triple negative PMF, which is associated with a poor prognosis.[60] In addition, other somatic mutations are frequently present in patients with PMF including *ASXL1*, *TET2*, *SRSF2*, *EZH2*, and *IDH1/IDH2*, among others.[62] (See Jakub Szybinski and Sara C. Meyer's article, "Genetics of Myeloproliferative Neoplasms," in this issue.)

In 2016, the WHO defined a new entity called pre-PMF pathologically characterized by megakaryocytic atypia without reticulin fibrosis greater than grade 1 and a hypercellular marrow (**Box 4**). Although this diagnostic entity was only recently incorporated was a WHO diagnostic category, pre-PMF was first described as a distinct clinical

---

Box 4
Diagnostic criteria for pre-PMF

Major criteria
- Megakaryocytic proliferation and atypia, without reticulin fibrosis > grade 1, accompanied by increased age-adjusted bone marrow cellularity, granulocytic proliferation, and often decreased erythropoiesis
- Not meeting the WHO criteria for BCR-ABL1[+] CML, PV, ET, myelodysplastic syndromes, or other myeloid neoplasms
- Presence of JAK2, CALR, or MPL mutation or in the absence of these mutations, presence of another clonal marker,[a] or absence of minor reactive bone marrow reticulin fibrosis[b]

Minor criteria
Presence of at least one of the following, confirmed in two consecutive determinations:
- Anemia not attributed to a comorbid condition
- Leukocytosis $\geq 11 \times 10^9$/L
- Palpable splenomegaly
- LDH increased to greater than upper normal limit of institutional reference range

Diagnosis of pre-PMF requires meeting all three major criteria, and at least one minor criterion.[a] In the absence of any of the three major clonal mutations, the search for the most frequent accompanying mutations (eg, ASXL1, EZH2, TET2, IDH1/IDH2, SRSF2, SF3B1) is of help in determining the clonal nature of the disease.[b] Minor (grade 1) reticulin fibrosis secondary to infection, autoimmune disorder or other chronic inflammatory conditions, hairy cell leukemia or other lymphoid neoplasm, metastatic malignancy, or toxic (chronic) myelopathies.

From Arber DA, Orazi A, Hasserjian R, et al. The 2016 revision to the World Health Organization classification of myeloid neoplasms and acute leukemia. Blood 2016;127(20):2391-2405. LDH, Lactate dehydrogenase

---

entity in 1976 and was formally introduced in the previous 2001 and 2008 WHO diagnostic criteria.[63–65] Clinically, pre-PMF is often associated with isolated thrombocytosis and is often misdiagnosed as ET. In fact, a review of more than 1000 cases of 2008 WHO-diagnosed ET demonstrated that nearly one in five meets criteria for pre-PMF instead of ET.[66] The pathologic considerations of MF are discussed Mohamed Salama, including the diagnosis of pre-PMF, in this issue. Although both disorders are characterized by an increased risk of developing thrombotic events, the distinction between ET and pre-PMF is key because pre-PMF carries a significantly elevated risk of transformation to leukemia and death.[66]

Survival among the classic MPNs is longest with ET, with an estimated median survival of approximately 20 years.[60] Patients with PV have a shorter estimated survival as compared with ET, with one study reporting a median overall survival 14.1 years after diagnosis.[52] Patients with pre-PMF have a median survival of approximately 14.7 years based on a large European series; however, survival is significant shorter in patients with adverse karyotypic or mutational profiles.[67] Overt MF portends the worse prognosis among the MPNs, with a median survival of 3.1 to 5.8 years.[67,68] However, the survival of all MPNs is highly dependent on many patient- and disease-specific factors.

Other WHO-recognized MPNs, including chronic neutrophilic leukemia, mastocytosis, and chronic eosinophilic leukemia, and MPNs not otherwise specified are not discussed in this issue. However, a group of disorders that have characteristics of MDS and MPNs, called MDS/MPN overlap syndrome, is detailed by Andrew T. Kuykendall and colleagues' article, "Traipsing Through Muddy Waters: A Critical Review of the Myelodysplastic Syndrome/Myeloproliferative Neoplasm (MDS/MPN) Overlap Syndromes," in this issue. These disorders include chronic myelomonocytic leukemia, juvenile myelomonocytic leukemia, and atypical CML.

PATHOGENESIS

The pathogenesis of MPNs is multifactorial and incompletely understood. However, substantial progress has been made over the last several decades toward understanding the biologic underpinnings of MPNs. It is important to recognize that all MPNs originate at the level of a pluripotent hematopoietic stem cell.[69,70] In murine models, even a single cell carrying the *JAK2V617F* mutation can initiate the MPN phenotype.[71] However, there are considerable complexities in MPN pathogenesis as it relates to the stem cell microenvironment. Interactions between hematopoietic stem cells and nonhematopoietic marrow cells in MF are responsible for bone marrow fibrosis, increased microvascular density, and production of inflammatory cytokines.[72] In particular, transforming growth factor-β (TGF-β) is a potent stimulator of fibroblast growth, which is not part of the malignant clone.[73] However, monocytes that belong to the malignant clone can acquire the properties that resemble fibroblasts and are termed fibrocytes. These fibrocytes along with fibroblasts contribute to bone marrow fibrosis in MF.[74] (See Gajalakshmi Ramanathan and Angela G. Fleischman's article, "The Microenvironment in Myeloproliferative Neoplasms," in this issue.)

A key pathogenetic event in all MPNs is constitutive activation of the JAK/STAT pathway. Seminal to this understanding was the identification of mutations *JAK2* in 98% of patients with PV, and 50% to 60% of patients with ET and PMF.[38–41] Additional somatic mutations, such as the thrombopoietin receptor *MPL* in *JAK2V617F*-negative patients with MPN suggest common genetic mutations resulting in overactivation of the JAK-STAT pathway.[75] In addition, a small subset of *JAK2V617F*-negative polycythemic patients harbor a mutation in *LNK*, which inhibits JAK2 phosphorylation and serves as a negative regulator of MPL signaling.[76,77] The *CALR* mutation, which is generally exclusive to *JAK2* and *MPL* mutations, creates a mutant protein that directly binds the thrombopoietin receptor (MPL) leading to constitutive activation of downstream signaling molecules in the JAK/STAT pathway.[78,79] The central role of the JAK-STAT pathway in the pathogenesis of MPNs was confirmed by a seminal study by Rampal and colleagues[10] using gene expression profiling. JAK/STAT target genes were upregulated, independent of JAK2 mutational status or clinical phenotype. Even triple-negative MPN cases were characterized by upregulation of this pathway affirming the central role of hyperactive JAK/STAT pathway.[10] This dependency on upregulated JAK/STAT signaling accounts for the success of JAK2 inhibitors as a cornerstone therapy in patients with MF regardless of driver mutation status.

Additional somatic mutations frequently occur in patients with MPNs, especially those involved in epigenetic regulation. In a study of 197 patients with MPN, after *JAK2* and *CALR*, the most commonly mutated genes were *TET2*, *ASXL1*, *DNMT3A*, and *EZH2*.[80] These mutations are likely involved in disease initiation and evolution.[80,81] Further details of epigenetic mechanisms of MF are included in Andrew Dunbar and colleagues' article, "Epigenetic Dysregulation of Myeloproliferative Neoplasms," in this issue.

It has long been recognized that inflammation is an important contributor to neoplastic development, sometimes referred to as "oncoinflammation."[82] In MPNs, there is biochemical, molecular, clinical, and epidemiologic evidence that links overactive inflammation and MPN development. Patients with MPNs have persistently elevated C-reactive protein, an acute phase reactant, and the degree of elevation is predictive of leukemic transformation.[83,84] Several genes involved in immune regulation and inflammation are upregulated, particularly interferon-related genes, such as interferon-inducible gene *IFI27*.[85] Upregulation of *IFI27* is step wise, with higher levels observed in MF as compared with ET or PV, suggesting a role of inflammation in disease progression.[86] Fisher and colleagues[87] showed that the increased production of cytokines in patients with MF, including tumor necrosis factor, was driven partly by each of the nuclear factor-κB, MAP kinase, and JAK-STAT pathways. Their observations indicated that an intact nuclear factor-κB pathway is necessary for maximal production of these cytokines in MF. Epidemiologic evidence also supports a link between inflammation and development of an MPN. Patients with an autoimmune disorder, including Crohn disease, polyarthritis rheumatica, and giant cell arthritis, carry an increased risk for subsequent development of an MPN.[88] Tobacco smoking has also been consistently associated with an increased risk of MPN development.[89]

Inflammatory cytokines are responsible for many of the clinical features of MF. TGF-β has been implicated in angiogenesis, tumor growth, and collagen fibrosis in several tumor types. In MF, TGF-β is more abundantly produced as compared with other fibrogenic cytokines, such as platelet-derived growth factor, and fibroblast growth factor-basic.[90] Cytokine overexpression is also thought to be related to constitutive mobilization of CD34+ cells into the peripheral blood of patients with MF.[91] In addition, splenomegaly and constitutional symptoms have been correlated with hepatocyte growth factor and interleukin (IL)-6, respectively. In addition, IL-8, IL-2R, IL-12, and IL-15 have been shown to be independently prognostic in patients with MF.[92] Adam Mead expands on these topics in his article, "Application of Single-Cell Approaches to Study Myeloproliferative Neoplasm Biology," in this issue.

COMPLICATIONS

The major complications experienced by patients with MPNs include thrombosis, bleeding, and progression of disease to overt phases of MF or MPN-blast phase (MPN-BP). In PV and ET, the primary contributor of morbidity and mortality is thrombosis, which is either arterial or venous. In a large population-based Swedish study, the hazard ratio for arterial thrombosis 3 months, 1 year, and 5 years after diagnosis was 3.0, 2.0, and 1.5, respectively, as compared with the general population. The corresponding hazard ratio for venous thrombosis was 9.7, 4.7, and 3.2, suggesting a significantly increased rate of thrombosis compared with patients without MPNs, particularly in the few months following diagnosis.[93] Another hallmark of MPN-related thrombosis is the development of clots in atypical locations, particularly the splanchnic bed.[94,95] Thrombosis of the hepatic vein (Budd-Chiari syndrome) and the portal vein are particularly prevalent and may be related to endothelial cells harboring JAK2V617F and increased P-selectin expression.[96,97] Erythromelalgia is another microvascular disorder caused by platelet microthrombi and activation, which is ameliorated by aspirin.[98]

Bleeding is also a concern for MPN patients, especially those with ET and PMF. In a meta-analysis, bleeding complications occurred in 8.9% of patients with MF, 7.3% in ET, and 6.9% in PV, with gastrointestinal and mucocutaneous locations being the most common sites.[99] Thrombocytosis is among the most important risk factors for bleeding, as demonstrated in a post hoc analysis of the PT1 trial.[100] In particular, significant elevations in platelets can lead to acquired von Willebrand syndrome.[101] Andrew I. Schafer describes these complications further in his article, "Thrombotic, Vascular, and Bleeding Complications of the Myeloproliferative Neoplasms," in this issue.

Progression from a proliferative disease (ie, ET or PV) to a fibrotic disease (ie, post-ET MF or post-PV MF) and MPN-BP is a primary concern for clinicians and patients alike.[11] The risk of progression varies depending on series and risk factors, such as age, mutational status, and other clinical factors. In one series, progression rate from ET and PV to post-ET MF and post-PV MF was 9.2% to 10.3% and 12.5% to

21%, respectively.[60] Transformation to MPN-BP is highest with PMF, with a 10-year risk of 10% to 20%, followed by PV (2%–4%) and ET (1%–2%).[102] Many clinical, laboratory, cytogenetic, and molecular risk factors have been identified. These factors have been incorporated into multiple risk scores.[103–105] Unlike de novo acute myeloid leukemia, MPN-BP is rarely associated with mutations in NPM1 or FLT3, highlighting its unique biology as compared with other forms of secondary leukemia.[106] Raajit K. Rampal delves further into leukemic transformation in his article, "Accelerated and Blast Phase Myeloproliferative Neoplasms," in this issue.

Infections are more common in patients with MPN as compared with the general population and remains one of the primary contributors toward mortality in patients with MPN.[107] Although the risk is highest in patients with PMF, there is still a significant increase in the risk of infection with ET and PV.[108] There is also growing evidence, albeit controversial, that ruxolitinib may increase the risk of infection in patients with MPNs.[109,110] In addition, patients with MPNs are at an increased risk of developing second primary malignancies, in particular skin cancer.[111] The reason for this observation is not known, but has been hypothesized to be related to the chronic inflammatory milieu in patients with MPNs.[112] A recent provocative study suggested that ruxolitinib was associated with the development of B-cell lymphomas.[113] However, this association has not been confirmed in subsequent studies.[114,115]

SUMMARY

MPNs represent a biologically related group of hematologic disorders with significant clinical consequences. Early work from pioneering hematologists established the relationships between this group of disorders and led to early understanding of its pathogenesis. Importantly, the 2005 identification of the JAK2V617F, which is present in most patients with MPNs, has established the central role of the JAK-STAT pathway in MPN biology. Inflammation is also a major contributor to disease initiation and progression. Further studies are needed to identify additional pathogenic mechanisms, including the role of epigenetics, additional signaling pathways, and megakaryocyte abnormalities.

Despite progress in the pathobiologic understanding of MPNs, significant advancement in therapeutically impacting the natural history of disease remains elusive. For patients with proliferative disease (ET and PV), cytoreduction is the mainstay of therapy. However, it is not clear if this intervention significantly impacts the thrombotic burden in ET and PV. In addition, the impact on progression of disease to MF or MPN-BP is lacking. Given the chronic nature of MPNs and the low event rate of disease transformation and thrombosis, which are key clinical outcomes, the performance of clinical trials in MPNs is extremely challenging, as detailed in Heidi E. Kosiorek and Amylou C. Dueck's article, "Advancing effective clinical trial designs for Myelofibrosis," in this issue. Despite significant improvement in symptom burden and spleen size with JAK inhibitor treatment of MF, these therapies are unlikely to significantly alter disease progression to MPN-BP. Additional therapies are urgently needed that can deplete the MPN stem cell and significantly impact the course of disease, with the ultimate goal of improving the quality and quantity of life of patients with MPN.

CLINICS CARE POINTS

- Evaluation of erythrocytosis and thrombocytosis must include work-up of secondary causes.
- A bone marrow biopsy is essential for establishing the diagnosis of ET as it can differentiate between ET and pre-PMF.

- The major complications experienced by patients with MPNs include thrombosis, bleeding, and progression of disease to overt phases of MF or MPN-blast phase.

DISCLOSURE

Dr R. Hoffman is a consultant for Protagonist and serves on Data Safety Monitoring Boards for Novartis and AbbVie. He also receives research support from Novartis, Dompe, Kartos, AbbVie, Scholar Rock, and Turning Point Therapeutics. Dr A. Yacoub is a consultant for Incyte and Novartis. He has stocks and ownership in Hylapharm.

REFERENCES

1. Dickstein JI, Vardiman JW. Hematopathologic findings in the myeloproliferative disorders. Semin Oncol 1995;22(4):355–73.
2. Barosi G, Mesa RA, Thiele J, et al. Proposed criteria for the diagnosis of post-polycythemia vera and post-essential thrombocythemia myelofibrosis: a consensus statement from the international working group for myelofibrosis research and treatment. Leukemia 2008;22(2):437–8.
3. Arber DA, Orazi A, Hasserjian R, et al. The 2016 revision to the World Health Organization classification of myeloid neoplasms and acute leukemia. Blood 2016; 127(20):2391–405.
4. Rowley JD. Letter: a new consistent chromosomal abnormality in chronic myelogenous leukaemia identified by quinacrine fluorescence and Giemsa staining. Nature 1973;243(5405):290–3.
5. Cortes JE, Talpaz M, Giles F, et al. Prognostic significance of cytogenetic clonal evolution in patients with chronic myelogenous leukemia on imatinib mesylate therapy. Blood 2003;101(10):3794–800.
6. Goldman JM, Apperley JF, Jones L, et al. Bone marrow transplantation for patients with chronic myeloid leukemia. N Engl J Med 1986;314(4):202–7.
7. Gratwohl A, Baldomero H, Horisberger B, et al. Current trends in hematopoietic stem cell transplantation in Europe. Blood 2002;100(7):2374–86.
8. Druker BJ, Sawyers CL, Kantarjian H, et al. Activity of a specific inhibitor of the BCR-ABL tyrosine kinase in the blast crisis of chronic myeloid leukemia and acute lymphoblastic leukemia with the Philadelphia chromosome. N Engl J Med 2001;344(14):1038–42.
9. Cohen MH, Williams G, Johnson JR, et al. Approval summary for imatinib mesylate capsules in the treatment of chronic myelogenous leukemia. Clin Cancer Res 2002;8(5):935–42.
10. Rampal R, Al-Shahrour F, Abdel-Wahab O, et al. Integrated genomic analysis illustrates the central role of JAK-STAT pathway activation in myeloproliferative neoplasm pathogenesis. Blood 2014;123(22):e123–33.
11. Mesa RA, Miller CB, Thyne M, et al. Differences in treatment goals and perception of symptom burden between patients with myeloproliferative neoplasms (MPNs) and hematologists/oncologists in the United States: findings from the MPN Landmark survey. Cancer 2017;123(3):449–58.
12. Mylonas E, Yoshida K, Frick M, et al. Single-cell analysis based dissection of clonality in myelofibrosis. Nat Commun 2020;11(1):73.
13. Verstovsek S, Mesa RA, Gotlib J, et al. Long-term treatment with ruxolitinib for patients with myelofibrosis: 5-year update from the randomized, double-blind, placebo-controlled, phase 3 COMFORT-I trial. J Hematol Oncol 2017;10(1):55.

14. Harrison CN, Vannucchi AM, Kiladjian JJ, et al. Long-term findings from COMFORT-II, a phase 3 study of ruxolitinib vs best available therapy for myelofibrosis. Leukemia 2016;30(8):1701–7.

15. Deeg HJ, Bredeson C, Farnia S, et al. Hematopoietic cell transplantation as curative therapy for patients with myelofibrosis: long-term success in all age groups. Biology of blood and marrow transplantation. Biol Blood Marrow Transplant 2015;21(11):1883–7.

16. Tremblay D, Marcellino B, Mascarenhas J. Pharmacotherapy of myelofibrosis. Drugs 2017;77(14):1549–63.

17. Asher S, McLornan DP, Harrison CN. Current and future therapies for myelofibrosis. Blood Rev 2020;42:100715.

18. Shallis RM, Wang R, Davidoff A, et al. Epidemiology of the classical myeloproliferative neoplasms: the four corners of an expansive and complex map. Blood Rev 2020;42:100706.

19. Passamonti F, Malabarba L, Orlandi E, et al. Polycythemia vera in young patients: a study on the long-term risk of thrombosis, myelofibrosis and leukemia. Haematologica 2003;88(1):13–8.

20. Cario H, Schwarz K, Herter JM, et al. Clinical and molecular characterisation of a prospectively collected cohort of children and adolescents with polycythemia vera. Br J Haematol 2008;142(4):622–6.

21. Srour SA, Devesa SS, Morton LM, et al. Incidence and patient survival of myeloproliferative neoplasms and myelodysplastic/myeloproliferative neoplasms in the United States, 2001-12. Br J Haematol 2016;174(3):382–96.

22. Cobb M. Reading and writing the book of nature: Jan Swammerdam (1637–1680). Endeavour 2000;24(3):122–8.

23. Hamarneh S. Measuring the invisible world. The life and works of Antoni van Leeuwenhoek. Science 1960;132(3422):289–90.

24. Piller G. Leukaemia: a brief historical review from ancient times to 1950. Br J Haematol 2001;112(2):282–92.

25. Donne AF. De l'origine des globules du sang, de leur mode de formatton et de leur fin. Prov Med Surg J 1840;3(77):498–9.

26. Bennett JH. Case of hypertrophy of the spleen and liver, in which death took place from suppuration of the blood. Edinburgh Med Sug J 1845;64:413–23.

27. Heuck G. Zwei fälle von Leukämie mit eigenthümlichem Blut-resp. Knochenmarksbefund. Archiv für pathologische Anatomie und Physiologie und für klinische Medicin 1879;78(3):475–96.

28. Vaquez H. Sur une forme spéciale de cyanose s' accompagnant d'hyperglobulie excessive et persistante. CR Soc Biol (Paris) 1892;44:384–8.

29. Osler W. Chronic cyanosis, with polycythæmia and enlarged spleen: a new clinical entity. Am J Med Sci 1903;126(2):187.

30. Epstein E, Goedel A. Hemorrhagic thrombocythemia with a cascular, sclerotic spleen. Virchows Arch 1934;293:233–48.

31. Dameshek W. Some speculations on the myeloproliferative syndromes. Blood 1951;6(4):372–5.

32. Adamson JW, Fialkow PJ, Murphy S, et al. Polycythemia vera: stem-cell and probable clonal origin of the disease. N Engl J Med 1976;295(17):913–6.

33. Fialkow PJ, Faguet GB, Jacobson RJ, et al. Evidence that essential thrombocythemia is a clonal disorder with origin in a multipotent stem cell. Blood 1981;58(5):916–9.

34. Jacobson RJ, Salo A, Fialkow PJ. Agnogenic myeloid metaplasia: a clonal proliferation of hematopoietic stem cells with secondary myelofibrosis. Blood 1978; 51(2):189–94.

35. Early approaches in the treatment of polycythemia vera. In: Wasserman LR, Berk PD, Berlin NI, editors. Polycythemia vera and the myeloproliferative disorders. Philadelphia: WB Saunders Company; 1995. p. 147–53.

36. Fruchtman SM, Mack K, Kaplan ME, et al. From efficacy to safety: a Polycythemia Vera Study group report on hydroxyurea in patients with polycythemia vera. Semin Hematol 1997;34(1):17–23.

37. Tartaglia AP, Goldberg JD, Berk PD, et al. Adverse effects of antiaggregating platelet therapy in the treatment of polycythemia vera. Semin Hematol 1986; 23(3):172–6.

38. Levine RL, Loriaux M, Huntly BJ, et al. The JAK2V617F activating mutation occurs in chronic myelomonocytic leukemia and acute myeloid leukemia, but not in acute lymphoblastic leukemia or chronic lymphocytic leukemia. Blood 2005; 106(10):3377–9.

39. James C, Ugo V, Le Couedic JP, et al. A unique clonal JAK2 mutation leading to constitutive signalling causes polycythaemia vera. Nature 2005;434(7037): 1144–8.

40. Kralovics R, Passamonti F, Buser AS, et al. A gain-of-function mutation of JAK2 in myeloproliferative disorders. N Engl J Med 2005;352(17):1779–90.

41. Baxter EJ, Scott LM, Campbell PJ, et al. Acquired mutation of the tyrosine kinase JAK2 in human myeloproliferative disorders. Lancet 2005;365(9464): 1054–61.

42. Biswas M, Prakash PK, Cossburn M, et al. Life-threatening thrombotic complications of relative polycythaemia. J Intern Med 2003;253(4):481–3.

43. Weinreb NJ, Shih CF. Spurious polycythemia. Semin Hematol 1975;12(4): 397–407.

44. Kremyanskaya M, Mascarenhas J, Hoffman R. Why does my patient have erythrocytosis? Hematol Oncol Clin North Am 2012;26(2):267–283, vii-viii.

45. Huang LJ, Shen YM, Bulut GB. Advances in understanding the pathogenesis of primary familial and congenital polycythaemia. Br J Haematol 2010;148(6): 844–52.

46. Sergeyeva A, Gordeuk VR, Tokarev YN, et al. Congenital polycythemia in Chuvashia. Blood 1997;89(6):2148–54.

47. Hoyer JD, Allen SL, Beutler E, et al. Erythrocytosis due to bisphosphoglycerate mutase deficiency with concurrent glucose-6-phosphate dehydrogenase (G-6-PD) deficiency. Am J Hematol 2004;75(4):205–8.

48. Formenti F, Beer PA, Croft QP, et al. Cardiopulmonary function in two human disorders of the hypoxia-inducible factor (HIF) pathway: von Hippel-Lindau disease and HIF-2alpha gain-of-function mutation. FASEB J 2011;25(6):2001–11.

49. Albiero E, Ruggeri M, Fortuna S, et al. Isolated erythrocytosis: study of 67 patients and identification of three novel germ-line mutations in the prolyl hydroxylase domain protein 2 (PHD2) gene. Haematologica 2012;97(1):123–7.

50. Gordeuk VR, Sergueeva AI, Miasnikova GY, et al. Congenital disorder of oxygen sensing: association of the homozygous Chuvash polycythemia VHL mutation with thrombosis and vascular abnormalities but not tumors. Blood 2004; 103(10):3924–32.

51. Percy MJ, McMullin MF, Jowitt SN, et al. Chuvash-type congenital polycythemia in 4 families of Asian and Western European ancestry. Blood 2003;102(3): 1097–9.

52. Tefferi A, Rumi E, Finazzi G, et al. Survival and prognosis among 1545 patients with contemporary polycythemia vera: an international study. Leukemia 2013; 27(9):1874–81.

53. Pardanani A, Lasho TL, Finke C, et al. Prevalence and clinicopathologic correlates of JAK2 exon 12 mutations in JAK2V617F-negative polycythemia vera. Leukemia 2007;21(9):1960–3.

54. Silver RT, Krichevsky S. Distinguishing essential thrombocythemia JAK2V617F from polycythemia vera: limitations of erythrocyte values. Haematologica 2019;104(11):2200–5.

55. Santhosh-Kumar CR, Yohannan MD, Higgy KE, et al. Thrombocytosis in adults: analysis of 777 patients. J Intern Med 1991;229(6):493–5.

56. Vannucchi AM, Barbui T. Thrombocytosis and thrombosis. Hematology Am Soc Hematol Educ Program 2007;363–70. https://doi.org/10.1182/asheducation-2007.1.363.

57. Wiestner A, Schlemper RJ, van der Maas AP, et al. An activating splice donor mutation in the thrombopoietin gene causes hereditary thrombocythaemia. Nat Genet 1998;18(1):49–52.

58. Ghilardi N, Wiestner A, Kikuchi M, et al. Hereditary thrombocythaemia in a Japanese family is caused by a novel point mutation in the thrombopoietin gene. Br J Haematol 1999;107(2):310–6.

59. Teofili L, Larocca LM. Advances in understanding the pathogenesis of familial thrombocythaemia. Br J Haematol 2011;152(6):701–12.

60. Tefferi A, Guglielmelli P, Larson DR, et al. Long-term survival and blast transformation in molecularly annotated essential thrombocythemia, polycythemia vera, and myelofibrosis. Blood 2014;124(16):2507–13 [quiz 2615].

61. Milosevic Feenstra JD, Nivarthi H, Gisslinger H, et al. Whole-exome sequencing identifies novel MPL and JAK2 mutations in triple-negative myeloproliferative neoplasms. Blood 2016;127(3):325–32.

62. Tefferi A, Lasho TL, Finke CM, et al. Targeted deep sequencing in primary myelofibrosis. Blood Adv 2016;1(2):105–11.

63. Thiele J, Georgii A, Vykoupil KF. Ultrastructure of chronic megakaryocytic-granulocytic myelosis. Blut 1976;32(6):433–8.

64. Vardiman JW, Harris NL, Brunning RD. The World Health Organization (WHO) classification of the myeloid neoplasms. Blood 2002;100(7):2292–302.

65. Vardiman JW, Thiele J, Arber DA, et al. The 2008 revision of the World Health Organization (WHO) classification of myeloid neoplasms and acute leukemia: rationale and important changes. Blood 2009;114(5):937–51.

66. Barbui T, Thiele J, Passamonti F, et al. Survival and disease progression in essential thrombocythemia are significantly influenced by accurate morphologic diagnosis: an international study. J Clin Oncol 2011;29(23):3179–84.

67. Guglielmelli P, Pacilli A, Rotunno G, et al. Presentation and outcome of patients with 2016 WHO diagnosis of prefibrotic and overt primary myelofibrosis. Blood 2017;129(24):3227–36.

68. Cervantes F, Dupriez B, Pereira A, et al. New prognostic scoring system for primary myelofibrosis based on a study of the International Working Group for Myelofibrosis Research and Treatment. Blood 2009;113(13):2895–901.

69. Skoda RC, Duek A, Grisouard J. Pathogenesis of myeloproliferative neoplasms. Exp Hematol 2015;43(8):599–608.

70. Kralovics R, Skoda RC. Molecular pathogenesis of Philadelphia chromosome negative myeloproliferative disorders. Blood Rev 2005;19(1):1–13.

71. Lundberg P, Takizawa H, Kubovcakova L, et al. Myeloproliferative neoplasms can be initiated from a single hematopoietic stem cell expressing JAK2-V617F. J Exp Med 2014;211(11):2213–30.

72. Zahr AA, Salama ME, Carreau N, et al. Bone marrow fibrosis in myelofibrosis: pathogenesis, prognosis and targeted strategies. Haematologica 2016;101(6):660–71.

73. Kimura A, Katoh O, Hyodo H, et al. Transforming growth factor-beta regulates growth as well as collagen and fibronectin synthesis of human marrow fibroblasts. Br J Haematol 1989;72(4):486–91.

74. Ozono Y, Shide K, Kameda T, et al. Neoplastic fibrocytes play an essential role in bone marrow fibrosis in Jak2V617F-induced primary myelofibrosis mice. Leukemia 2020. https://doi.org/10.1038/s41375-020-0880-3.

75. Pardanani AD, Levine RL, Lasho T, et al. MPL515 mutations in myeloproliferative and other myeloid disorders: a study of 1182 patients. Blood 2006;108(10):3472–6.

76. Lasho TL, Pardanani A, Tefferi A. LNK mutations in JAK2 mutation-negative erythrocytosis. N Engl J Med 2010;363(12):1189–90.

77. Tong W, Lodish HF. Lnk inhibits Tpo-mpl signaling and Tpo-mediated megakaryocytopoiesis. J Exp Med 2004;200(5):569–80.

78. Marty C, Pecquet C, Nivarthi H, et al. Calreticulin mutants in mice induce an MPL-dependent thrombocytosis with frequent progression to myelofibrosis. Blood 2016;127(10):1317–24.

79. Klampfl T, Gisslinger H, Harutyunyan AS, et al. Somatic mutations of calreticulin in myeloproliferative neoplasms. N Engl J Med 2013;369(25):2379–90.

80. Lundberg P, Karow A, Nienhold R, et al. Clonal evolution and clinical correlates of somatic mutations in myeloproliferative neoplasms. Blood 2014;123(14):2220–8.

81. Vannucchi AM, Lasho TL, Guglielmelli P, et al. Mutations and prognosis in primary myelofibrosis. Leukemia 2013;27(9):1861–9.

82. Colotta F, Allavena P, Sica A, et al. Cancer-related inflammation, the seventh hallmark of cancer: links to genetic instability. Carcinogenesis 2009;30(7):1073–81.

83. Barbui T, Carobbio A, Finazzi G, et al. Inflammation and thrombosis in essential thrombocythemia and polycythemia vera: different role of C-reactive protein and pentraxin 3. Haematologica 2011;96(2):315–8.

84. Barbui T, Carobbio A, Finazzi G, et al. Elevated C-reactive protein is associated with shortened leukemia-free survival in patients with myelofibrosis. Leukemia 2013;27(10):2084–6.

85. Skov V, Larsen TS, Thomassen M, et al. Molecular profiling of peripheral blood cells from patients with polycythemia vera and related neoplasms: identification of deregulated genes of significance for inflammation and immune surveillance. Leuk Res 2012;36(11):1387–92.

86. Skov V, Larsen TS, Thomassen M, et al. Whole-blood transcriptional profiling of interferon-inducible genes identifies highly upregulated IFI27 in primary myelofibrosis. Eur J Haematol 2011;87(1):54–60.

87. Fisher DAC, Miner CA, Engle EK, et al. Cytokine production in myelofibrosis exhibits differential responsiveness to JAK-STAT, MAP kinase, and NFkappaB signaling. Leukemia 2019;33(8):1978–95.

88. Kristinsson SY, Landgren O, Samuelsson J, et al. Autoimmunity and the risk of myeloproliferative neoplasms. Haematologica 2010;95(7):1216–20.

89. Pedersen KM, Bak M, Sorensen AL, et al. Smoking is associated with increased risk of myeloproliferative neoplasms: a general population-based cohort study. Cancer Med 2018;7(11):5796–802.

90. Wang JC, Chang TH, Goldberg A, et al. Quantitative analysis of growth factor production in the mechanism of fibrosis in agnogenic myeloid metaplasia. Exp Hematol 2006;34(12):1617–23.

91. Cho SY, Xu M, Roboz J, et al. The effect of CXCL12 processing on CD34+ cell migration in myeloproliferative neoplasms. Cancer Res 2010;70(8):3402–10.

92. Tefferi A, Vaidya R, Caramazza D, et al. Circulating interleukin (IL)-8, IL-2R, IL-12, and IL-15 levels are independently prognostic in primary myelofibrosis: a comprehensive cytokine profiling study. J Clin Oncol 2011;29(10):1356–63.

93. Hultcrantz M, Bjorkholm M, Dickman PW, et al. Risk for arterial and venous thrombosis in patients with myeloproliferative neoplasms: a population-based cohort study. Ann Intern Med 2018;168(5):317–25.

94. Sekhar M, McVinnie K, Burroughs AK. Splanchnic vein thrombosis in myeloproliferative neoplasms. Br J Haematol 2013;162(6):730–47.

95. Tremblay D, Vogel AS, Moshier E, et al. Outcomes of splanchnic vein thrombosis in patients with myeloproliferative neoplasms in a single center experience. Eur J Haematol 2019;104(1):72–3.

96. Sozer S, Fiel MI, Schiano T, et al. The presence of JAK2V617F mutation in the liver endothelial cells of patients with Budd-Chiari syndrome. Blood 2009;113(21):5246–9.

97. Guy A, Gourdou-Latyszenok V, Le Lay N, et al. Vascular endothelial cell expression of JAK2(V617F) is sufficient to promote a pro-thrombotic state due to increased P-selectin expression. Haematologica 2019;104(1):70–81.

98. van Genderen PJ, Lucas IS, van Strik R, et al. Erythromelalgia in essential thrombocythemia is characterized by platelet activation and endothelial cell damage but not by thrombin generation. Thromb Haemost 1996;76(3):333–8.

99. Rungjirajittranon T, Owattanapanich W, Ungprasert P, et al. A systematic review and meta-analysis of the prevalence of thrombosis and bleeding at diagnosis of Philadelphia-negative myeloproliferative neoplasms. BMC cancer 2019;19(1):184.

100. Campbell PJ, MacLean C, Beer PA, et al. Correlation of blood counts with vascular complications in essential thrombocythemia: analysis of the prospective PT1 cohort. Blood 2012;120(7):1409–11.

101. Mital A, Prejzner W, Bieniaszewska M, et al. Prevalence of acquired von Willebrand syndrome during essential thrombocythemia: a retrospective analysis of 170 consecutive patients. Pol Arch Med Wewn 2015;125(12):914–20.

102. Dunbar AJ, Rampal RK, Levine R. Leukemia secondary to myeloproliferative neoplasms. Blood 2020;136(1):61–70.

103. Vallapureddy RR, Mudireddy M, Penna D, et al. Leukemic transformation among 1306 patients with primary myelofibrosis: risk factors and development of a predictive model. Blood Cancer J 2019;9(2):12.

104. Vannucchi AM, Guglielmelli P, Rotunno G, et al. Mutation-enhanced international prognostic scoring system (MIPSS) for primary myelofibrosis: an AGIMM & IWG-MRT Project. Blood 2014;124(21):405.

105. Tefferi A, Guglielmelli P, Nicolosi M, et al. GIPSS: genetically inspired prognostic scoring system for primary myelofibrosis. Leukemia 2018;32(7):1631–42.

106. Tefferi A, Lasho TL, Guglielmelli P, et al. Targeted deep sequencing in polycythemia vera and essential thrombocythemia. Blood Adv 2016;1(1):21–30.

107. Hultcrantz M, Wilkes SR, Kristinsson SY, et al. Risk and cause of death in patients diagnosed with myeloproliferative neoplasms in sweden between 1973 and 2005: a population-based study. J Clin Oncol 2015;33(20):2288–95.
108. Landtblom AR, Andersson TM, Dickman PW, et al. Risk of infections in patients with myeloproliferative neoplasms-a population-based cohort study of 8363 patients. Leukemia 2020. https://doi.org/10.1038/s41375-020-0909-7.
109. Lussana F, Cattaneo M, Rambaldi A, et al. Ruxolitinib-associated infections: a systematic review and meta-analysis. Am J Hematol 2018;93(3):339–47.
110. Tremblay D, King A, Li L, et al. Risk factors for infections and secondary malignancies in patients with a myeloproliferative neoplasm treated with ruxolitinib: a dual-center, propensity score-matched analysis. Leuk Lymphoma 2019;1–8.
111. Frederiksen H, Farkas DK, Christiansen CF, et al. Chronic myeloproliferative neoplasms and subsequent cancer risk: a Danish population-based cohort study. Blood 2011;118(25):6515–20.
112. Hasselbalch HC. Chronic inflammation as a promotor of mutagenesis in essential thrombocythemia, polycythemia vera and myelofibrosis. A human inflammation model for cancer development? Leuk Res 2013;37(2):214–20.
113. Porpaczy E, Tripolt S, Hoelbl-Kovacic A, et al. Aggressive B-cell lymphomas in patients with myelofibrosis receiving JAK1/2 inhibitor therapy. Blood 2018; 132(7):694–706.
114. Pemmaraju N, Kantarjian H, Nastoupil L, et al. Characteristics of patients with myeloproliferative neoplasms with lymphoma, with or without JAK inhibitor therapy. Blood 2019;133(21):2348–51.
115. Hong J, Lee JH, Byun JM, et al. Risk of disease transformation and second primary solid tumors in patients with myeloproliferative neoplasms. Blood Adv 2019;3(22):3700–8.

Epidemiology of the Philadelphia Chromosome-Negative Classical Myeloproliferative Neoplasms

Rory M. Shallis, MD[a], Amer M. Zeidan, MBBS, MHS[a],
Rong Wang, PhD[b], Nikolai A. Podoltsev, MD, PhD[a],*

KEYWORDS

• Epidemiology • Incidence • Myeloproliferative neoplasms • Prevalence • Survival

KEY POINTS

• The classical myeloproliferative neoplasms (MPNs) are characterized by the absence of the Philadelphia chromosome and include polycythemia vera (PV), essential thrombocythemia (ET), and primary myelofibrosis (PMF).
• The incidence of PV, ET, and PMF is estimated to be 0.5 to 4.0, 1.1 to 2.0, and 0.3 to 2.0, respectively.
• PV and ET patients have overall survival rates that approach, but are not equal to, the general population; a diagnosis of PMF predicts the shortest survival, with a median of 4 to 7 years.
• Germline predispositions constitute an underappreciated determinant in the development of MPN.
• Age, sex, ethnicity, and limited number of identified modifiable risk factors contribute to MPN risk.

INTRODUCTION

Polycythemia vera (PV), essential thrombocythemia (ET), and primary myelofibrosis (PMF) constitute the classical myeloproliferative neoplasms (MPNs), which are relatively uncommon and characterized by the absence of the reciprocal translocation between chromosomes 9 and 22 (or Philadelphia chromosome) creating the *BCR-ABL1* fusion gene.[1] Throughout this article, reference to MPN specifically refers to classical

[a] Section of Hematology, Department of Internal Medicine, Yale University School of Medicine and Yale Cancer Center, 333 Cedar Street, P.O. Box 208028, New Haven, CT 06520-8028, USA;
[b] Department of Chronic Disease Epidemiology, Yale School of Public Health, Yale University, 333 Cedar Street, P.O. Box 208028, New Haven, CT 06520-8028, USA
* Corresponding author.
E-mail address: nikolai.podoltsev@yale.edu

Hematol Oncol Clin N Am 35 (2021) 177–189
https://doi.org/10.1016/j.hoc.2020.11.005
0889-8588/21/© 2020 Elsevier Inc. All rights reserved.

hemonc.theclinics.com

MPN or the diseases PV, ET, and PMF. The molecular pathogenesis of the MPNs is rooted in hematopoietic progenitor cell JAK-STAT signaling pathway perturbations and consequent disruption of otherwise tightly regulated cellular proliferation.[2] PV is universally associated with mutations in the *JAK2* gene, including the most common *JAK2*-V617F, which are also frequently found in cases of ET and PMF; mutations in calreticulin (*CALR*) or thrombopoietin receptor (*MPL*) genes drive most of the non-*JAK2*-mutated MPNs.[2] Sequelae from the uncontrolled intramedullary cellular proliferation observed in the MPNs not only include blood count abnormalities, but also significant symptomatology, risk of thrombosis, and acquired bone marrow failure states such as terminal myelofibrosis, myelodysplastic syndrome (MDS), or MPN-blast phase (MPN-BP). These substantial disease-related events occur at varying frequencies predicated upon disease biology and risk, which together influence the prevalence and survival of patients with MPN.[3]

In discussing the epidemiology of the MPNs, one must consider the evolution of their classification and the relatively recent and piecemeal identification of their molecular drivers that now serve as diagnostic criteria; these issues influence the accuracy of case ascertainment methods that are frequently employed to define disease incidence, prevalence, and survival. MPNs were originally described as myeloproliferative disorders in 1951.[4] Eventual recognition of the malignant nature of the MPNs was not systematically established until 2000 when the International Classification of Diseases for Oncology, 3rd edition (ICD-O-3) changed their status from uncertain/borderline to malignant.[5] Recharacterizing the MPNs as malignant diseases has allowed for greater case capture through registry-based analyses, which have been further facilitated by the identification of MPN-specific driver mutations. The *JAK2* V617F mutation was only discovered in 2005[6]; the *JAK2* exon 12 mutation, harbored in the remaining 5% of PV cases, was discovered in 2007.[6–8]

These seminal events persuaded the World Health Organization (WHO) in 2008 to revise the description of these entities from myeloproliferative disorders to MPNs and also incorporate the *JAK2*-V617F mutation as a major criterion for PV diagnosis.[9,10] The other JAK-STAT pathway activating mutations in *MPL*, exon 10 (found in about 5% of ET and PMF patients)[11,12] and *CALR* (found in about 25% of ET and PMF patients), were discovered in 2006 and 2013, respectively.[13,14] With these revelations, in 2016 the presence of either a *CALR* or *MPL* mutation was included as a WHO major criterion for the diagnosis of ET and PMF; further, this revision separated PMF into the 2 biologically and prognostically distinct entities, prefibrotic/early PMF (prePMF) and fibrotic/overt PMF.[15,16] This evolution of classification and diagnostic criteria has undoubtedly influenced the epidemiologic study of the MPNs over time.

ETIOLOGY

Beyond the identification of a driver mutation in *JAK2, CALR,* or *MPL*, the pathogenesis of the MPNs is not fully understood. Tobacco smoking is among a limited number of exposures consistently associated with an increased risk of developing an MPN.[17–19] One study noted that, when compared with never-smokers, a higher risk of MPN was observed for current smokers (hazard ratio [HR] = 2.5, 95% confidence interval [CI]: 1.3–5.0), particularly those smoking more than 15 g of tobacco/day, generally equivalent to less than or equal to 15 cigarettes/d (HR = 3.4, 95%CI: 1.4–8.2); a monotonic relationship was observed with increasing cumulative exposure (HR = 1.14 for every 10 pack-years smoking, 95%CI: 1.06–1.22; p_{trend}=.0005).[19] Studies attempting to isolate which specific event is responsible for this increased risk observed for all MPNs have offered conflicting results. One prospective study demonstrated an increased risk of PV and not ET for female current smokers,[20] but another case-control study only observed an increased risk of ET among ever-smokers.[17] To reduce bias, the latter study employed a comparator group comprised of patients with chronic lymphocytic leukemia, who have a similarly chronic malignant disease with no evidence of protective impact of tobacco smoking from multivariable analyses.[17] These 2 studies, however, had differing methodology and specifically qualitative exposure categories (eg, current, former, and ever-smokers). The NIH-AARP Diet and Health Study evaluated a large cohort of over 460,000 individuals, of whom 236 developed either PV or ET; active tobacco smoking was found to increase the risk of PV/ET in women (HR = 1.71, 95% CI: 1.08–2.71).[21] Interestingly, this study also demonstrated that increased caffeine intake was associated with a lower risk of PV (p_{trend}<.01), but not ET.[21] In another study using the same NIH-AARP cohort, fruit consumption was associated with an increased risk of MPN overall (third tertile vs first tertile, HR = 1.32, 95% CI: 1.04–1.67; p_{trend}=.02) and PV (third tertile vs first tertile, HR = 2.00, 95% CI: 1.35–2.95; p_{trend}<0.01).[22] High sugar intake was also associated with the development of PV (HR = 1.77, 95% CI: 1.12–2.79).[22]

Intrinsic risk factors have a more established role in the risk of MPN. Despite the slight male predominance among patients with MPN (discussed in more in detail in the following section), a history of autoimmune disease (in which 85% of cases affect females[23]) is shown to increase the risk of MPN. One registry-based study using age- and sex-matched controls reported an odds ratio (OR) of 1.2 (95% CI: 1.0–1.3; P=.021) for individuals with an autoimmune disease to develop MPN; analyses by specific MPN subtype were not performed.[24] A similar registry-based analysis reported ORs of 1.29 and 1.50 for acute myeloid leukemia (AML) and MDS, respectively.[25] It is unclear if a common upstream mechanism increases the risk of MPN and autoimmune disease. Alternatively, a biologic mechanism linking autoimmune disease or its immunosuppressive therapies (that may influence marrow immunosurveillance for abnormal proliferative clones) to downstream MPN development is unknown. Although a debated example of an underlying inflammatory state,[26] obesity has been weakly associated with an increased risk of developing an MPN.[27,28]

Not all individuals with MPN are felt to have disease resulting from exclusively acquired phenomena; inherited genetic abnormalities may serve as the substrate for a greater risk of their development. One of the most illustrative examples in support of this assertion is the observation that individuals with a first-degree relative affected by an MPN are up to 7 times more likely than unaffected controls to develop an MPN.[29] The exact proportion of MPNs arising out of a familial syndrome or germline predisposition is unknown, but estimated to be 5% to 10%.[30] Given the significant proportion of MPNs driven by mutations in *JAK2, CALR,* and *MPL,* much of the research evaluating the burden of congenital MPNs has centered on these genes. Inherited driver mutations in *JAK2* (specifically the non-V617F mutations R564Q, V617I, and H608N) have been uncommonly detected in individuals with MPNs.[31–33] Germline *MPL* mutations have been reported, and particularly in cases of triple-negative ET and PMF.[34] Because mutations in *CALR* as they relate to MPN have only been studied since 2013, a smaller body of data exists on germline variants, currently limited to case reports.[35]

Congenital predispositions to acquire an MPN have been associated with specific polymorphisms. The *JAK2* 46/1 or GGCC haplotype is the most well described and is found in up to 25% of the general population.[36–38] The *JAK2* 46/1 haplotype is hypothesized to increase *JAK2* locus hypermutability.[39] Population level data from patients on multiple continents have supported this hypothesis and shown that individuals with the *JAK2* 46/1 haplotype have an increased risk of developing a

JAK2-V617F-mutated MPN when compared with normal controls with ORs ranging from 2.0 to 6.3.[37,40–42] The influence of the JAK2 46/1 haplotype on the risk of non-JAK2-V617F-mutated MPNs has been debated.[37,40–43] Germline variants in TERT, HBS1L-MYB, MECOM have also been identified in familial MPN studies as predisposing to a higher risk of sporadic canonical driver mutations and triple-negative disease.[36,44–47]

Similar to the more penetrant germline mutations and less penetrant single nucleotide polymorphisms already described, not all of the acquired somatic canonical MPN driver mutations will lead to the development of MPN. Mutations in JAK2 have been reported to occur in 0.1% to 3% of the general population.[48–51] The majority of these mutations will occur in the absence of MPN and represent clonal hematopoiesis of indeterminate potential (CHIP). However, individuals with JAK2-V617F CHIP are found to have higher erythrocyte, platelet, and leukocyte counts and ultimately a higher risk of coronary events and thromboembolism when compared with their nonmutated counterparts.[48,52] These data suggest that, despite being described as having an entity of indeterminate potential, these patients exhibit clinical sequelae consistent with MPN. In fact, similar to the risk of progression from monoclonal gammopathy of undetermined significance (MGUS) to multiple myeloma or CHIP otherwise to MDS, individuals with JAK2-V617F CHIP have an increased risk (up to 75% of individuals) of progression to overt MPN.[50]

INCIDENCE

Most published data estimating the incidence of MPNs were obtained either through registry-based or claims-based analyses. The largest cancer registry in the United States is the Surveillance, Epidemiology, and End Results (SEER) program, which began collecting data in 1973 and is most recently estimated to encompass 35% of the US population.[53] After the MPNs were formally recognized as malignant and assigned ICD-O-3 codes in 2000, the initial SEER estimate in 2001 for the age-adjusted incidence of the MPNs collectively was 1.6 cases per 100,000 population per year.[54] In evaluating the diseases individually, PV was the most incident at 0.8 cases per 100,000 population per year, with ET and myelosclerosis with myeloid metaplasia (describing what would later be called PMF in 2008) having initial incidence estimates of 0.5 and 0.3 cases per 100,000 population per year, respectively.[54] The SEER-based estimated incidences of the MPNs collectively have slightly increased since 2001, with the most recent data in 2016 demonstrating an incidence of 2.7 cases per 100,000 population per year.[55] This increase appears to be largely driven by an increase in the incidence of ET, which had a 1.1 case per 100,000 population per year incidence rate as of 2016 (**Table 1**).[55] The incidence of PV and PMF as of 2016 has remained unchanged from initial estimates.[55] The reason for the relative increase in the incidence of ET as per SEER from 2001 to 2016 is unclear, but has been corroborated by other analyses using Norwegian and Australian registry-based data, which also report generally similar incidence rates.[56,57] The advent of peripheral blood testing for driver mutations, namely those in JAK2 and MPL during this timeframe, may have caused some providers to erroneously abandon the required bone marrow evaluations to establish a correct diagnosis; for instance, a diagnosis of ET may be incorrectly assigned to a patient with masked PV or PMF that would have likely been revealed if the bone marrow evaluation had been performed.

Although registries are robust cancer incidence data sources, they are prone to under-reporting because of incomplete case ascertainment. Many cases of MPN are not identified in the hospital setting, and, as mentioned, pathologic confirmation

Table 1 Summary of epidemiologic data for the classical myeloproliferative neoplasia			
	Incidence (per 100,000 Person-Years)	Median Age at Diagnosis (Years)	Prevalence (per 100,000 Person-Years)	Survival
Polycythemia vera	0.5–4.0	65	22–57	5-y relative survival: 84%–89% Median OS: 12–14 y
Essential thrombocythemia	1.1–2.0	67	24–58	5-y relative survival: 86%–91% Median OS: 13–23 y
Primary myelofibrosis	0.3–2.0	69	0.5–6.0	5-y relative survival: 35%–46% Median OS: 4–7 y

of the diagnosis is sometimes not performed. Furthermore, many cases may be subject to delayed reporting that significantly underestimates the true incidence of MPNs. For instance, 1 SEER-based analysis found that about 35% and 50% of PV and ET cases, respectively, are reported with delay.[58] The same study found that after accounting for this delayed reporting, the estimated incidences of these disease increased more than tenfold, with PV, ET, and PMF having an incidence of 10.9, 9.6, and 3.1, respectively.[58] These estimates are notably higher than those offered by claims-based analyses, which provide an alternative means of evaluating disease epidemiology. Claims-based analyses have demonstrated an approximately 2.0 to 4.0, 1.0 to 2.0, and 0.5 to 2.0 incidence of PV, ET and PMF, respectively (see Table 1).[59–62] An informative example of the disconnect between registry- and claims-based estimates was provided by Mehta and colleagues,[60] who noted a three-fold higher PMF incidence for those aged at least 65 years at time of case capture using Medicare claims when compared with SEER data for the same age group. However, like registry-based analyses, claims-based studies may be affected by a lack of pathologic confirmation of the diagnosis and coding errors. In addition, incident patients may be inaccurately included within the prevalent population under the scenario when the disease develops or is diagnosed before a relevant claim is eventually filed.

The incidence of the MPNs is also influenced by several unmodifiable patient-specific factors, particularly age, sex and ethnicity. The MPNs are diseases of the elderly; the incidence of PV (Fig. 1), ET (Fig. 2), and PMF (Fig. 3) increases with increasing age. The median age at diagnosis of PV, ET and PMF ranges from 61 to 65, 54 to 73, and 65 to 76, respectively, based on US, European, and Australian studies.[55,56,63–68] Significant heterogeneity exists in the studied populations to suggest substantial differences in median age at diagnoses between individual MPNs. However, among patients with ET, those with CALR-mutated (49 vs 58 years, P<.0001) and triple-negative disease (47 vs 58 years, P=.004) are found to be diagnosed at an earlier age compared to those with JAK2-mutated disease.[69] The MPNs are also largely observed to be a disease of males with male:female incidence rate ratios of 1.3 to 1.6 and 1.3 to 4.0 for PV and PMF, respectively (see Figs. 1 and 3).[55,57,65,70–72] The exception to the male predominance within MPNs is patients with ET, among whom there is a male:female IRR of 0.5 to 0.7 (see Fig. 2).[56–58,65,71,72] Males are also found to have a higher rate of transformation to

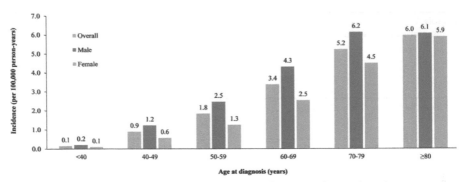

Fig. 1. Age-adjusted incidence of polycythemia vera by age at diagnosis and sex as per Surveillance, Epidemiology, and End Results (SEER) Program data, 2001 to 2016.

post-PV/ET myelofibrosis and MPN-BP after accounting for age at MPN at diagnosis and mutations with known prognostic significance.[73] In evaluating differences in MPN incidence by race/ethnicity, patients diagnosed with PV are more likely to be white, and those diagnosed with ET are more likely to be black.[55] When compared with their white or black counterparts, individuals of Latino, Asian/Pacific Islander, and American Indian/Alaskan Native descent have a lower incidence of each of these MPNs.[55]

PREVALENCE

The issues that trouble incidence estimates also limit the identification of the true prevalence of the MPNs. More recent estimates of both incidence and prevalence are likely the more accurate representations given the widespread knowledge and availability of driver mutation testing to aid disease recognition and accurate diagnosis. The estimated prevalence of PV and ET immediately prior to the discovery of the *JAK2*-V617F mutation was 22 and 24 cases per 100,000 population, respectively, based on claims-based analyses; this corresponded to approximately 65,000 and 71,000 active cases of PV and ET in the Unite States, respectively at that time.[74] Early estimates of PMF prevalence were limited by its rare nature, lack of prior mutation testing, and relatively poor prognosis.

More recent US claims-based analyses in the era of testing for *JAK2*-V617F, *JAK2* exon 12 and *MPL* exon 10 and using both different data sources and methodology

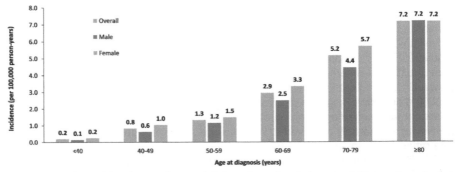

Fig. 2. Age-adjusted incidence of essential thrombocythemia by age at diagnosis and sex as per Surveillance, Epidemiology, and End Results (SEER) Program data, 2001 to 2016.

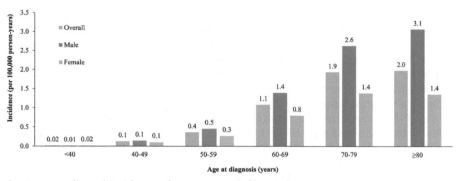

Fig. 3. Age-adjusted incidence of primary myelofibrosis by age at diagnosis and sex as per Surveillance, Epidemiology, and End Results (SEER) Program data, 2001 to 2016.

have offered higher estimates (see **Table 1**). During 2008 to 2010, the claims-based estimated prevalence of PV and ET in the US was 44 to 57 and 38 to 58 per 100,000, respectively.[60] European and Scandinavian registry-based studies during the same time period and including data up to 2012 have estimated the PV and ET prevalence to be lower in the 5 to 30 and 4 to 24 per 100,000, respectively.[57,65] The prevalence of PMF has been difficult to assess until recently. Claims-based and registry-based analyses in the United States and Europe have estimated the age-standardized prevalence of PMF to be 0.5 to 6.0 cases per 100,000 population, corresponding to up to 18,000 patients currently living with the disease in the United States.[57,60,65] Similar to incidence estimates, the range of MPN prevalence estimates observed is likely because of heterogeneity in the data sources and methodology employed in studies as well as possible ethnic differences that affect incidence and survival, the 2 determinants of prevalence.

SURVIVAL

Although studies prior to the use of molecular testing reported a normal life expectancy for patients with PV or ET when compared to the general population,[75,76] later data support a detrimental effect on long-term survival. The median survival of patients in the United States, Europe, and Australia after a diagnosis of PV is estimated to be 12 to 14 years (see **Table 1**).[55,68] When considering the older age at time of diagnosis for patients with MPNs, relative survival is a more meaningful description of survival. Studies have demonstrated that, when compared with the general population, the estimated 5-year relative survival of PV patients ranges from 84% to 89%.[55,56,68,77,78]

The median survival of ET patients mostly mirrors that of PV patients, although longer survival for patients with ET has been suggested. ET patients diagnosed in the United States, Europe, and Australia are reported to have a median survival ranging from 13 to 23 years.[55,63,64] Five-year relative survival ranges from 86% to 91% for patients diagnosed up to 2011 (see **Table 1**).[55,56,77,78] It is important to note that the distinction between prePMF and fibrotic/overt PMF since 2016 has allowed one to realize that many previous patients with these early histologic findings may have been misclassified as ET. Consistent with this concern, 1 large study of patients diagnosed with ET reported that 16% were ultimately reclassified as prePMF and were noted to have an inferior survival when compared with patients with true ET.[79]

Patients with PMF have been found to have shortest survival of all MPNs. In contrast to the near-normal survival observed for patients with PV or ET, the median survival for all PMF patients diagnosed in the United States, Europe, and Australia is estimated to be 4 to 7 years, with a 5-year relative survival of 35% to 46% (see **Table 1**).[55,66,69,77,78,80,81] The survival of PMF patients appears to be unchanged since the JAK 1/2 inhibitor ruxolitinib became available in 2011.[55]

Survival variance is noted within each of these MPN groups, and several factors are at play. PMF patients perhaps serve as the most informative example of the heterogeneity in prognosis and survival for the MPNs. Patient-specific factors, like age and symptomatology, and disease-specific factors like cytopenias, transfusion-dependence, and karyotypic/mutational profiles, assist in stratifying PMF patient prognosis. Risk stratification tools, like the International Prognostic Scoring System (IPSS), the Dynamic IPSS (DIPSS), the DIPSS-plus, the genetically inspired prognostic scoring system (GIPSS), and more recently the mutation-enhanced IPSS (MIPSS)70+ version 2.0 are able to identify PMF patients with a predicted median survival as short as 2.6 years or as long as 26.4 years.[82,83] When accounting for sex and karyotype among other relevant covariates, increasing age at diagnosis of PV, ET, and PMF is associated with shorter survival.[63,68,84–86] This is likely explained by increasing risk of post-PV or post-ET myelofibrosis and/or transformation to MPN-BP. The independent impact of age at diagnosis is still accounted for in newer prognostic scoring systems that incorporate mutational profiles.[83] The male sex also appears to independently confer slightly shorter survival for patients with MPNs, with most of this disparity driven by PV and ET.[56,64,80,84]

SUMMARY

The MPNs are a collection of entities that, despite having distinct WHO definitions, often share similar biology and clinical sequelae. The etiology of these diseases is not clear, but is rooted in the acquisition of a driver mutation that consequently activates the JAK-STAT pathway; these genetic abnormalities have been progressively discovered and understood, although many cases have undefined drivers of disease. Germline predispositions, including highly penetrant mutations and weakly penetrant single nucleotide polymorphisms, have been described and may be responsible for up to 10% of all cases of MPN. The incidence of the MPNs has remained relatively unchanged over time, except for ET, where a slight increase has been observed for unclear reasons. Similarly, the survival of patents with the MPNs has been static, mostly owing to the lack of effective disease-modifying therapies other than allogeneic stem cell transplantation. An unchanged incidence and survival for MPN patients over time explains a stable estimated prevalence, although the methodology of epidemiologic studies has been heterogeneous. Slight differences in incidence and survival for MPN subtypes are noted by age, sex, and ethnicity among other weaker factors. Better understanding of MPN pathogenesis and the development of disease-modifying therapies are needed to significantly impact the lives of affected patients.

CLINICS CARE POINTS

- Not all identified MPN-associated mutations represent disease, but these patients should be closely observed over time for disease development.
- A family history of MPN should always be examined to evaluate the possibility of hereditary associations; suspicion for a patient to have an MPN should be heightened if a first-degree relative is affected.

- A bone marrow evaluation is required for most patients undergoing a work-up for MPN to confirm the diagnosis and subclassify the disease type.
- Expert hematopathologic consultation is necessary to establish the appropriate diagnosis and avoid misclassification such as that encountered in distinguishing between ET and prePMF.

DISCLOSURES/COMPETING INTERESTS

A.M. Zeidan received research funding (institutional) from Celgene, Acceleron, Abbvie, Otsuka, Pfizer, Medimmune/AstraZeneca, Boehringer Ingelheim, Trovagene, Incyte, Takeda, and ADC Therapeutics. A.M. Zeidan had a consultancy with and received honoraria from AbbVie, Otsuka, Pfizer, Celgene, Ariad, Incyte, Agios, Boehringer-Ingelheim, Novartis, Acceleron, Astellas, Daiichi Sankyo, Cardinal Health, Seattle Genetics, BeyondSpring, and Takeda. N.A. Podoltsev consulted for and received honoraria from Alexion, Pfizer, Agios Pharmaceuticals, Blueprint Medicines, Incyte, Novartis, Celgene, Bristol-Myers Squib, CTI BioPharma, and PharmaEssentia. N.A. Podoltsev received research funding (all to the institution) from Boehringer Ingelheim, Astellas Pharma, Daiichi-Sankyo, Sunesis Pharmaceuticals, Jazz Pharmaceuticals, Pfizer, Astex Pharmaceuticals, CTI biopharma, Celgene, Genentech, AI Therapeutics, Samus Therapeutics, Arog Pharmaceuticals, and Kartos Therapeutics. None of these relationships were related to the development of this article. All other authors report no relevant disclosures/competing interests.

REFERENCES

1. Swerdlow SH, Campo E, Harris NL, et al, editors. WHO classification of tumours of haematopoietic and lymphoid tissues. Lyon (France): IARC; 2017.
2. Vainchenker W, Kralovics R. Genetic basis and molecular pathophysiology of classical myeloproliferative neoplasms. Blood 2017;129(6):667–79.
3. Barbui T, Tefferi A, Vannucchi AM, et al. Philadelphia chromosome-negative classical myeloproliferative neoplasms: revised management recommendations from European LeukemiaNet. Leukemia 2018;32(5):1057–69.
4. Dameshek W. Some speculations on the myeloproliferative syndromes. Blood 1951;6(4):372–5.
5. Fritz APC, Jack A, Shanmugaratnam K, et al, editors. International classification of diseases for oncology. Geneva (Switzerland): World Health Organization; 2000.
6. Kralovics R, Passamonti F, Buser AS, et al. A gain-of-function mutation of JAK2 in myeloproliferative disorders. N Engl J Med 2005;352(17):1779–90.
7. Passamonti F, Elena C, Schnittger S, et al. Molecular and clinical features of the myeloproliferative neoplasm associated with JAK2 exon 12 mutations. Blood 2011;117(10):2813–6.
8. Scott LM, Tong W, Levine RL, et al. JAK2 exon 12 mutations in polycythemia vera and idiopathic erythrocytosis. N Engl J Med 2007;356(5):459–68.
9. Vardiman JW, Thiele J, Arber DA, et al. The 2008 revision of the World Health Organization (WHO) classification of myeloid neoplasms and acute leukemia: rationale and important changes. Blood 2009;114(5):937–51.
10. Xu Z, Gale RP, Zhang Y, et al. Unique features of primary myelofibrosis in Chinese. Blood 2012;119(11):2469–73.

11. Pardanani AD, Levine RL, Lasho T, et al. MPL515 mutations in myeloproliferative and other myeloid disorders: a study of 1182 patients. Blood 2006;108(10): 3472–6.
12. Pikman Y, Lee BH, Mercher T, et al. MPLW515L is a novel somatic activating mutation in myelofibrosis with myeloid metaplasia. PLoS Med 2006;3(7):e270.
13. Klampfl T, Gisslinger H, Harutyunyan AS, et al. Somatic mutations of calreticulin in myeloproliferative neoplasms. N Engl J Med 2013;369(25):2379–90.
14. Nangalia J, Massie CE, Baxter EJ, et al. Somatic CALR mutations in myeloproliferative neoplasms with nonmutated JAK2. N Engl J Med 2013;369(25):2391–405.
15. Arber DA, Orazi A, Hasserjian R, et al. The 2016 revision to the World Health Organization classification of myeloid neoplasms and acute leukemia. Blood 2016; 127(20):2391–405.
16. Kashofer K, Gornicec M, Lind K, et al. Detection of prognostically relevant mutations and translocations in myeloid sarcoma by next generation sequencing. Leuk Lymphoma 2018;59(2):501–4.
17. Lindholm Sorensen A, Hasselbalch HC. Smoking and Philadelphia-negative chronic myeloproliferative neoplasms. Eur J Haematol 2016;97(1):63–9.
18. Musselman JR, Blair CK, Cerhan JR, et al. Risk of adult acute and chronic myeloid leukemia with cigarette smoking and cessation. Cancer Epidemiol 2013;37(4):410–6.
19. Pedersen KM, Bak M, Sorensen AL, et al. Smoking is associated with increased risk of myeloproliferative neoplasms: a general population-based cohort study. Cancer Med 2018;7(11):5796–802.
20. Leal AD, Thompson CA, Wang AH, et al. Anthropometric, medical history and lifestyle risk factors for myeloproliferative neoplasms in the Iowa Women's Health Study cohort. Int J Cancer 2014;134(7):1741–50.
21. Podoltsev NA, Wang X, Wang R, et al. Lifestyle factors and risk of myeloproliferative neoplasms in the NIH-AARP diet and health study. Int J Cancer 2020;147(4): 948–57.
22. Podoltsev NA, Wang X, Wang R, et al. Diet and risk of myeloproliferative neoplasms in older individuals from the NIH-AARP Cohort. Cancer Epidemiol Biomarkers Prev 2020;29(11):2343–50.
23. Cooper GS, Stroehla BC. The epidemiology of autoimmune diseases. Autoimmun Rev 2003;2(3):119–25.
24. Kristinsson SY, Landgren O, Samuelsson J, et al. Autoimmunity and the risk of myeloproliferative neoplasms. Haematologica 2010;95(7):1216–20.
25. Anderson LA, Pfeiffer RM, Landgren O, et al. Risks of myeloid malignancies in patients with autoimmune conditions. Br J Cancer 2009;100(5):822–8.
26. Reilly SM, Saltiel AR. Adapting to obesity with adipose tissue inflammation. Nat Rev Endocrinol 2017;13(11):633–43.
27. Duncombe AS, Anderson LA, James G, et al. Modifiable lifestyle and medical risk factors associated with myeloproliferative neoplasms. Hemasphere 2020;4(1): e327.
28. Leiba A, Duek A, Afek A, et al. Obesity and related risk of myeloproliferative neoplasms among Israeli adolescents. Obesity (Silver Spring) 2017;25(7):1187–90.
29. Sud A, Chattopadhyay S, Thomsen H, et al. Familial risks of acute myeloid leukemia, myelodysplastic syndromes, and myeloproliferative neoplasms. Blood 2018; 132(9):973–6.
30. Rumi E, Passamonti F, Della Porta MG, et al. Familial chronic myeloproliferative disorders: clinical phenotype and evidence of disease anticipation. J Clin Oncol 2007;25(35):5630–5.

31. Mead AJ, Chowdhury O, Pecquet C, et al. Impact of isolated germline JAK2V617I mutation on human hematopoiesis. Blood 2013;121(20):4156–65.
32. Etheridge SL, Cosgrove ME, Sangkhae V, et al. A novel activating, germline JAK2 mutation, JAK2R564Q, causes familial essential thrombocytosis. Blood 2014; 123(7):1059–68.
33. Rumi E, Harutyunyan AS, Casetti I, et al. A novel germline JAK2 mutation in familial myeloproliferative neoplasms. Am J Hematol 2014;89(1):117–8.
34. Milosevic Feenstra JD, Nivarthi H, Gisslinger H, et al. Whole-exome sequencing identifies novel MPL and JAK2 mutations in triple-negative myeloproliferative neoplasms. Blood 2016;127(3):325–32.
35. Szuber N, Lamontagne B, Busque L. Novel germline mutations in the calreticulin gene: implications for the diagnosis of myeloproliferative neoplasms. J Clin Pathol 2016. https://doi.org/10.1136/jclinpath-2016-203940.
36. Hinds DA, Barnholt KE, Mesa RA, et al. Germ line variants predispose to both JAK2 V617F clonal hematopoiesis and myeloproliferative neoplasms. Blood 2016;128(8):1121–8.
37. Jones AV, Chase A, Silver RT, et al. JAK2 haplotype is a major risk factor for the development of myeloproliferative neoplasms. Nat Genet 2009;41(4):446–9.
38. Kilpivaara O, Mukherjee S, Schram AM, et al. A germline JAK2 SNP is associated with predisposition to the development of JAK2(V617F)-positive myeloproliferative neoplasms. Nat Genet 2009;41(4):455–9.
39. Rumi E, Cazzola M. Advances in understanding the pathogenesis of familial myeloproliferative neoplasms. Br J Haematol 2017;178(5):689–98.
40. Macedo LC, Santos BC, Pagliarini-e-Silva S, et al. JAK2 46/1 haplotype is associated with JAK2 V617F–positive myeloproliferative neoplasms in Brazilian patients. Int J Lab Hematol 2015;37(5):654–60.
41. Tanaka M, Yujiri T, Ito S, et al. JAK2 46/1 haplotype is associated with JAK2 V617F-positive myeloproliferative neoplasms in Japanese patients. Int J Hematol 2013;97(3):409–13.
42. Wang J, Xu Z, Liu L, et al. JAK2V617F allele burden, JAK2 46/1 haplotype and clinical features of Chinese with myeloproliferative neoplasms. Leukemia 2013; 27(8):1763–7.
43. Alvarez-Larran A, Angona A, Martinez-Aviles L, et al. Influence of JAK2 46/1 haplotype in the natural evolution of JAK2V617F allele burden in patients with myeloproliferative neoplasms. Leuk Res 2012;36(3):324–6.
44. Chiang YH, Chang YC, Lin HC, et al. Germline variations at JAK2, TERT, HBS1L-MYB and MECOM and the risk of myeloproliferative neoplasms in Taiwanese population. Oncotarget 2017;8(44):76204–13.
45. Jager R, Harutyunyan AS, Rumi E, et al. Common germline variation at the TERT locus contributes to familial clustering of myeloproliferative neoplasms. Am J Hematol 2014;89(12):1107–10.
46. Oddsson A, Kristinsson SY, Helgason H, et al. The germline sequence variant rs2736100_C in TERT associates with myeloproliferative neoplasms. Leukemia 2014;28(6):1371–4.
47. Tapper W, Jones AV, Kralovics R, et al. Genetic variation at MECOM, TERT, JAK2 and HBS1L-MYB predisposes to myeloproliferative neoplasms. Nat Commun 2015;6:6691.
48. Nielsen C, Birgens HS, Nordestgaard BG, et al. Diagnostic value of JAK2 V617F somatic mutation for myeloproliferative cancer in 49 488 individuals from the general population. Br J Haematol 2013;160(1):70–9.

49. Nielsen C, Birgens HS, Nordestgaard BG, et al. The JAK2 V617F somatic mutation, mortality and cancer risk in the general population. Haematologica 2011; 96(3):450–3.
50. Nielsen C, Bojesen SE, Nordestgaard BG, et al. JAK2V617F somatic mutation in the general population: myeloproliferative neoplasm development and progression rate. Haematologica 2014;99(9):1448–55.
51. Cordua S, Kjaer L, Skov V, et al. Prevalence and phenotypes of JAK2 V617F and calreticulin mutations in a Danish general population. Blood 2019;134(5):469–79.
52. Jaiswal S, Natarajan P, Silver AJ, et al. Clonal hematopoiesis and risk of atherosclerotic cardiovascular disease. N Engl J Med 2017;377(2):111–21.
53. About SEER. Surveillance, epidemiology, and end results program. National Cancer Insistute. Available at: https://seer.cancer.gov/registries/cancer_registry/index.html. Accessed June 11, 2020.
54. Rollison DE, Howlader N, Smith MT, et al. Epidemiology of myelodysplastic syndromes and chronic myeloproliferative disorders in the United States, 2001-2004, using data from the NAACCR and SEER programs. Blood 2008;112(1):45–52.
55. Shallis RM, Wang R, Davidoff A, et al. Epidemiology of the classical myeloproliferative neoplasms: the four corners of an expansive and complex map. Blood Rev 2020;42:100706.
56. Baade PD, Ross DM, Anderson LA, et al. Changing incidence of myeloproliferative neoplasms in Australia, 2003-2014. Am J Hematol 2019;94(4):E107–9.
57. Roaldsnes C, Holst R, Frederiksen H, et al. Myeloproliferative neoplasms: trends in incidence, prevalence and survival in Norway. Eur J Haematol 2017;98(1):85–93.
58. Srour SA, Devesa SS, Morton LM, et al. Incidence and patient survival of myeloproliferative neoplasms and myelodysplastic/myeloproliferative neoplasms in the United States, 2001-12. Br J Haematol 2016;174(3):382–96.
59. Selinger HA, Ma X. Jakking up tumor registry reporting of the myeloproliferative neoplasms. Am J Hematol 2009;84(2):124–6.
60. Mehta J, Wang H, Iqbal SU, et al. Epidemiology of myeloproliferative neoplasms in the United States. Leuk Lymphoma 2014;55(3):595–600.
61. Johansson P. Epidemiology of the myeloproliferative disorders polycythemia vera and essential thrombocythemia. Semin Thromb Hemost 2006;32(3):171–3.
62. Byun JM, Kim YJ, Youk T, et al. Real world epidemiology of myeloproliferative neoplasms: a population based study in Korea 2004-2013. Ann Hematol 2017; 96(3):373–81.
63. Wolanskyj AP, Schwager SM, McClure RF, et al. Essential thrombocythemia beyond the first decade: life expectancy, long-term complication rates, and prognostic factors. Mayo Clin Proc 2006;81(2):159–66.
64. Passamonti F, Rumi E, Pungolino E, et al. Life expectancy and prognostic factors for survival in patients with polycythemia vera and essential thrombocythemia. Am J Med 2004;117(10):755–61.
65. Moulard O, Mehta J, Fryzek J, et al. Epidemiology of myelofibrosis, essential thrombocythemia, and polycythemia vera in the European Union. Eur J Haematol 2014;92(4):289–97.
66. Penna D, Lasho TL, Finke CM, et al. 20+ Years and alive with primary myelofibrosis: phenotypic signature of very long-lived patients. Am J Hematol 2019; 94(3):286–90.
67. Tefferi A, Lasho TL, Jimma T, et al. One thousand patients with primary myelofibrosis: the mayo clinic experience. Mayo Clin Proc 2012;87(1):25–33.

68. Tefferi A, Rumi E, Finazzi G, et al. Survival and prognosis among 1545 patients with contemporary polycythemia vera: an international study. Leukemia 2013; 27(9):1874–81.
69. Tefferi A, Guglielmelli P, Larson DR, et al. Long-term survival and blast transformation in molecularly annotated essential thrombocythemia, polycythemia vera, and myelofibrosis. Blood 2014;124(16):2507–13 [quiz 2615].
70. Titmarsh GJ, Duncombe AS, McMullin MF, et al. How common are myeloproliferative neoplasms? A systematic review and meta-analysis. Am J Hematol 2014;89(6):581–7.
71. Zhang L, Lan Q, Guo W, et al. Chromosome-wide aneuploidy study (CWAS) in workers exposed to an established leukemogen, benzene. Carcinogenesis 2011;32(4):605–12.
72. Price GL, Davis KL, Karve S, et al. Survival patterns in United States (US) medicare enrollees with non-CML myeloproliferative neoplasms (MPN). PLoS One 2014;9(3):e90299.
73. Karantanos T, Chaturvedi S, Braunstein EM, et al. Sex determines the presentation and outcomes in MPN and is related to sex-specific differences in the mutational burden. Blood Adv 2020;4(12):2567–76.
74. Ma X, Vanasse G, Cartmel B, et al. Prevalence of polycythemia vera and essential thrombocythemia. Am J Hematol 2008;83(5):359–62.
75. Rozman C, Giralt M, Feliu E, et al. Life expectancy of patients with chronic non-leukemic myeloproliferative disorders. Cancer 1991;67(10):2658–63.
76. Tefferi A, Fonseca R, Pereira DL, et al. A long-term retrospective study of young women with essential thrombocythemia. Mayo Clin Proc 2001;76(1):22–8.
77. Visser O, Trama A, Maynadie M, et al. Incidence, survival and prevalence of myeloid malignancies in Europe. Eur J Cancer 2012;48(17):3257–66.
78. Maynadie M, De Angelis R, Marcos-Gragera R, et al. Survival of European patients diagnosed with myeloid malignancies: a HAEMACARE study. Haematologica 2013;98(2):230–8.
79. Barbui T, Thiele J, Passamonti F, et al. Survival and disease progression in essential thrombocythemia are significantly influenced by accurate morphologic diagnosis: an international study. J Clin Oncol 2011;29(23):3179–84.
80. Hultcrantz M, Kristinsson SY, Andersson TM, et al. Patterns of survival among patients with myeloproliferative neoplasms diagnosed in Sweden from 1973 to 2008: a population-based study. J Clin Oncol 2012;30(24):2995–3001.
81. Cervantes F, Dupriez B, Passamonti F, et al. Improving survival trends in primary myelofibrosis: an international study. J Clin Oncol 2012;30(24):2981–7.
82. Tefferi A. Primary myelofibrosis: 2019 update on diagnosis, risk-stratification and management. Am J Hematol 2018;93(12):1551–60.
83. Tefferi A, Guglielmelli P, Nicolosi M, et al. GIPSS: genetically inspired prognostic scoring system for primary myelofibrosis. Leukemia 2018;32(7):1631–42.
84. Tefferi A, Betti S, Barraco D, et al. Gender and survival in essential thrombocythemia: a two-center study of 1,494 patients. Am J Hematol 2017;92(11):1193–7.
85. Cervantes F, Dupriez B, Pereira A, et al. New prognostic scoring system for primary myelofibrosis based on a study of the International Working Group for Myelofibrosis Research and Treatment. Blood 2009;113(13):2895–901.
86. Passamonti F, Cervantes F, Vannucchi AM, et al. A dynamic prognostic model to predict survival in primary myelofibrosis: a study by the IWG-MRT (International Working Group for Myeloproliferative Neoplasms Research and Treatment). Blood 2010;115(9):1703–8.

The Role of Megakaryocytes in Myelofibrosis

Johanna Melo-Cardenas, PhD[a], Anna Rita Migliaccio, PhD[b], John D. Crispino, PhD[a],*

KEYWORDS

• Megakaryocyte • Myeloproliferative neoplasms • JAK/STAT

KEY POINTS

• Megakaryocyte abnormalities are a common feature of the myeloproliferative neoplasms.
• Activation of JAK/STAT signaling owing to mutations in JAK2, MPL, or CALR lead to an overproduction of megakaryocytes.
• Atypical megakaryocytes in myelofibrosis show defects in maturation and release profibrotic and proinflammatory factors.
• Inducing the differentiation of megakaryocytes shows clinical activity in myeloproliferative neoplasms.

INTRODUCTION

The myeloproliferative neoplasms (MPNs) constitute a heterogenous group of related hematologic disorders affecting different myeloid lineages.[1] Activating mutations in Janus Kinase 2 (*JAK2*), the thrombopoietin receptor (myeloproliferative leukemia protein [*MPL*]), and Calreticulin (*CALR*) have been found in more than 95% of patients with polycythemia vera (PV), essential thrombocythemia (ET), and myelofibrosis (including primary myelofibrosis [PMF] pre-PMF, post-PV MF, and post-ET MF).[2–9] Each of these mutations lead to constitutive activation of the JAK2/STAT pathway, but through different mechanisms.[10,11] MF is the most aggressive of the JAK2/CALR/MPL-mutated MPNs, whereas patients with PV or ET can progress to myelofibrosis with a 15-year cumulative incidence rate of 19% and 9%, respectively.[1,12,13]

PV is characterized by erythrocytosis and ET by thrombocytosis. Patients with MF can present with thrombocytosis or thrombocytopenia, anemia, and leukocytosis or leukopenia.[13] Bone marrow histopathologic changes in MF include megakaryocytic proliferation and atypia with clustering that is accompanied by fibrosis. By contrast,

[a] Division of Experimental Hematology, St. Jude Children's Research Hospital, 262 Danny Thomas Place, MC341, Memphis, TN 38105, USA; [b] Department of Biomedical and Neuromotor Sciences, University of Bologna, Via Irnerio, 48 - I 40126, Bologna, Italy
* Corresponding author.
E-mail address: john.crispino@stjude.org
Twitter: @melo_cardenas1 (J.M.-C.)

Hematol Oncol Clin N Am 35 (2021) 191–203
https://doi.org/10.1016/j.hoc.2020.11.004
0889-8588/21/© 2020 Elsevier Inc. All rights reserved.

in ET there are increased numbers of mature, enlarged megakaryocytes with hyperlobulated nuclei. Finally, the bone marrow is characterized by mature pleomorphic megakaryocytes in PV.[13]

BACKGROUND
Normal Megakaryopoiesis

Megakaryocytes are derived from hematopoietic stem cells (HSCs) through a stepwise process that depends on thrombopoietin (TPO). The traditional view of megakaryopoiesis begins with HSCs giving rise to multipotent progenitors, which generate the common myeloid progenitor. These common myeloid progenitors then produce the megakaryocyte erythrocyte progenitor (MEP), which gives rise to both erythroid cells and megakaryocytes.[14,15] Upon commitment, immature megakaryocytes undergo multiple rounds of endomitosis and cytoskeletal rearrangements to generate proplatelets, which enter the peripheral blood and generate platelets. Recent studies have redefined this traditional view by showing that megakaryocytes can also be generated directly from HSCs or multipotent progenitors without the canonical common myeloid progenitor or MEP intermediate.[16] Megakaryopoiesis is controlled by a number of transcription factors, including RUNX1, GATA1, GFI1B, and several ETS factors. Their importance in this process is highlighted by the presence of mutations in these factors in individuals with congenital amegakaryocytic thrombocytopenia, bleeding disorders, and Gray platelet syndrome, as well as by ineffective megakaryopoiesis in induced pluripotent stem cells and animal models.[17,18]

Megakaryopoiesis in myelofibrosis

As mentioned, megakaryocytes in MF are atypical in that they display morphologic abnormalities such as hypolobulated nuclei and clustering (**Fig. 1**). Studies with CD34+ cells from patients with MF revealed their increased capacity to generate megakaryocytes in culture, albeit immature ones with decreased ploidy.[19–21] MPN megakaryocytes have higher proliferative capacity and decreased apoptosis rate. More recently, by using single cell approaches, 2 groups demonstrated that HSCs from

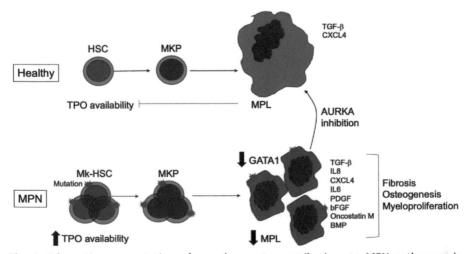

Fig. 1. Schematic representation of megakaryocyte contributions to MPN pathogenesis. Upon acquisition of an MPN driver mutation, megakaryocytes in MF display impaired differentiation, decreased GATA1 expression and enhanced cytokine/chemokine secretion. A number of these secreted factors promote fibrosis, osteogenesis, and myeloproliferation.

patients with ET and patients with MF express megakaryocytic genes indicating their bias toward this lineage, consistent with the directed differentiation model of HSC specification to megakaryocytes.[22,23]

In 2005, Migliaccio and Vannucchi reported that MF megakaryocytes express low levels of the transcription factor GATA1.[24,25] This finding was confirmed and extended by the demonstration that restoration of GATA1 protein levels could restore normal differentiation.[26] This GATA1 deficiency is specific for megakaryocytes in MF, because it is not observed in patients with PV or ET.[27] Furthermore, a mouse model expressing low levels of GATA1, the $Gata1^{low}$ strain, displays similar megakaryocytic defects and, with time, these mice uniformly develop bone marrow fibrosis.[28,29] In MF, the decrease in GATA1 expression has been attributed to a ribosomal deficiency[27]; similarly, the megakaryocyte defects in $Gata1^{low}$ mice show abnormalities in ribosomes.[26,30] Finally, it has been shown that Aurora Kinase A inhibitors, which induce polyploidization and partial differentiation of MF megakaryocytes, increases expression of GATA1.[31,32]

Driver mutations in *JAK2*, *MPL*, and *CALR* have been detected in different hematopoietic cell types, suggesting their acquisition in a primitive hematopoietic cell.[22,33–36] The acquisition of additional somatic mutations has been associated with progression of ET, PV, or pre-PMF into overt PMF and acute myeloid leukemia.[37–41] Typically, these mutations can be detected in bulk preparations of leukocytes or CD34$^+$ cells. Interestingly, a study by Guo and colleagues[42] arrived at a different conclusion. By comparing the mutation profile of bone marrow megakaryocytes with megakaryocyte-depleted bone marrow cells from the same patients in MF, they found that, although megakaryocytes had the expected driver mutations, they also had a unique somatic mutational profile. MF megakaryocytes harbored mutations in genes involved in chromatin remodeling and chromosome alignment, some of which were not previously reported in MPNs. The extent to which these somatic mutations play a role in disease pathogenesis or are passenger mutations needs further study. Finally, with the advent of single cell DNA sequencing technologies, it would be interesting to investigate the clonal evolution in megakaryocytes as they undergo multiple rounds of endomitosis to determine whether they accumulate more genomic defects than other lineages.

THROMBOPOIETIN SIGNALING

TPO, a key regulator of megakaryopoiesis, binds to its receptor, MPL, and induces JAK/STAT, MAPK/ERK, and PI3K/AKT activation in HSCs, megakaryocytes, and platelets.[43] Mice lacking TPO or MPL are viable, but are thrombocytopenic with decreased numbers of HSCs and megakaryocytes.[44,45] MPL expression on megakaryocytes and platelets is essential to prevent myeloproliferation and megakaryocyte expansion by limiting the availability of TPO from HSCs and progenitors.[46–48] JAK2 binds MPL stimulating its recycling and enhancing its protein stability.[49] Mice lacking *Jak2* in megakaryocytes and platelets are characterized by thrombocytosis and expansion of HSCs,[50] similar to the phenotype of mice lacking MPL in megakaryocytes.[48] These data indicate that the thrombocytopenia often observed in patients treated with JAK2 inhibitors is due to the inhibition of JAK2 in HSCs rather than in megakaryocytes or platelets.

Numerous reports have highlighted the role of the enhanced TPO–MPL signaling axis in MPNs. Patients with ET and PV have normal to elevated levels of serum TPO, whereas patients with MF have increased levels.[51–53] More recent studies have shown that MPL expression in bone marrow cells from patients with MPN is heterogenous and that megakaryocytes and platelets express low MPL levels.[54–56]

The overexpression of TPO in the bone marrow has been shown to induce fibrosis in mice.[57] The constitutively active JAK2^{V617F} mutation in patients with MPN has been shown to decrease MPL expression by enhancing MPL degradation and decreasing its recycling.[58] In patients with MPN, an inverse correlation between the JAK2^{V617F} allele burden and MPL expression has been reported.[59] The dependency of MPN cells on the TPO–MPL signaling axis to initiate and maintain the disease has been shown in vivo in murine models and in vitro in human samples. Decreasing the expression of MPL in murine and xenograft MPN models decreased the disease burden and fibrosis.[60–62] The exciting potential of therapeutically targeting this pathway will be important to test in future clinical trials.

JAK/STAT SIGNALING

The specific contribution of megakaryocytes in MPNs was studied by conditionally expressing JAK2^{V617F} using the PF4-Cre mouse line. In PF4-Cre mice, Cre is expressed in the megakaryocytic lineage and to a low extent in other myeloid cells.[63–65] It has been shown that megakaryocytic restricted expression of JAK2^{V617F} in mice induces polycythemia or thrombocytosis, although with a longer latency compared with mice expressing JAK2^{V617F} in all hematopoietic cells.[66–68] Importantly, these phenotypes were not accompanied by the activation of JAK/STAT in the erythroid lineage, confirming that the disease was not caused by the activation of Cre in erythroid cells.[67,68] The depletion of megakaryocytes using the Cre-inducible diphtheria toxin receptor transgenic mice decreased the disease burden.[67]

Although studies have not to date been published addressing the role of mutant CALR specifically in megakaryocytes in murine models, several studies have shown the pronounced effect of mutant CALR on megakaryocytes. CALR is a multifunctional protein found with different subcellular localizations where it plays diverse functions.[69] In MPNs, mutations in CALR result in the expression of a protein with a novel amino acid sequence at the C-terminus.[70] By using antibodies that recognize mutant CALR, 2 groups have shown that MPN megakaryocytes preferentially express the mutant variant, unlike other cells in the bone marrow.[71,72] The expression of CALR^{del52} in the germline or in hematopoietic cells in mice predominantly affects the megakaryocyte lineage; these mice have thrombocytosis with megakaryocytic expansion.[73–77]

Mutant CALR has been shown to be an important regulator of TPO-MPL signaling. CALR mutants bind MPL receptors, leading to the cytokine-independent activation of JAK/STAT signaling, which in turn induces megakaryocyte proliferation.[76–81] CALR^{del52} also binds FLI1, a transcription factor important for megakaryopoiesis, leading to an increased expression of MPL.[82] Similarly, the expression of mutant CALR in cell lines increases the expression of MPL, CD41, and NF-E2.[83] More recently, Di Buduo and colleagues[84] showed that megakaryocytes from patients with a CALR^{del52} mutation lose the interaction with the store-operated calcium entry machinery, leading to increased TPO signaling and abnormal proliferation.

With regard to 2 downstream effectors of JAK2 signaling, STAT3 and STAT5, it has been shown that STAT3 acts as a negative regulator in MPNs. The absence of STAT3 in JAK2^{V617F} mice led to disease acceleration with an increase in dysplastic megakaryocytes.[85,86] This condition was attributed to an increase in STAT1 phosphorylation, which has been shown to promote megakaryocyte differentiation in mice and in samples from patients with JAK2^{V617F}.[87,88] By contrast, a loss of STAT5 in JAK2^{V617F} mice prevents MPN development, but is curiously dispensable for normal hematopoiesis.[89,90]

MEGAKARYOCYTE SECRETOME

A wide variety of substances, including coagulation factors, cytokines, neurotransmitters, and metalloproteinases, are secreted by megakaryocytes.[91–94] Megakaryocyte-derived transforming growth factor-β (TGF-β), C-X-C motif ligand 4 (CXCL4), and FGF1 have been shown critical to maintaining HSC quiescence and facilitating hematopoietic recovery upon stress in vivo.[95–97]

In MPNs, abnormal megakaryocytes secrete a number of factors, including platelet-derived growth factor, basic fibroblast growth factor, TGF-β, IL8, CXCL4, IL6, oncostatin M, and bone morphogenic protein. Moreover, megakaryocytes release extracellular matrix components and crosslinking enzymes important in the pathology of MPNs. A detailed review of each of these factors was published by Malara and colleagues,[98] therefore, we provide a brief overview of only some of these entities.

Transforming Growth Factor Beta

TGF-β is the main driver of fibrosis in different organs.[99] TGF-β directly stimulates fibroblasts among other cells to produce extracellular matrix. TGF-β levels are increased in patients with MPN and in mouse models.[100,101] Abnormal megakaryocytes and monocytes have been shown to be the main source.[25,92,102–106] Chagraoui and colleagues[107] showed for the first time that the genetic ablation of TGF-β in an MPN mouse model driven by TPO overexpression decreases bone marrow fibrosis. Further studies have shown that TGF-β inhibition in MPN mouse models decreases bone marrow fibrosis, although the effect on other aspects of the disease are less clear.[101,107–110] The effect of a TGF-β receptor inhibitor, AVID200, is currently being tested in a clinical trial in MF (NCT03895112).

C-X-C Motif Ligand 4

CXCL4, also known as platelet factor 4, has been implicated in fibrotic processes in the liver and in systemic sclerosis.[111–113] Patients with MF have elevated CXCL4 levels, although its levels do not correlate with bone marrow fibrosis.[114] Studies in MPN models showed that CXCL4 derived from megakaryocytes is key in promoting bone marrow fibrosis by inducing the myofibroblastic differentiation of stromal cells.[115] The absence of CXCL4 in MPN murine models decreases disease burden and bone marrow fibrosis.[116]

IL-6

IL-6 is a proinflammatory cytokine implicated in several types of diseases.[117] IL-6 levels are increased in patients with MPN and in murine models.[67,118–120] Increased IL-6 levels in the platelet factor 4–Cre/JAK2^{V617F} animal model was shown to promote erythropoiesis.[67] Furthermore, MEPs in the MPNs have been found to release high amounts of IL-6.[118] Fibronectin, a component of the extracellular matrix that is increased in patients with MF was shown to stimulate megakaryocytic secretion of IL-6.[121] Despite the important role of IL-6 in MPNs, targeting this cytokine has had a modest effect in mice; the blockade of IL-6 with neutralizing antibodies or by genetic deletion decreased erythropoiesis and myeloproliferation without a prominent improvement in the overall MPN phenotype.[67,118]

INFLAMMATION

Inflammation is one of the key features in MPNs. Although a number of inflammatory cytokines are increased in the serum of patients with MPN,[122,123] few studies have addressed the effect of proinflammatory cytokines on megakaryopoiesis in this disease. IL8 and TGF-β have been shown to promote the expansion megakaryocytes in samples from patients with MF.[92,124] Recent reports have demonstrated that inflammation associated with aging induces changes in metabolic and signaling pathways in the megakaryocytic lineage. Older mice show increased megakaryocyte-biased HSCs, mature megakaryocytes, and platelet counts compared with young mice.[125–127] Aging-related changes induced mitochondrial dysfunction and altered inflammatory pathways in megakaryocytes. These changes were mediated by tumor necrosis factor-α, which was found at high levels in the serum of old mice.[127] In MPNs, Rao and colleagues[128] recently showed that MEPs have a decreased mitochondrial mass and increased oxidative phosphorylation. Inflammatory signaling has been shown to promote megakaryopoiesis by increasing the protein expression of megakaryocytic genes in megakaryocyte-biased HSCs and progenitors.[129] MPNs are chronic diseases that are more common in the elderly, indicating that age-related changes might have a prominent role in the initiation and maintenance of the disease. Further studies on the effect of inflammation and aging in megakaryopoiesis in MPNs will improve our understanding of the disease.

SUMMARY

Megakaryocytes play a key role in the *JAK2*, *MPL*, and *CALR* mutated MPNs by promoting myeloproliferation and fibrosis. Recent studies have shown that the aberrant expansion in the megakaryocytic lineage results from increased numbers of megakaryocyte-biased HSCs. An expansion of megakaryocyte-biased HSCs is also observed with aging, indicating that microenvironmental factors and inflammation might influence the initiation and progression of MPNs. Furthermore, megakaryocyte-specific somatic mutations might influence the disease. Although there is an expansion of the megakaryocyte lineage in MPNs, the resulting megakaryocytes are immature and release large amounts of proinflammatory and profibrotic cytokines. Targeting MPN megakaryocytes with the Aurora Kinase A inhibitor alisertib, which promotes megakaryocytic differentiation, showed clinical benefit in a phase I study. Future studies of Aurora Kinase A inhibitors or other modulators of megakaryopoiesis should be considered.

ACKNOWLEDGMENTS

This work was supported by a grant from the National Institutes of Health (P01 CA108671). The content is solely the responsibility of the authors and does not necessarily represent the official views of the NIH. Additional support was provided by St. Jude/ ALSAC and the Associazione Italiana Ricerca Cancro (AIRC IG23525).

DISCLOSURE

The authors have nothing to disclose.

REFERENCES

1. Barbui T, Thiele J, Gisslinger H, et al. The 2016 WHO classification and diagnostic criteria for myeloproliferative neoplasms: document summary and in-depth discussion. Blood Cancer J 2018;8(2):15.
2. Baxter EJ, Scott LM, Campbell PJ, et al. Acquired mutation of the tyrosine kinase JAK2 in human myeloproliferative disorders. Lancet 2005;365(9464): 1054–61.

3. James C, Ugo V, Le Couedic JP, et al. A unique clonal JAK2 mutation leading to constitutive signalling causes polycythaemia vera. Nature 2005;434(7037): 1144–8.
4. Levine RL, Wadleigh M, Cools J, et al. Activating mutation in the tyrosine kinase JAK2 in polycythemia vera, essential thrombocythemia, and myeloid metaplasia with myelofibrosis. Cancer Cell 2005;7(4):387–97.
5. Kralovics R, Passamonti F, Buser AS, et al. A gain-of-function mutation of JAK2 in myeloproliferative disorders. N Engl J Med 2005;352(17):1779–90.
6. Pikman Y, Lee BH, Mercher T, et al. MPLW515L is a novel somatic activating mutation in myelofibrosis with myeloid metaplasia. PLoS Med 2006;3(7):e270.
7. Pardanani AD, Levine RL, Lasho T, et al. MPL515 mutations in myeloproliferative and other myeloid disorders: a study of 1182 patients. Blood 2006;108(10): 3472–6.
8. Klampfl T, Gisslinger H, Harutyunyan AS, et al. Somatic mutations of calreticulin in myeloproliferative neoplasms. N Engl J Med 2013;369(25):2379–90.
9. Nangalia J, Massie CE, Baxter EJ, et al. Somatic CALR mutations in myeloproliferative neoplasms with nonmutated JAK2. N Engl J Med 2013;369(25): 2391–405.
10. Jia R, Kralovics R. Progress in elucidation of molecular pathophysiology of myeloproliferative neoplasms and its application to therapeutic decisions. Int J Hematol 2020;111(2):182–91.
11. Schieber M, Crispino JD, Stein B. Myelofibrosis in 2019: moving beyond JAK2 inhibition. Blood Cancer J 2019;9(9):74.
12. Tefferi A, Guglielmelli P, Larson DR, et al. Long-term survival and blast transformation in molecularly annotated essential thrombocythemia, polycythemia vera, and myelofibrosis. Blood 2014;124(16):2507–13 [quiz 2615].
13. Arber DA, Orazi A, Hasserjian R, et al. The 2016 revision to the World Health Organization classification of myeloid neoplasms and acute leukemia. Blood 2016; 127(20):2391–405.
14. Dore LC, Crispino JD. Transcription factor networks in erythroid cell and megakaryocyte development. Blood 2011;118(2):231–9.
15. Guo T, Wang X, Qu Y, et al. Megakaryopoiesis and platelet production: insight into hematopoietic stem cell proliferation and differentiation. Stem Cell Investig 2015;2:3.
16. Woolthuis CM, Park CY. Hematopoietic stem/progenitor cell commitment to the megakaryocyte lineage. Blood 2016;127(10):1242–8.
17. Bianchi E, Norfo R, Pennucci V, et al. Genomic landscape of megakaryopoiesis and platelet function defects. Blood 2016;127(10):1249–59.
18. Antony-Debre I, Manchev VT, Balayn N, et al. Level of RUNX1 activity is critical for leukemic predisposition but not for thrombocytopenia. Blood 2015;125(6): 930–40.
19. Ciurea SO, Merchant D, Mahmud N, et al. Pivotal contributions of megakaryocytes to the biology of idiopathic myelofibrosis. Blood 2007;110(3):986–93.
20. Juvonen E. Megakaryocyte colony formation in chronic myeloid leukemia and myelofibrosis. Leuk Res 1988;12(9):751–6.
21. Balduini A, Badalucco S, Pugliano MT, et al. In vitro megakaryocyte differentiation and proplatelet formation in Ph-negative classical myeloproliferative neoplasms: distinct patterns in the different clinical phenotypes. PLoS One 2011; 6(6):e21015.
22. Nam AS, Kim KT, Chaligne R, et al. Somatic mutations and cell identity linked by Genotyping of Transcriptomes. Nature 2019;571(7765):355–60.

23. Psaila B, Wang G, Rodriguez-Meira A, et al. Single-cell analyses reveal megakaryocyte-biased hematopoiesis in myelofibrosis and identify mutant clone-specific targets. Mol Cell 2020;78(3):477–492 e478.

24. Vannucchi AM, Pancrazzi A, Guglielmelli P, et al. Abnormalities of GATA-1 in megakaryocytes from patients with idiopathic myelofibrosis. Am J Pathol 2005;167(3):849–58.

25. Vannucchi AM, Bianchi L, Paoletti F, et al. A pathobiologic pathway linking thrombopoietin, GATA-1, and TGF-beta1 in the development of myelofibrosis. Blood 2005;105(9):3493–501.

26. Gilles L, Arslan AD, Marinaccio C, et al. Downregulation of GATA1 drives impaired hematopoiesis in primary myelofibrosis. J Clin Invest 2017;127(4): 1316–20.

27. Lally J, Boasman K, Brown L, et al. GATA-1 a potential novel biomarker for the differentiation of essential thrombocythaemia and myelofibrosis. J Thromb Haemost 2019;17(6):896–900.

28. Vyas P, Ault K, Jackson CW, et al. Consequences of GATA-1 deficiency in megakaryocytes and platelets. Blood 1999;93(9):2867–75.

29. Vannucchi AM, Bianchi L, Cellai C, et al. Development of myelofibrosis in mice genetically impaired for GATA-1 expression (GATA-1(low) mice). Blood 2002; 100(4):1123–32.

30. Zingariello M, Sancillo L, Martelli F, et al. The thrombopoietin/MPL axis is activated in the Gata1(low) mouse model of myelofibrosis and is associated with a defective RPS14 signature. Blood Cancer J 2017;7(6):e572.

31. Gangat N, Marinaccio C, Swords R, et al. Aurora kinase a inhibition provides clinical benefit, normalizes megakaryocytes, and reduces bone marrow fibrosis in patients with myelofibrosis: a phase I trial. Clin Cancer Res 2019;25(16): 4898–906.

32. Wen QJ, Yang Q, Goldenson B, et al. Targeting megakaryocytic-induced fibrosis in myeloproliferative neoplasms by AURKA inhibition. Nat Med 2015; 21(12):1473–80.

33. Mylonas E, Yoshida K, Frick M, et al. Single-cell analysis based dissection of clonality in myelofibrosis. Nat Commun 2020;11(1):73.

34. Ishii T, Bruno E, Hoffman R, et al. Involvement of various hematopoietic-cell lineages by the JAK2V617F mutation in polycythemia vera. Blood 2006;108(9): 3128–34.

35. Pardanani A, Lasho TL, Finke C, et al. Prevalence and clinicopathologic correlates of JAK2 exon 12 mutations in JAK2V617F-negative polycythemia vera. Leukemia 2007;21(9):1960–3.

36. Delhommeau F, Dupont S, Tonetti C, et al. Evidence that the JAK2 G1849T (V617F) mutation occurs in a lymphomyeloid progenitor in polycythemia vera and idiopathic myelofibrosis. Blood 2007;109(1):71–7.

37. Guglielmelli P, Pacilli A, Rotunno G, et al. Presentation and outcome of patients with 2016 WHO diagnosis of prefibrotic and overt primary myelofibrosis. Blood 2017;129(24):3227–36.

38. Tefferi A, Lasho TL, Guglielmelli P, et al. Targeted deep sequencing in polycythemia vera and essential thrombocythemia. Blood Adv 2016;1(1):21–30.

39. Bartels S, Faisal M, Busche G, et al. Mutations associated with age-related clonal hematopoiesis in PMF patients with rapid progression to myelofibrosis. Leukemia 2020;34(5):1364–72.

40. Bartels S, Faisal M, Busche G, et al. Fibrotic progression in Polycythemia vera is associated with early concomitant driver-mutations besides JAK2. Leukemia 2018;32(2):556–8.
41. Masarova L, Verstovsek S. The evolving understanding of prognosis in post-essential thrombocythemia myelofibrosis and post-polycythemia vera myelofibrosis vs primary myelofibrosis. Clin Adv Hematol Oncol 2019;17(5):299–307.
42. Guo BB, Allcock RJ, Mirzai B, et al. Megakaryocytes in myeloproliferative neoplasms have unique somatic mutations. Am J Pathol 2017;187(7):1512–22.
43. de Sauvage FJ, Hass PE, Spencer SD, et al. Stimulation of megakaryocytopoiesis and thrombopoiesis by the c-Mpl ligand. Nature 1994;369(6481):533–8.
44. Gurney AL, Carver-Moore K, de Sauvage FJ, et al. Thrombocytopenia in c-mpl-deficient mice. Science 1994;265(5177):1445–7.
45. Alexander WS, Roberts AW, Nicola NA, et al. Deficiencies in progenitor cells of multiple hematopoietic lineages and defective megakaryocytopoiesis in mice lacking the thrombopoietic receptor c-Mpl. Blood 1996;87(6):2162–70.
46. Lannutti BJ, Epp A, Roy J, et al. Incomplete restoration of Mpl expression in the mpl-/- mouse produces partial correction of the stem cell-repopulating defect and paradoxical thrombocytosis. Blood 2009;113(8):1778–85.
47. Tiedt R, Coers J, Ziegler S, et al. Pronounced thrombocytosis in transgenic mice expressing reduced levels of Mpl in platelets and terminally differentiated megakaryocytes. Blood 2009;113(8):1768–77.
48. Ng AP, Kauppi M, Metcalf D, et al. Mpl expression on megakaryocytes and platelets is dispensable for thrombopoiesis but essential to prevent myeloproliferation. Proc Natl Acad Sci U S A 2014;111(16):5884–9.
49. Royer Y, Staerk J, Costuleanu M, et al. Janus kinases affect thrombopoietin receptor cell surface localization and stability. J Biol Chem 2005;280(29):27251–61.
50. Meyer SC, Keller MD, Woods BA, et al. Genetic studies reveal an unexpected negative regulatory role for Jak2 in thrombopoiesis. Blood 2014;124(14):2280–4.
51. Griesshammer M, Hornkohl A, Nichol JL, et al. High levels of thrombopoietin in sera of patients with essential thrombocythemia: cause or consequence of abnormal platelet production? Ann Hematol 1998;77(5):211–5.
52. Wang JC, Chen C, Lou LH, et al. Blood thrombopoietin, IL-6 and IL-11 levels in patients with agnogenic myeloid metaplasia. Leukemia 1997;11(11):1827–32.
53. Wang JC, Chen C, Novetsky AD, et al. Blood thrombopoietin levels in clonal thrombocytosis and reactive thrombocytosis. Am J Med 1998;104(5):451–5.
54. Moliterno AR, Hankins WD, Spivak JL. Impaired expression of the thrombopoietin receptor by platelets from patients with polycythemia vera. N Engl J Med 1998;338(9):572–80.
55. Panteli KE, Hatzimichael EC, Bouranta PK, et al. Serum interleukin (IL)-1, IL-2, sIL-2Ra, IL-6 and thrombopoietin levels in patients with chronic myeloproliferative diseases. Br J Haematol 2005;130(5):709–15.
56. Tefferi A, Yoon SY, Li CY. Immunohistochemical staining for megakaryocyte c-mpl may complement morphologic distinction between polycythemia vera and secondary erythrocytosis. Blood 2000;96(2):771–2.
57. Villeval JL, Cohen-Solal K, Tulliez M, et al. High thrombopoietin production by hematopoietic cells induces a fatal myeloproliferative syndrome in mice. Blood 1997;90(11):4369–83.

58. Pecquet C, Diaconu CC, Staerk J, et al. Thrombopoietin receptor down-modulation by JAK2 V617F: restoration of receptor levels by inhibitors of pathologic JAK2 signaling and of proteasomes. Blood 2012;119(20):4625–35.

59. Moliterno AR, Williams DM, Rogers O, et al. Molecular mimicry in the chronic myeloproliferative disorders: reciprocity between quantitative JAK2 V617F and Mpl expression. Blood 2006;108(12):3913–5.

60. Sangkhae V, Etheridge SL, Kaushansky K, et al. The thrombopoietin receptor, MPL, is critical for development of a JAK2V617F-induced myeloproliferative neoplasm. Blood 2014;124(26):3956–63.

61. Wang X, Haylock D, Hu CS, et al. A thrombopoietin receptor antagonist is capable of depleting myelofibrosis hematopoietic stem and progenitor cells. Blood 2016;127(26):3398–409.

62. Spivak JL, Merchant A, Williams DM, et al. Thrombopoietin is required for full phenotype expression in a JAK2V617F transgenic mouse model of polycythemia vera. PLoS One 2020;15(6):e0232801.

63. Tiedt R, Schomber T, Hao-Shen H, et al. Pf4-Cre transgenic mice allow the generation of lineage-restricted gene knockouts for studying megakaryocyte and platelet function in vivo. Blood 2007;109(4):1503–6.

64. Calaminus SD, Guitart AV, Sinclair A, et al. Lineage tracing of Pf4-Cre marks hematopoietic stem cells and their progeny. PLoS One 2012;7(12):e51361.

65. Nagy Z, Vogtle T, Geer MJ, et al. The Gp1ba-Cre transgenic mouse: a new model to delineate platelet and leukocyte functions. Blood 2019;133(4):331–43.

66. Mansier O, Kilani B, Guitart AV, et al. Description of a knock-in mouse model of JAK2V617F MPN emerging from a minority of mutated hematopoietic stem cells. Blood 2019;134(26):2383–7.

67. Woods B, Chen W, Chiu S, et al. Activation of JAK/STAT Signaling in Megakaryocytes Sustains Myeloproliferation In Vivo. Clin Cancer Res 2019;25(19):5901–12.

68. Zhan H, Ma Y, Lin CH, et al. JAK2(V617F)-mutant megakaryocytes contribute to hematopoietic stem/progenitor cell expansion in a model of murine myeloproliferation. Leukemia 2016;30(12):2332–41.

69. Varricchio L, Falchi M, Dall'Ora M, et al. Calreticulin: challenges posed by the intrinsically disordered nature of calreticulin to the study of its function. Front Cell Dev Biol 2017;5:96.

70. How J, Hobbs GS, Mullally A. Mutant calreticulin in myeloproliferative neoplasms. Blood 2019;134(25):2242–8.

71. Vannucchi AM, Rotunno G, Bartalucci N, et al. Calreticulin mutation-specific immunostaining in myeloproliferative neoplasms: pathogenetic insight and diagnostic value. Leukemia 2014;28(9):1811–8.

72. Stein H, Bob R, Durkop H, et al. A new monoclonal antibody (CAL2) detects CALRETICULIN mutations in formalin-fixed and paraffin-embedded bone marrow biopsies. Leukemia 2016;30(1):131–5.

73. Li J, Prins D, Park HJ, et al. Mutant calreticulin knockin mice develop thrombocytosis and myelofibrosis without a stem cell self-renewal advantage. Blood 2018;131(6):649–61.

74. Shide K, Kameda T, Kamiunten A, et al. Mice with Calr mutations homologous to human CALR mutations only exhibit mild thrombocytosis. Blood Cancer J 2019;9(4):42.

75. Balligand T, Achouri Y, Pecquet C, et al. Knock-in of murine Calr del52 induces essential thrombocythemia with slow-rising dominance in mice and reveals key role of Calr exon 9 in cardiac development. Leukemia 2020;34(2):510–21.

76. Elf S, Abdelfattah NS, Chen E, et al. Mutant calreticulin requires both its mutant c-terminus and the thrombopoietin receptor for oncogenic transformation. Cancer Discov 2016;6(4):368–81.
77. Marty C, Pecquet C, Nivarthi H, et al. Calreticulin mutants in mice induce an MPL-dependent thrombocytosis with frequent progression to myelofibrosis. Blood 2016;127(10):1317–24.
78. Balligand T, Achouri Y, Pecquet C, et al. Pathologic activation of thrombopoietin receptor and JAK2-STAT5 pathway by frameshift mutants of mouse calreticulin. Leukemia 2016;30(8):1775–8.
79. Chachoua I, Pecquet C, El-Khoury M, et al. Thrombopoietin receptor activation by myeloproliferative neoplasm associated calreticulin mutants. Blood 2016; 127(10):1325–35.
80. Masubuchi N, Araki M, Yang Y, et al. Mutant calreticulin interacts with MPL in the secretion pathway for activation on the cell surface. Leukemia 2020;34(2): 499–509.
81. Araki M, Yang Y, Imai M, et al. Homomultimerization of mutant calreticulin is a prerequisite for MPL binding and activation. Leukemia 2019;33(1):122–31.
82. Pronier E, Cifani P, Merlinsky TR, et al. Targeting the CALR interactome in myeloproliferative neoplasms. JCI Insight 2018;3(22):e122703.
83. Han L, Schubert C, Kohler J, et al. Calreticulin-mutant proteins induce megakaryocytic signaling to transform hematopoietic cells and undergo accelerated degradation and Golgi-mediated secretion. J Hematol Oncol 2016;9(1):45.
84. Di Buduo CA, Abbonante V, Marty C, et al. Defective interaction of mutant calreticulin and SOCE in megakaryocytes from patients with myeloproliferative neoplasms. Blood 2020;135(2):133–44.
85. Yan D, Jobe F, Hutchison RE, et al. Deletion of Stat3 enhances myeloid cell expansion and increases the severity of myeloproliferative neoplasms in Jak2V617F knock-in mice. Leukemia 2015;29(10):2050–61.
86. Grisouard J, Shimizu T, Duek A, et al. Deletion of Stat3 in hematopoietic cells enhances thrombocytosis and shortens survival in a JAK2-V617F mouse model of MPN. Blood 2015;125(13):2131–40.
87. Huang Z, Richmond TD, Muntean AG, et al. STAT1 promotes megakaryopoiesis downstream of GATA-1 in mice. J Clin Invest 2007;117(12):3890–9.
88. Chen E, Beer PA, Godfrey AL, et al. Distinct clinical phenotypes associated with JAK2V617F reflect differential STAT1 signaling. Cancer Cell 2010;18(5):524–35.
89. Yan D, Hutchison RE, Mohi G. Critical requirement for Stat5 in a mouse model of polycythemia vera. Blood 2012;119(15):3539–49.
90. Walz C, Ahmed W, Lazarides K, et al. Essential role for Stat5a/b in myeloproliferative neoplasms induced by BCR-ABL1 and JAK2(V617F) in mice. Blood 2012;119(15):3550–60.
91. Noetzli LJ, French SL, Machlus KR. New insights into the differentiation of megakaryocytes from hematopoietic progenitors. Arterioscler Thromb Vasc Biol 2019; 39(7):1288–300.
92. Badalucco S, Di Buduo CA, Campanelli R, et al. Involvement of TGFbeta1 in autocrine regulation of proplatelet formation in healthy subjects and patients with primary myelofibrosis. Haematologica 2013;98(4):514–7.
93. Mohle R, Green D, Moore MA, et al. Constitutive production and thrombin-induced release of vascular endothelial growth factor by human megakaryocytes and platelets. Proc Natl Acad Sci U S A 1997;94(2):663–8.
94. Saulle E, Guerriero R, Petronelli A, et al. Autocrine role of angiopoietins during megakaryocytic differentiation. PLoS One 2012;7(7):e39796.

95. Zhao M, Perry JM, Marshall H, et al. Megakaryocytes maintain homeostatic quiescence and promote post-injury regeneration of hematopoietic stem cells. Nat Med 2014;20(11):1321–6.

96. Zhao M, Ross JT, Itkin T, et al. FGF signaling facilitates postinjury recovery of mouse hematopoietic system. Blood 2012;120(9):1831–42.

97. Bruns I, Lucas D, Pinho S, et al. Megakaryocytes regulate hematopoietic stem cell quiescence through CXCL4 secretion. Nat Med 2014;20(11):1315–20.

98. Malara A, Abbonante V, Zingariello M, et al. Megakaryocyte contribution to bone marrow fibrosis: many arrows in the quiver. Mediterr J Hematol Infect Dis 2018; 10(1):e2018068.

99. Meng XM, Nikolic-Paterson DJ, Lan HY. TGF-beta: the master regulator of fibrosis. Nat Rev Nephrol 2016;12(6):325–38.

100. Campanelli R, Rosti V, Villani L, et al. Evaluation of the bioactive and total transforming growth factor beta1 levels in primary myelofibrosis. Cytokine 2011; 53(1):100–6.

101. Zingariello M, Martelli F, Ciaffoni F, et al. Characterization of the TGF-beta1 signaling abnormalities in the Gata1low mouse model of myelofibrosis. Blood 2013;121(17):3345–63.

102. Bock O, Loch G, Schade U, et al. Aberrant expression of transforming growth factor beta-1 (TGF beta-1) per se does not discriminate fibrotic from non-fibrotic chronic myeloproliferative disorders. J Pathol 2005;205(5):548–57.

103. Yoon SY, Tefferi A, Li CY. Cellular distribution of platelet-derived growth factor, transforming growth factor-beta, basic fibroblast growth factor, and their receptors in normal bone marrow. Acta Haematol 2000;104(4):151–7.

104. Ponce CC, de Lourdes FCM, Ihara SS, et al. The relationship of the active and latent forms of TGF-beta1 with marrow fibrosis in essential thrombocythemia and primary myelofibrosis. Med Oncol 2012;29(4):2337–44.

105. Schmitt A, Jouault H, Guichard J, et al. Pathologic interaction between megakaryocytes and polymorphonuclear leukocytes in myelofibrosis. Blood 2000;96(4): 1342–7.

106. Zingariello M, Ruggeri A, Martelli F, et al. A novel interaction between megakaryocytes and activated fibrocytes increases TGF-beta bioavailability in the Gata1(low) mouse model of myelofibrosis. Am J Blood Res 2015;5(2):34–61.

107. Chagraoui H, Komura E, Tulliez M, et al. Prominent role of TGF-beta 1 in thrombopoietin-induced myelofibrosis in mice. Blood 2002;100(10):3495–503.

108. Yue L, Bartenstein M, Zhao W, et al. Efficacy of ALK5 inhibition in myelofibrosis. JCI Insight 2017;2(7):e90932.

109. Gastinne T, Vigant F, Lavenu-Bombled C, et al. Adenoviral-mediated TGF-beta1 inhibition in a mouse model of myelofibrosis inhibit bone marrow fibrosis development. Exp Hematol 2007;35(1):64–74.

110. Ceglia I, Dueck AC, Masiello F, et al. Preclinical rationale for TGF-beta inhibition as a therapeutic target for the treatment of myelofibrosis. Exp Hematol 2016; 44(12):1138–1155 e1134.

111. Vandercappellen J, Van Damme J, Struyf S. The role of the CXC chemokines platelet factor-4 (CXCL4/PF-4) and its variant (CXCL4L1/PF-4var) in inflammation, angiogenesis and cancer. Cytokine Growth Factor Rev 2011;22(1):1–18.

112. Zaldivar MM, Pauels K, von Hundelshausen P, et al. CXC chemokine ligand 4 (Cxcl4) is a platelet-derived mediator of experimental liver fibrosis. Hepatology 2010;51(4):1345–53.

113. van Bon L, Affandi AJ, Broen J, et al. Proteome-wide analysis and CXCL4 as a biomarker in systemic sclerosis. N Engl J Med 2014;370(5):433–43.

114. Burstein SA, Malpass TW, Yee E, et al. Platelet factor-4 excretion in myeloprolif-erative disease: implications for the aetiology of myelofibrosis. Br J Haematol 1984;57(3):383–92.
115. Schneider RK, Mullally A, Dugourd A, et al. Gli1(+) mesenchymal stromal cells are a key driver of bone marrow fibrosis and an important cellular therapeutic target. Cell Stem Cell 2017;20(6):785–800 e788.
116. Gleitz HFE, Dugourd AJF, Leimkuhler NB, et al. Increased CXCL4 expression in hematopoietic cells links inflammation and progression of bone marrow fibrosis in MPN. Blood 2020;136(18):2051–64.
117. Liu X, Jones GW, Choy EH, et al. The biology behind interleukin-6 targeted in-terventions. Curr Opin Rheumatol 2016;28(2):152–60.
118. Kleppe M, Kwak M, Koppikar P, et al. JAK-STAT pathway activation in malignant and nonmalignant cells contributes to MPN pathogenesis and therapeutic response. Cancer Discov 2015;5(3):316–31.
119. Cokic VP, Mitrovic-Ajtic O, Beleslin-Cokic BB, et al. Proinflammatory Cytokine IL-6 and JAK-STAT Signaling Pathway in Myeloproliferative Neoplasms. Mediators Inflamm 2015;2015:453020.
120. Cacemiro MDC, Cominal JG, Tognon R, et al. Philadelphia-negative myelopro-liferative neoplasms as disorders marked by cytokine modulation. Hematol Transfus Cell Ther 2018;40(2):120–31.
121. Malara A, Gruppi C, Abbonante V, et al. EDA fibronectin-TLR4 axis sustains megakaryocyte expansion and inflammation in bone marrow fibrosis. J Exp Med 2019;216(3):587–604.
122. Mondet J, Hussein K, Mossuz P. Circulating cytokine levels as markers of inflam-mation in Philadelphia negative myeloproliferative neoplasms: diagnostic and prognostic interest. Mediators Inflamm 2015;2015:670580.
123. Tefferi A, Vaidya R, Caramazza D, et al. Circulating interleukin (IL)-8, IL-2R, IL-12, and IL-15 levels are independently prognostic in primary myelofibrosis: a comprehensive cytokine profiling study. J Clin Oncol 2011;29(10):1356–63.
124. Emadi S, Clay D, Desterke C, et al. IL-8 and its CXCR1 and CXCR2 receptors participate in the control of megakaryocytic proliferation, differentiation, and ploidy in myeloid metaplasia with myelofibrosis. Blood 2005;105(2):464–73.
125. Grover A, Sanjuan-Pla A, Thongjuea S, et al. Single-cell RNA sequencing re-veals molecular and functional platelet bias of aged haematopoietic stem cells. Nat Commun 2016;7:11075.
126. Davizon-Castillo P, McMahon B, Aguila S, et al. TNF-alpha-driven inflammation and mitochondrial dysfunction define the platelet hyperreactivity of aging. Blood 2019;134(9):727–40.
127. Gekas C, Graf T. CD41 expression marks myeloid-biased adult hematopoietic stem cells and increases with age. Blood 2013;121(22):4463–72.
128. Rao TN, Hansen N, Hilfiker J, et al. JAK2-mutant hematopoietic cells display metabolic alterations that can be targeted to treat myeloproliferative neoplasms. Blood 2019;134(21):1832–46.
129. Haas S, Hansson J, Klimmeck D, et al. Inflammation-induced emergency mega-karyopoiesis driven by hematopoietic stem cell-like megakaryocyte progenitors. Cell Stem Cell 2015;17(4):422–34.

The Microenvironment in Myeloproliferative Neoplasms

Gajalakshmi Ramanathan, PhD[a],
Angela G. Fleischman, MD, PhD[a,b,*]

KEYWORDS

- Inflammation • Microenvironment • Cytokines • Myeloproliferative neoplasm
- Prognosis • Myeloid cells

KEY POINTS

- The inflammatory microenvironment in myeloproliferative neoplasms (MPNs) encompasses soluble cytokines and associated cellular players.
- A self-sustained inflammatory loop results in a milieu that supports the clonal expansion of the neoplastic clone.
- Cytokine profiles in MPN can be leveraged for diagnosis, disease monitoring, and prognostication, which will help to obtain more favorable patient outcomes.

INTRODUCTION

Myeloproliferative neoplasms (MPNs) are a classic example of a group of diseases in which inflammation and the neoplastic clone are so intimately entwined that it is difficult to ascertain which is the "chicken" and which is the "egg." MPNs are typified by a chronic inflammatory milieu that provides a permissive microenvironment for disease progression and severity. Inflammatory signaling involving the malignant and nonmalignant cells contribute to the MPN symptom burden, thrombotic risk, and disease evolution and transformation to acute myeloid leukemia. Chronic inflammation is characterized by elevated levels of circulating inflammatory cytokines and chemokines,

Financial Support: This research was supported by funds from the Tobacco-Related Disease Research Program of the University of California, Grant Numbers T29FT0267 (G. Ramanathan) and T29IP0414 (A.G. Fleischman). G. Ramanathan was supported by the NCI T32CA009054.
[a] Division of Hematology/Oncology, Department of Medicine, University of California, 839 Health Sciences Road, Sprague Hall B100, Irvine, CA 92617, USA; [b] Department of Biological Chemistry, Irvine Chao Family Comprehensive Cancer Center, University of California, 839 Health Sciences Road, Sprague Hall 126, Irvine, CA 92617, USA
* Corresponding author. Department of Biological Chemistry, Irvine Chao Family Comprehensive Cancer Center, University of California, 839 Health Sciences Road, Sprague Hall 126, Irvine, CA 92617.
E-mail address: agf@hs.uci.edu

Hematol Oncol Clin N Am 35 (2021) 205–216
https://doi.org/10.1016/j.hoc.2020.11.003
0889-8588/21/

whereas inflammatory cells and soluble mediators of inflammation constitute the inflammatory microenvironment in the MPNs. In addition to the presence of MPN driver mutations, disease heterogeneity suggests that host factors likely shape the pathologic consequences of the presence of the MPN neoplastic clone.

Plasma/serum measurements of various cytokines and other soluble proteins reflect inflammatory processes and could serve as noninvasive diagnostic or prognostic tools for predicting disease evolution in patients with MPNs.[1] Considerable progress has been made on better understanding the genetic basis of the MPNs since the discovery of major driver somatic mutations in Janus kinase 2 (JAK2),[2–5] calreticulin (CALR),[6,7] and myeloproliferative leukemia virus oncogene (MPL).[8–10] Despite this, mutation-targeted and selective MPN therapies have been slow to exploit this knowledge and remain challenging. One reason for this is significant disease heterogeneity due to the effect of an altered microenvironment on disease pathogenesis. Thus, applying broader approaches toward identifying novel biomarkers for disease monitoring and combined therapies will hopefully lead to better outcomes.

This review discusses the role of an inflammatory microenvironment as a driver of clonal evolution in the MPNs, cytokine production in the MPNs, use of inflammatory cytokines as diagnostic and prognostic tools, and the use of the inflammatory microenvironment as a therapeutic target.

CHRONIC INFLAMMATION AS A CONTRIBUTOR TO THE DEVELOPMENT OF MYELOPROLIFERATIVE NEOPLASMS

There is evidence supporting the notion that chronic inflammation precedes the development of MPNs, thus creating a permissive environment for the expansion of the mutant MPN driver clone. A prior history of an autoimmune disease is associated with an increased risk of developing an MPN (odds ratio [OR] = 1.2).[11] A history of inflammation mediated by an infection has also been associated with an increased risk of myeloid malignancies; however, only a history of cellulitis was associated with a significantly increased risk of an MPN (OR 1.34).[12] Modifiable lifestyle factors that lead to chronic inflammation may also play a role in the development of MPNs. For example, smoking increases the risk of MPNs.[13,14] Obesity has been associated with an increased risk for multiple malignancies, including MPNs.[14–16] This suggests that aggressive treatment of autoimmune and inflammatory conditions and lifestyle modifications aimed at reducing inflammation may be impactful to reduce one's risk of developing an MPN.

Nonmodifiable factors such as the patient's germline predisposition also likely contribute to the development of an MPN. Although MPN driver mutations are clearly not inheritable, the predisposition to develop a somatic MPN driver mutation is. Interestingly, first-degree relatives of patients with MPN have a 4- to 5-fold higher risk of developing an MPN.[17] The single nucleotide polymorphisms identified as being associated with MPN include inflammasome-related genes[18] and monocyte chemoattractant protein-1 (MCP-1),[19] suggesting that the host's immune milieu may contribute to the genetic predisposition to acquire an MPN.

MYELOPROLIFERATIVE NEOPLASM SUBTYPE–SPECIFIC CYTOKINE SIGNATURES

Although MPN subtypes can share identical driver mutations such as $JAK2^{V617F}$, the resulting phenotype is variable. Just as other clinical MPN subtype–specific clinical features, there seems to be subtype-specific cytokine signatures. A recent longitudinal study of more than 400 patients[20] identified specific inflammatory cytokine signatures according to disease subtypes. Ten cytokines, including interferon gamma

(INF-γ), interleukin-1 receptor antagonist (IL-1RA), IL-6, IL-8, IFN-γ–inducible protein 10 (IP-10), epidermal growth factor (EGF), eotaxin (CCL11), tumor necrosis factor-alpha (TNF-α), transforming growth factor-alpha (TGF-α), and growth-regulated onco-gene (GRO-α or CXCL1), were significantly altered and showed strong disease sub-type specificity (**Fig. 1**). Specifically, primary myelofibrosis (PMF) was associated with increased levels of TNF-α, IP-10, and IL-8, whereas TGF-α was unique to polycy-themia vera (PV) and essential thrombocythemia (ET) presented with higher eotaxin, EGF, and GRO-α levels.[20]

Another study measured plasma cytokine levels in patients with MPN, younger than 35 years, to identify possible subtype-specific biomarkers. Dickkopf-related protein 1 (Dkk-1) was found to be the most significantly increased protein in patients with MPN compared with healthy donors.[21] Plasma Dkk-1 levels normalized to platelet counts were not significantly different between controls and ET but could discriminate ET from pre-PMF, in both $JAK2^{V617F}$ and CALR mutant patients (**Fig. 2**).

The patients with PV exhibit an altered cytokine milieu with significantly higher levels of IL-1RA, IL-5, IL-6, IL-7, IL-8, IL-12, IL-13, IFN-γ, granulocyte-macrophage colony-stimulating factor (GM-CSF), macrophage inflammatory protein-1alpha (MIP-1α), MIP-1β, hepatocyte growth factor (HGF), IP-10, monokine induced by IFN-gamma (MIG), MCP-1, and vascular endothelial growth factor (VEGF) compared with normal controls.[22] A comparative study of plasma cytokine profiles in PV and ET MPN sub-types showed differentially elevated levels of IL-4, IL-8, GM-CSF, IFN-γ, MCP-1, platelet-derived growth factor (PDGF), and VEGF in ET as compared with PV.[23]

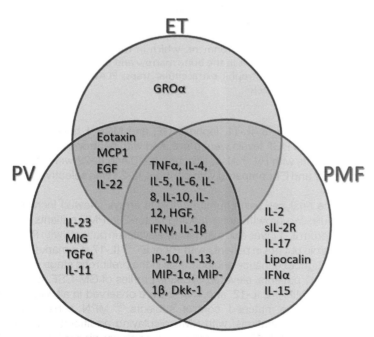

Fig. 1. MPN-associated cytokines and chemokines according to subtype. Dkk-1, Dickkopf-related protein 1; EGF, epidermal growth factor; GRO-α, growth-regulated oncogene; HGF, hepatocyte growth factor; IFNα, interferon alpha; IFNγ, interferon gamma; IL-1RA, interleukin-1 receptor antagonist; IP-10, IFN-γ–inducible protein 10; MIG, monokine induced by IFN-gamma; MIP, macrophage inflammatory protein-1; TGF-α, transforming growth factor alpha; TNFα, tumor necrosis factor alpha.

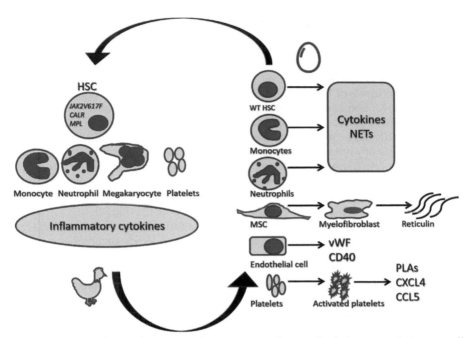

Fig. 2. Overview of the inflammatory loop in MPNs. The neoplastic hematopoietic stem cell (HSC) clone carrying the *JAK2^V617F^*, *CALR*, or *MPL* mutation secretes cytokines involved in inflammation and differentiate into malignant cells of the myeloid lineage such as megakaryocytes, monocytes, and granulocytes. Together, these cells produce a host of cytokines creating an inflammatory microenvironment, which in turn results in aberrant activation and function of nonmalignant cells in the bone marrow and peripheral blood. MSC, mesenchymal stromal cell; NETs, neutrophil extracellular traps; PLAs, platelet-leukocyte aggregates; vWF, von Willebrand factor.

High levels of serum IL-8, IL-11, leptin, HGF, and MCP-1 have been reported in PV,[24,25] and IL-11 and HGF levels were correlated with neutrophil counts and hematocrit levels in patients with PV.[25] Also, although IL-10 and IL-22 were increased in patients with both PV and ET compared with controls, IL-23 was selectively elevated only in PV.[26]

Global cytokine analyses using human cytokine arrays showed increased TIMP-1, MIP-1β, and insulin-like growth factor binding factor-2 in PMF patients with PMF but not ET or PV.[27] Serum IL-17 was also exclusively elevated in patients with PMF compared with healthy controls but not in patients with PV or ET.[28] IL-17 is a marker of angiogenic activity and is thought to enhance angiogenesis in the prefibrotic stage of PMF.[28]

In treatment naïve patients, elevated cytokine profiles of GM-CSF, IL-1β, IL-4, IL-5, IL-6, IL-10, IFN-α2, MIP-1α, IL-12, and TNF-α were observed in all 3 MPN categories as compared with age-matched control subjects.[29] MPN subset analysis also revealed intra-disease variations, with PMF displaying additional cytokine modulations such as increased IL-17A compared with controls; higher levels of IFN-γ, IL-12, IL-17A, and IP-10 in comparison to patients with ET; and elevated plasma levels of IL-12, IL-4, and GM-CSF compared with patients with PV.[29] *JAK2^V617F^* mutational status was also associated with higher IP-10 levels in MF. Subsequently, although all patients with MPN displayed an inflammatory status, PMF emerged as the highest producer of cytokines and chemokines.[29]

ASSOCIATION OF CYTOKINES WITH SPECIFIC DISEASE OUTCOMES

Specific cytokines are associated with specific disease outcomes, suggesting that cytokine profiling could be useful clinically as predictive tools. A study involving 127 patients with PMF showed increased IL-1β, IL-1RA, IL-2R, IL-6, IL-8, IL-10, IL-12, IL-13, IL-15, TNF-α, granulocyte colony-stimulating factor, IFN-α, MIP-1α, MIP-1β, HGF, IP-10, MIG, MCP-1, and VEGF levels as well as decreased IFN-γ levels compared with normal controls. Treatment-naïve subjects with PMF displayed increased levels of IL-8, IL-2R, IL-12, IL-15, and IP-10, which predicted inferior survival. Association of phenotypic clinical features with cytokines included IL-8 with constitutional symptoms, leukocytosis and leukemia-free survival, IL-2R and IL-12 with transfusion need; IP-10 correlated with thrombocytopenia, whereas HGF, MIG, and IL-1RA corresponded with marked splenomegaly.[30]

Vaidya and colleagues[22] assessed the disease phenotypic and prognostic relevance of cytokine levels in PV and found that IL-12 levels correlated with hematocrit levels, IL-1β with leukocytosis, and IFNα/IFNγ with thrombocytosis. MIP-1β was significantly associated with an inferior overall survival. A recent study found that high levels of GRO-α was associated with an increased risk of transformation of ET to MF. In addition, longitudinal sampling indicated decreasing EGF levels in patients with ET strongly correlated with disease transformation risk.[20]

Bourantas and colleagues[31] demonstrated increased serum beta-2-microglobulin, IL-2, and soluble IL-2 receptor alpha (sIL-2RA) in patients with MPNs progressing to advanced clinical stages. Panteli and colleagues[32] observed that serum levels of IL-2, sIL-2RA, and IL-6 were increased when PMF progressed to MPN-blast phase (MPN-BP) and positively correlated with bone marrow (BM) angiogenesis, hence indicating that disease progression is coupled with amplified inflammation and that cytokine levels can be useful biomarkers to predict disease progression such as BM angiogenesis.

Thus, measuring cytokines could potentially be leveraged as a tool for disease monitoring and to provide parallel information in addition to genomic and clinical data to predict disease progression/transformation.

CELLULAR COMPONENTS OF INFLAMMATION IN MYELOPROLIFERATIVE NEOPLASM

Emerging evidence indicates that inflammation in the BM microenvironment and systemic inflammation contribute to the development and progression of MPNs. Different cell types act as mediators of inflammation in MPNs, including mutant and normal hematopoietic stem and progenitor cells, mesenchymal stromal cells, megakaryocytes, monocytes, platelets, and endothelial cells. These cells produce numerous inflammatory cytokines that act in an autocrine and paracrine fashion to provide a self-perpetuating and permissive microenvironment for disease evolution, ultimately resulting in BM fibrosis and transformation to MPN-BP.

Bone Marrow Hematopoietic Cells

The effect of MPN-driven mutations on inflammatory transcriptional programs and cytokine secretion in hematopoietic stem and progenitor cells (HSPCs) can lead to an inflammatory BM niche that supports the proliferation of mutant cells. The authors observed increased circulating TNF-α in patients with MPN in comparison to healthy controls and also demonstrated that mononuclear cells and CD34+ cells from patients with $JAK2^{V617F}$ MPN unlike normal controls are resistant to the growth suppressive effects of TNF-α while colony formation.[33] Thus, the presence of $JAK2^{V617F}$ not only increases TNF-α secretion but also creates a favorable environment for MPN mutant cell expansion.[33] Similarly, lipocalin-2 is another molecule that has been shown to be increased in the serum and conditioned media of BM mononuclear cells from patients with MPN compared with controls.[34] The presence of lipocalin-2 also reduced the proliferation and colony-forming capacity of BM CD34[+] cells from patients without MPN or normal controls but not patients with MPN, thus providing a relative growth advantage to MPN clones.[34,35] Lipocalin was expressed by MF marrow myeloid cells and not erythroid or megakaryocytic cells.[35] BM neural death has been associated with IL-1β released from mutant HSCs-reduced mesenchymal stromal cells and allowed the uncontrolled expansion of mutant HSCs and disease progression.[36]

Using single-cell technology to understand disease pathology in MF, Psaila and colleagues[37] identified a megakaryocyte differentiation bias in early human multipotent stem cells and strong expression of fibrotic mediators in megakaryocyte progenitors. Furthermore, cell surface expression of G6B was specific to mutant HSPCs from patients with MF, thus identifying a potential selective target for MF HSPCs.[37] CD34[+] cells from patients with *CALR*-mutations were profiled by integrating target genotyping with single-cell RNA sequencing. This technology revealed that the frequency of *CALR*-mutated cells was higher in committed myeloid progenitors and megakaryocyte progenitors, indicating increased fitness of the *CALR* mutation with myeloid differentiation. Compared with wild-type HSPCs, an upregulation of NF-κB pathway genes in undifferentiated mutant HSCs supports a cell-intrinsic role for *CALR* mutation in NF-κB activation.[38]

Megakaryocytes in PMF possess an inflammatory and profibrotic secretome, which is a major driver of BM fibrosis.[39] The role of megakaryocytes in promoting inflammation has been reviewed separately in this edition and is not discussed here.

Mesenchymal Stromal Cells

BM mesenchymal stromal cells (also mesenchymal stem cells or multipotent stromal cells (MSCs)) contribute to the maintenance of HSCs and normal hematopoiesis. Leukemic myeloid cells remodel the BM niche into a "self-reinforcing leukemic niche" that favorably supports leukemic stem cells but not healthy stem cells.[40] Nestin-positive MSC reduction was observed in the BM of patients with MPN and MPN mouse models carrying the human *JAK2^V617F* mutation due to IL-1β released by mutant HSCs, resulting in a favorable environment for mutant HSC expansion.[36]

MSCs from patients with PMF are characterized by an increased secretion of TGFB, BMP, and glycosaminoglycans and specific impairment of osteogenic abilities. Transcriptome analysis identified a TGF-β signature in primary MF MSCs.[41] Differentiation of glioma-associated oncogene positive (Gli1+) MSCs toward fibrosis-driving myofibroblasts was shown in mouse models of MF. Similarly, BM samples from patients with MPN also showed an increased frequency of Gli1+ cells and corresponded to the severity of fibrosis by reticulin staining irrespective of JAK2V617 F or CALR mutation status.[42] Leptin receptor–expressing MSCs were also found to be expanded and fibrogenic in a mouse model of MF.[43]

Monocytes

Mature hematopoietic cells in the peripheral blood are pivotal sources of increased systemic cytokines in MPN. Classic CD14+CD16− monocytes are a strongest producers of cytokines including TNF- α, IL-6, IL-8, and IL-10 in MF.[44] TNF-α is consistently increased in all MPN subtypes and has an integral role in the clonal expansion of *JAK2^V617F* cells.[33] The authors recently showed that primary monocytes from patients with MPN have extensive TNF-α production compared with normal controls in response to stimulation due to a dampened response to the antiinflammatory cytokine, IL-10.[45] IL-10 receptor signaling via suppressor of cytokine signaling-3 was found to be downregulated in patients with MPN. Interestingly, persistent TNF-α production was observed in both unmutated and $JAK2^{V617F}$ monocytes indicating a noncell autonomous role for monocytes in MPN inflammation.[45] Very recently, CD56+CD14+ proinflammatory monocytes have been identified as a pivotal source of GRO-α in patients with ET, thus creating an environment suitable for MPN disease evolution.[20]

Granulocytes

Single-cell cytokine profiling of circulating granulocytes from patients with PMF showed that several cytokines, including IL-6, IL-8, IL-10, IL-12, TNF-α, CCL2, CCL3, and CCL5, were significantly increased compared with healthy controls.[46] This was the result of an increased fraction of cytokine-secreting cells and the level of individual cytokines per cell. The proportion of cytokine-secreting myeloid cells was higher than the $JAK2^{V617F}$-mutant allele burden, which suggested that nonmalignant cells also contribute to cytokine production. Thus, aberrant inflammatory signaling in MPN is not restricted to cell-intrinsic effects but also noncell autonomous processes.[46]

The formation of neutrophil extracellular traps by neutrophils not only contributes to innate immunity and host defense but also promotes thrombosis.[47] Increased neutrophil activation has been reported in ET and PV with increased cell-surface CD11b expression and circulating myeloperoxidase levels.[48] Recently, Wolach and colleagues[49] demonstrated that neutrophils from patients with MPN show increased NET formation with a prothrombotic phenotype, which can be blocked by ruxolitinib. Increased NET formation was associated with PAD4 overexpression in $JAK2^{V617F}$ PV patient samples.[49] Thus, premature neutrophil activation in MPN is a cell-intrinsic effect of the $JAK2^{V617F}$ mutation and is associated with thrombotic events. The authors also demonstrated that N-acetylcysteine reduces NET formation in patients with MPN and could be used as a potential antithrombotic in MPN.[50]

Platelets

Platelets play a role in innate immunity and inflammation in addition to their hemostatic function and contribute to thrombo-inflammation in MPN.[51] Thrombosis is a major cause of mortality and morbidity in patients with MPN with several underlying mechanisms, including membrane alterations on red blood cells, activated platelets, activated leukocytes, platelet-leukocyte aggregates, and dysfunctional endothelium. Systemic inflammation also plays a critical role in the development of vascular events, as elevated high-sensitivity C-reactive protein is significantly associated with thrombosis risk in patients with PV and ET.[52]

Platelet interactions with neutrophils and monocytes in MPN triggers activation of both cell types and stimulates inflammatory and thrombotic processes. We and others have reported increased platelet-leukocyte aggregates in patients with MPN.[50,53] We also observed that MPN platelets can induce NET formation with normal and MPN neutrophils without an external stimulus indicating that MPN platelets generate a prothrombotic microenvironment.[50] Platelet crosstalk with monocytes can also increase cytokine synthesis and release because monocytes are already known to play an important role in MPN inflammation.[44,45] Inflammatory cytokines and reactive oxygen species result in an activated and prothrombotic endothelium as observed by increased von Willebrand factor and E-selectin levels.[54] Recruitment of platelets and leukocytes to an activated endothelium results in a prothrombotic phenotype in patients with MPN. Activated platelets themselves can act as immune cells by releasing proinflammatory cytokines such as CCL5 and platelet factor 4 (PF4 or CXCL4) stored in α-granules.[55] Elevated cytokine levels lead to reciprocal activation of platelets, thus driving the thrombo-inflammatory loop in MPN.

LOOKING AHEAD—HOW COULD WE INCORPORATE KNOWLEDGE OF THE MICROENVIRONMENT TO AID IN THE CLINICAL CARE OF PATIENTS WITH MYELOPROLIFERATIVE NEOPLASM?

Although our knowledge of the role of inflammation in patients with MPN is rapidly expanding, we have yet to fully harness this knowledge toward improvements in diagnosis, prognostication, monitoring of disease progression or treatment, and use as a therapeutic target.

Cytokine profiling remains relatively untapped as a clinical tool. MPN subtypes seem to have unique cytokine profile signatures (see discussed earlier), and it is conceivable that sometime in the future cytokine profiling could be incorporated as a diagnostic tool to aid in delineating the MPN subtype. Moreover, cytokine profiling could also possibly increase the accuracy of our prognostic scoring tools in MPN. Not only could cytokines be leveraged to help predict general prognosis but may be most helpful to identify patients at highest risk of specific outcomes such as thrombosis. Moreover, cytokines could also possibly be used to help aid in selection of drugs, for example, those who are most likely to benefit from JAK 1/2 inhibitors.

Targeting of specific microenvironmental offender cell types could be applied therapeutically in MPNs. An example of targeting specific microenvironmental cell subtypes involved in fibrosis is the drug PRM-151, which targets the differentiation of fibrocytes, a cell type important for fibrosis.[56] There are a multitude of other potential targets, including GLI1 proteins on MSCs by GANT61,[42] G6B on mutant HSCs,[37] PDGFRA signaling pathway in fibrosis,[43] and reducing NETs and platelet-leukocyte aggregates.[50] A greater understanding of the intricate relationship between inflammation and MPN disease pathogenesis will allow for more accurate therapeutic targeting to achieve the much-desired goal of disease-modifying therapy in MPN.

DISCLOSURES

The authors declare that they have no conflict of interests. Research reported in this publication was supported by the National Cancer Institute of the National Institutes of Health under Award Number T32CA009054. The content is solely the responsibility of the authors and does not necessarily represent the official views of the National Institutes of Health.

CLINICS CARE POINTS

- Chronic inflammation is a characteristic feature of myeloproliferative neoplasm (MPN).
- Reduction of inflammation is of clinical utility in MPN.

REFERENCES

1. Reikvam H, Fredly H, Kittang AO, et al. The possible diagnostic and prognostic use of systemic chemokine profiles in clinical medicine—the experience in acute

myeloid leukemia from disease development and diagnosis via conventional chemotherapy to allogeneic stem cell transplantation. Toxins (Basel) 2013;5(2): 336–62.

2. Levine RL, Wadleigh M, Cools J, et al. Activating mutation in the tyrosine kinase JAK2 in polycythemia vera, essential thrombocythemia, and myeloid metaplasia with myelofibrosis. Cancer Cell 2005;7(4):387–97.

3. James C, Ugo V, Le Couédic JP, et al. A unique clonal JAK2 mutation leading to constitutive signalling causes polycythaemia vera. Nature 2005;434(7037): 1144–8.

4. Kralovics R, Passamonti F, Buser AS, et al. A gain-of-function mutation of JAK2 in myeloproliferative disorders. N Engl J Med 2005;352(17):1779–90.

5. Baxter EJ, Scott LM, Campbell PJ, et al. Acquired mutation of the tyrosine kinase JAK2 in human myeloproliferative disorders. Lancet 2005;365(9464):1054–61.

6. Nangalia J, Massie CE, Baxter EJ, et al. Somatic CALR mutations in myeloproliferative neoplasms with nonmutated JAK2. N Engl J Med 2013;369(25):2391–405.

7. Klampfl T, Gisslinger H, Harutyunyan AS, et al. Somatic mutations of calreticulin in myeloproliferative neoplasms. N Engl J Med 2013;369(25):2379–90.

8. Pikman Y, Lee BH, Mercher T, et al. MPLW515L is a novel somatic activating mutation in myelofibrosis with myeloid metaplasia. PLoS Med 2006;3(7):e270.

9. Pardanani AD, Levine RL, Lasho T, et al. MPL515 mutations in myeloproliferative and other myeloid disorders: a study of 1182 patients. Blood 2006;108(10): 3472–6.

10. Beer PA, Campbell PJ, Scott LM, et al. MPL mutations in myeloproliferative disorders: analysis of the PT-1 cohort. Blood 2008;112(1):141–9.

11. Kristinsson SY, Landgren O, Samuelsson J, et al. Autoimmunity and the risk of myeloproliferative neoplasms. Haematologica 2010;95(7):1216–20.

12. Titmarsh GJ, McMullin MF, McShane CM, et al. Community-acquired infections and their association with myeloid malignancies. Cancer Epidemiol 2014;38(1): 56–61.

13. Pedersen KM, Bak M, Sørensen AL, et al. Smoking is associated with increased risk of myeloproliferative neoplasms: a general population-based cohort study. Cancer Med 2018;7(11):5796–802.

14. Duncombe AS, Anderson LA, James G, et al. Modifiable lifestyle and medical risk factors associated with myeloproliferative neoplasms. Hemasphere 2020;4(1): e327.

15. Murphy F, Kroll ME, Pirie K, et al. Body size in relation to incidence of subtypes of haematological malignancy in the prospective Million Women Study. Br J Cancer 2013;108(11):2390–8.

16. Leal AD, Thompson CA, Wang AH, et al. Anthropometric, medical history and lifestyle risk factors for myeloproliferative neoplasms in the Iowa Women's Health Study cohort. Int J Cancer 2014;134(7):1741–50.

17. Sud A, Chattopadhyay S, Thomsen H, et al. Familial risks of acute myeloid leukemia, myelodysplastic syndromes, and myeloproliferative neoplasms. Blood 2018; 132(9):973–6.

18. Huang Y, Wang H, Hao Y, et al. Myeloid PTEN promotes chemotherapy-induced NLRP3-inflammasome activation and antitumour immunity. Nat Cell Biol 2020; 22(6):716–27.

19. Masselli E, Carubbi C, Cambò B, et al. The -2518 A/G polymorphism of the monocyte chemoattractant protein-1 as a candidate genetic predisposition factor for secondary myelofibrosis and biomarker of disease severity. Leukemia 2018; 32(10):2266–70.

20. Øbro NF, Grinfeld J, Belmonte M, et al. Longitudinal cytokine profiling identifies GRO-α and EGF as potential biomarkers of disease progression in essential thrombocythemia. Hemasphere 2020;4(3):e371.
21. Mambet C, Necula L, Mihai S, et al. Increased Dkk-1 plasma levels may discriminate disease subtypes in myeloproliferative neoplasms. J Cell Mol Med 2018. https://doi.org/10.1111/jcmm.13753.
22. Vaidya R, Gangat N, Jimma T, et al. Plasma cytokines in polycythemia vera: phenotypic correlates, prognostic relevance, and comparison with myelofibrosis. Am J Hematol 2012;87(11):1003–5.
23. Pourcelot E, Trocme C, Mondet J, et al. Cytokine profiles in polycythemia vera and essential thrombocythemia patients: clinical implications. Exp Hematol 2014;42(5):360–8.
24. Hermouet S, Godard A, Pineau D, et al. Abnormal production of interleukin (IL)-11 and IL-8 in polycythaemia vera. Cytokine 2002;20(4):178–83.
25. Boissinot M, Cleyrat C, Vilaine M, et al. Anti-inflammatory cytokines hepatocyte growth factor and interleukin-11 are over-expressed in Polycythemia vera and contribute to the growth of clonal erythroblasts independently of JAK2V617F. Oncogene 2011;30(8):990–1001.
26. Gangemi S, Allegra A, Pace E, et al. Evaluation of interleukin-23 plasma levels in patients with polycythemia vera and essential thrombocythemia. Cell Immunol 2012;278(1–2):91–4.
27. Ho CL, Lasho TL, Butterfield JH, et al. Global cytokine analysis in myeloproliferative disorders. Leuk Res 2007;31(10):1389–92.
28. Allegra A, Alonci A, Bellomo G, et al. Evaluation of interleukin-17 serum levels in patients with chronic myeloproliferative diseases. Tumori 2009;95(3):404–5.
29. Cacemiro MDC, Cominal JG, Tognon R, et al. Philadelphia-negative myeloproliferative neoplasms as disorders marked by cytokine modulation. Hematol Transfus Cell Ther 2018;40(2):120–31.
30. Tefferi A, Vaidya R, Caramazza D, et al. Circulating interleukin (IL)-8, IL-2R, IL-12, and IL-15 levels are independently prognostic in primary myelofibrosis: a comprehensive cytokine profiling study. J Clin Oncol 2011;29(10):1356–63.
31. Bourantas KL, Hatzimichael EC, Makis AC, et al. Serum beta-2-microglobulin, TNF-alpha and interleukins in myeloproliferative disorders. Eur J Haematol 1999;63(1):19–25.
32. Panteli KE, Hatzimichael EC, Bouranta PK, et al. Serum interleukin (IL)-1, IL-2, sIL-2Ra, IL-6 and thrombopoietin levels in patients with chronic myeloproliferative diseases. Br J Haematol 2005;130(5):709–15.
33. Fleischman AG, Aichberger KJ, Luty SB, et al. TNFα facilitates clonal expansion of JAK2V617F positive cells in myeloproliferative neoplasms. Blood 2011; 118(24):6392–8.
34. Kagoya Y, Yoshimi A, Tsuruta-Kishino T, et al. JAK2V617F+ myeloproliferative neoplasm clones evoke paracrine DNA damage to adjacent normal cells through secretion of lipocalin-2. Blood 2014;124(19):2996–3006.
35. Lu M, Xia L, Liu YC, et al. Lipocalin produced by myelofibrosis cells affects the fate of both hematopoietic and marrow microenvironmental cells. Blood 2015; 126(8):972–82.
36. Arranz L, Sánchez-Aguilera A, Martín-Pérez D, et al. Neuropathy of haematopoietic stem cell niche is essential for myeloproliferative neoplasms. Nature 2014;512(7512):78–81.

37. Psaila B, Wang G, Rodriguez-Meira A, et al. Single-cell analyses reveal megakaryocyte-biased hematopoiesis in myelofibrosis and identify mutant clone-specific targets. Mol Cell 2020;78(3):477–92.e8.

38. Nam AS, Kim KT, Chaligne R, et al. Somatic mutations and cell identity linked by genotyping of transcriptomes. Nature 2019;571(7765):355–60.

39. Ciurea SO, Merchant D, Mahmud N, et al. Pivotal contributions of megakaryocytes to the biology of idiopathic myelofibrosis. Blood 2007;110(3):986–93.

40. Schepers K, Pietras EM, Reynaud D, et al. Myeloproliferative neoplasia remodels the endosteal bone marrow niche into a self-reinforcing leukemic niche. Cell Stem Cell 2013;13(3):285–99.

41. Martinaud C, Desterke C, Konopacki J, et al. Osteogenic potential of mesenchymal stromal cells contributes to primary myelofibrosis. Cancer Res 2015; 75(22):4753–65.

42. Schneider RK, Mullally A, Dugourd A, et al. Gli1 + Mesenchymal stromal cells are a key driver of bone marrow fibrosis and an important cellular therapeutic target. Cell Stem Cell 2017;20(6):785–800.e8.

43. Decker M, Martinez-Morentin L, Wang G, et al. Leptin-receptor-expressing bone marrow stromal cells are myofibroblasts in primary myelofibrosis. Nat Cell Biol 2017;19(6):677–88.

44. Fisher DAC, Miner CA, Engle EK, et al. Cytokine production in myelofibrosis exhibits differential responsiveness to JAK-STAT, MAP kinase, and NFκB signaling. Leukemia 2019;33(8):1978–95.

45. Lai HY, Brooks SA, Craver BM, et al. Defective negative regulation of Toll-like receptor signaling leads to excessive TNF-α in myeloproliferative neoplasm. Blood Adv 2019;3(2):122–31.

46. Kleppe M, Kwak M, Koppikar P, et al. JAK-STAT pathway activation in malignant and nonmalignant cells contributes to MPN pathogenesis and therapeutic response. Cancer Discov 2015;5(3):316–31.

47. Fuchs TA, Brill A, Duerschmied D, et al. Extracellular DNA traps promote thrombosis. Proc Natl Acad Sci U S A 2010;107(36):15880–5.

48. Falanga A, Marchetti M, Evangelista V, et al. Polymorphonuclear leukocyte activation and hemostasis in patients with essential thrombocythemia and polycythemia vera. Blood 2000;96(13):4261–6.

49. Wolach O, Sellar RS, Martinod K, et al. Increased neutrophil extracellular trap formation promotes thrombosis in myeloproliferative neoplasms. Sci Transl Med 2018;10:436.

50. Craver BM, Ramanathan G, Hoang S, et al. N-acetylcysteine inhibits thrombosis in a murine model of myeloproliferative neoplasm. Blood Adv 2020; 4(2):312–21.

51. Marin Oyarzún CP, Heller PG. Platelets as mediators of thromboinflammation in chronic myeloproliferative neoplasms. Front Immunol 2019;10:1373.

52. Barbui T, Carobbio A, Finazzi G, et al. Inflammation and thrombosis in essential thrombocythemia and polycythemia vera: different role of C-reactive protein and pentraxin 3. Haematologica 2011;96(2):315–8.

53. Falanga A, Marchetti M, Vignoli A, et al. Leukocyte-platelet interaction in patients with essential thrombocythemia and polycythemia vera. Exp Hematol 2005;33(5): 523–30.

54. Arellano-Rodrigo E, Alvarez-Larrán A, Reverter JC, et al. Platelet turnover, coagulation factors, and soluble markers of platelet and endothelial activation in

essential thrombocythemia: relationship with thrombosis occurrence and JAK2 V617F allele burden. Am J Hematol 2009;84(2):102–8.

55. Koupenova M, Clancy L, Corkrey HA, et al. Circulating platelets as mediators of immunity, inflammation, and thrombosis. Circ Res 2018;122(2):337–51.

56. Verstovsek S, Manshouri T, Pilling D, et al. Role of neoplastic monocyte-derived fibrocytes in primary myelofibrosis. J Exp Med 2016;213(9):1723–40.

Genetics of Myeloproliferative Neoplasms

Jakub Szybinski, PhD[a], Sara C. Meyer, MD, PhD[a,b,*]

KEYWORDS

- Myeloproliferative neoplasms • Genetics • Genomics • JAK2 • Calreticulin • MPL
- Genetic alterations

KEY POINTS

- Phenotypic driver mutations in JAK2, calreticulin, and MPL are present in 85% to 90% of myeloproliferative neoplasms and induce constitutive activation of JAK2-STAT signaling.
- Modern sequencing efforts have revealed large parts of the genomic landscape of myeloproliferative neoplasms with additional genetic alterations mainly in epigenetic modifiers and splicing factors.
- Genetic alterations in myeloproliferative neoplasms are subject to clonal evolution as myeloproliferative neoplasms progress, with high molecular risk mutations impacting dynamics and outcome.
- Because JAK2 V617F is not specific to myeloproliferative neoplasms and is seen in other myeloid malignancies, it is important to note JAK2 V617F is recurrently detected in clonal hematopoiesis of indeterminate potential.
- The expanding insight into the genetic basis has facilitated diagnosis and prognostication of myeloproliferative neoplasms and poses novel candidates for targeted therapeutic intervention.

BACKGROUND

Myeloproliferative neoplasms (MPN) are hematopoietic stem cell disorders with dysregulated production of mature myeloid blood cells including polycythemia vera (PV), essential thrombocythemia (ET), and primary myelofibrosis (PMF). They were first grouped together as an entity in 1951 by William Dameshek, suggesting that they are driven by a so far undiscovered stimulus.[1] Over the last 15 years, constitutive

Conflicts of interest: S.C. Meyer has consulted for and received honoraria from Celgene/BMS.
Funded by: Swiss National Science Foundation and others.
[a] Department of Biomedicine, University Hospital Basel and University of Basel, Hebelstrasse 20, Basel CH-4031, Switzerland; [b] Division of Hematology, University Hospital Basel, Petersgraben 4, Basel CH-4031, Switzerland
* Corresponding author. Division of Hematology, University Hospital Basel, Petersgraben 4, Basel CH-4031, Switzerland
E-mail address: sara.meyer@unibas.ch

Hematol Oncol Clin N Am 35 (2021) 217–236
https://doi.org/10.1016/j.hoc.2020.12.002
hemonc.theclinics.com
0889-8588/21/© 2020 The Author(s). Published by Elsevier Inc. This is an open access article under the CC BY-NC-ND license (http://creativecommons.org/licenses/by-nc-nd/4.0/).

activation of JAK2-STAT signaling has been revealed as a common characteristic of MPN owing to somatic mutations in the tyrosine kinase JAK2, the chaperone protein calreticulin (CALR) or the thrombopoietin receptor MPL in the majority of patients[2] (**Fig. 1**). In addition, the advent of modern sequencing technologies has enabled detailed investigation of the genomic landscape of MPN. A set of additional mutations frequently seen also in other myeloid malignancies, often co-occurs contributing to the clinical phenotype, disease dynamics, and overall outcome[3] (**Fig. 2**). In this review, we provide an overview of the genetics in MPN, which by now provides us with helpful diagnostic biomarkers[4] and contributes to refined prognostication of several MPN subsets.[5,6] Importantly, the extensive characterization of the genetic basis has revealed several promising candidates, which could serve as targets for novel, mechanism-based therapeutic approaches, which represents a current need of patients with MPN.

SOMATIC DRIVER MUTATIONS MEDIATING CONSTITUTIVE JAK2-STAT ACTIVATION

The discovery of the JAK2 V617F mutation in 2005 by several groups using different methodologies was a breakthrough for the field and initiated the era of genetic characterization of MPN, which has progressed at a rapid pace.[7–10] A somatic JAK2 V617F

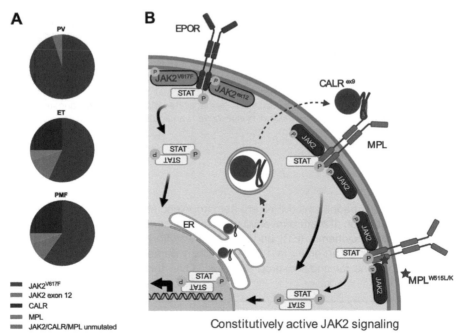

Fig. 1. Somatic driver mutations in MPN activating JAK2-STAT signaling. (*A*) Approximate frequencies of JAK2 V617F, JAK2 exon 12, CALR and MPL mutations in PV, ET, and PMF. JAK2/CALR/MPL unmutated cases are referred to as triple negative MPN. (*B*) JAK2 V617F mutations occur in association with EPOR and MPL in all MPN subtypes including PV, ET, and PMF. JAK2 exon 12 mutations exclusively occur in association with EPOR in PV. CALR mutations locate to exon 9 and occur in ET and PMF. MPL mutations are in exon 10 with missense mutations affecting mostly residue W515 and occur in ET and PMF. Somatic driver mutations in JAK2, CALR, and MPL converge on constitutively activated JAK2-STAT signaling. EPOR, erythropoietin receptor; ER, endoplasmic reticulum; MPL, thrombopoietin receptor.

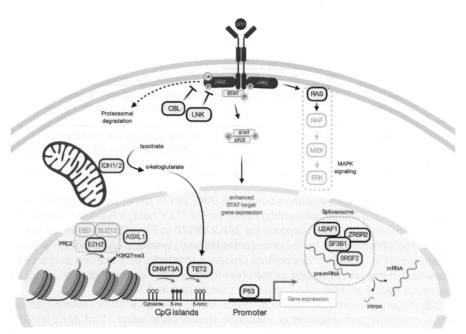

Fig. 2. Somatic mutations in genes broadly affected in myeloid malignancies occurring in MPN. Somatic mutations in myeloid cancer genes are often co-mutated in MPN, particularly in PMF. Epigenetic regulators involved in DNA methylation (DNMT3A), demethylation (TET2), and in histone modification relating to the PRC2 complex (EZH2, ASXL1), as well as factors involved in messenger RNA splicing (SRSF2, U2AF1, SF3B1, ZRSR2) are most frequently affected. IDH1 and IDH2 mutations lead to accumulation of the oncometabolite 2-hydroxyglutarate instead of physiologic α-ketoglutarate, which interferes with TET2 function. Factors activating (RAS) or regulating (CBL, LNK/SH2B3) signaling as well as factors involved in transcriptional regulation/DNA repair (TP53) are also found mutated. Mutations in ASXL1, EZH2, IDH1/2, and SRSF2 (highlighted in *red*) are considered high molecular risk (HMR) mutations, because they confer adverse prognosis, whereas mutations in TP53, IDH1/2, and SRSF2 are enriched in blast-phase MPN. 5-hmc, 5-hydroxymethylcytosine; 5-mc, 5-methylcytosine; EPO erythropoietin; PRC2, polycomb repressive complex 2.

mutation is present in the majority of patients with MPN, including 95% of PV and 50% to 60% of ET and PMF (see **Fig. 1**, **Table 1**). The JAK2 non–receptor tyrosine kinase essential for hematopoietic cytokine signaling via erythropoietin, thrombopoietin and granulocyte colony stimulating factor receptors is constitutively activated by a G to T transition in exon 14 mediating a valine to phenylalanine substitution at position 617 of the protein. Functionally, the inhibitory effect of the JAK2 pseudokinase domain on the kinase domain is abrogated.[11] It results in the constitutive activation of JAK2-driven signaling pathways, including STAT1, STAT3, and STAT5 transcription factors, as well as the PI3K/AKT and the MAPK signaling pathway promoting proliferation, differentiation, and survival of myeloid progenitor cells.[12] The JAK2 V617F mutation acquired at the level of hematopoietic stem cells is in line with the occurrence of erythrocytosis, thrombocytosis, and/or leukocytosis in the peripheral blood.[13] However, the question how JAK2 V617F may induce the differential phenotypes of PV with predominant erythrocytosis, ET with isolated thrombocytosis, and PMF with increased megakaryocytes, bone marrow fibrosis, and progressing cytopenias in patients displaying the same V617F missense mutation in JAK2 is incompletely understood. It has been shown that gene dosage and mutant allele frequency impact on the clinical

Table 1
Approximate frequencies of somatic driver mutations in MPN

Mutation		Frequency (%)			
Gene	Location	PV	ET	PMF	Molecular Function
JAK2	V617F exon 14	95	50–60	50–60	Non–receptor tyrosine kinase mediating hematopoietic cytokine signaling
JAK2	exon 12	2–3	-	-	
CALR	exon 9	<1	26	18–32	ER chaperone protein interacting with thrombopoietin receptor MPL
MPL	exon 10	<1	4	5–9	Thrombopoietin receptor

presentation, because a low allele burden of JAK2 V617F rather presents as ET versus higher mutational burden presenting rather as PV.[14] Of note, it has been shown that the MPN clone is often homozygous for JAK2 V617F in PV owing to a loss of heterozygosity at chromosome 9p by uniparental disomy, whereas JAK2 V617F is mostly heterozygous in ET.[15] The concomitant presence of additional mutations as discussed elsewhere in this article, as well as the order in which the mutations are occurring during clonal evolution, may also impact the clinical picture.[3,16]

Subsequent sequencing efforts in JAK2 V617F–negative MPN revealed several small insertions and deletions or missense mutations in exon 12 of JAK2 in 2007, which occur exclusively in PV, accounting for 2% to 3% of patients, but not in ET and PMF.[17] Interestingly, JAK2 exon 12 mutated patients with PV preferentially present with pronounced erythrocytosis in the absence of concomitant thrombocytosis or leukocytosis, whereas JAK2 V617F rather is associated with an older age at diagnosis and erythrocytosis, often accompanied by neutrophilia and/or thrombocytosis.[18] The association of these specific JAK2 genotypes with differential PV phenotypes has been recapitulated in preclinical models as well.[19]

Although JAK2 V617F or exon 12 mutations provide a genetic basis for the constitutive activation of JAK-STAT signaling in the vast majority of patients with PV, a large proportion of patients with ET and patients with myelofibrosis are negative for genetic alterations in JAK2.[12] In 2006, missense mutations in the thrombopoietin receptor MPL, which signals through JAK2, were identified at position 515 in 4% of patients with ET and 5% to 9% of patients with PMF, but not in patients with PV.[20] Although W515L represents the most frequent alteration in the MPL gene, W515K and rarely others have also been reported and similarly induce constitutive activation of JAK2 signaling.[21]

After these exciting discoveries in 2005 to 2007, the genetic basis of JAK2- and MPL-unmutated ET and PMF remained elusive for several years, leaving 30% to 40% of patients without a known driver mutation. The adaptor protein LNK (SH2B3) and the Casitas B-lineage lymphoma proto-oncogene CBL, negative regulators of JAK2, were found mutated in a relatively small proportion of patients, also leading to JAK-STAT activation.[22,23] Although LNK, an inhibitor of erythropoietin and thrombopoietin signaling, is mutated in 0% to 9% of patients with MPN, inactivating CBL mutations interfere with ubiquitin ligase activity and induce prolonged activation of JAK2 signaling in up to 6% of PMF or secondary acute myeloid leukemia (AML). It was only in 2013 that 2 groups reported another breakthrough discovery identifying a putative driver mutation in 67% to 88% of the JAK2 and MPL wild-type MPN patients. By applying whole exome sequencing to individuals with wild-type genotypes for JAK2 and MPL, both groups independently identified somatic mutations in CALR, an endoplasmic reticulum (ER) chaperone protein that has not been previously implicated in cancer development.[24,25] Under physiologic conditions, CALR is involved in the appropriate folding of glycoproteins in the lumen of the ER containing a C-terminal ER retention signal with a characteristic KDEL sequence.

CALR is also implicated in calcium homeostasis given its negatively charged C-terminus facilitating calcium binding. Of the more than 35 CALR mutations identified, all localize to C-terminal exon 9 and result in a 1 bp frameshift inducing a novel C-terminal sequence. The 2 most frequent mutations accounting for 85% of the alterations include a 52 bp deletion (CALR^{del52}, type 1) with 44% to 53% of patients and a 5 bp insertion (CALR^{ins5}, type 2) in 32% to 42% of patients. Alternative insertions or deletions with lower frequencies account for the remainder (type 1 like or type 2 like). It rapidly became clear that the observed CALR mutations all interfere with the distal ER retention signal via the altered C-terminal sequence, with the loss of the typical negative charge and that activation of JAK2-STAT signaling as a common feature of MPN was preserved also in CALR mutant MPN. Intense research efforts over the last years have delineated how JAK2-STAT activation from mutated CALR may occur and how the CALR chaperone may function as an oncogene in MPN. Several elegant studies have shown that ER-located mutant CALR associates with MPL, inducing aberrant activation of MPL-JAK2 signaling, whereas mutant CALR would also leave the ER and associate with MPL at the cell surface.[26-28] These findings provide a plausible explanation as to why CALR mutant MPN phenocopy MPL mutant MPN to large extents. Differential aspects relating to CALR as a driver include the findings of more pronounced thrombocytosis, slightly lower hemoglobin levels, presentation at a younger age, and a lesser incidence of thromboembolic events in CALR versus JAK2 V617F mutant ET, which has implications for prognostication and clinical management.[29] In PMF, patients with a CALR mutant show a more favorable prognosis as compared with patients with JAK2 V617F and MPL mutations, which primarily relates to type 1 CALR mutations, with a significantly prolonged survival, making them a relevant parameter for modern, molecularly based prognostication schemes in myelofibrosis.[5,6,30,31]

Although JAK2, CALR, and MPL mutations are mostly mutually exclusive in MPN given their redundant effects with constitutive activation of JAK-STAT signaling, "double hits" with 2 concomitant JAK2 mutations as, for example, JAK2 V617F and a JAK2 exon 12 mutation or JAK2 V617F with a concomitant JAK2 R1063H mutation, have been reported, albeit rarely.[3,32,33] Alternatively, concomitant CALR or MPL mutations may also rarely occur, mostly in the setting of low allele burden JAK2 V617F. The clonal architecture of such cases is not entirely clarified.

The insight into the genetic basis of MPN in the last 15 years now provides us with information on somatic driver mutations in a majority of patients, because only approximately 2% of PV and approximately 10% of ET and PMF are unmutated for JAK2, CALR, or MPL. These "triple-negative" MPN require a particularly diligent diagnostic workup, because reactive causes for a phenotype suggestive of MPN as well as alternative myeloid malignancies need to be carefully excluded. It has been reported that triple-negative MPN tested positive for typical somatic driver mutations at low mutant allele burden when resequenced using methodologies with greater sensitivity.[3,32,33] In addition, noncanonical somatic mutations in JAK2 and MPL have also been identified, as well as germline variants, implying a familial basis of thrombocytosis or erythrocytosis of nonclonal origin.[32-34] Truly triple-negative ET have typically been found in young, female patients with a benign prospect.[3] In contrast, triple-negative PMF associates with significantly poorer outcome as compared with CALR, JAK2, or MPL mutant PMF, which show a more favorable prognosis in decreasing order. An adverse prognosis of triple-negative PMF implies increased risk of progression as well as shortened overall survival and should be considered for decisions on clinical manage-ment.[30] With sequencing technologies rapidly moving forward, somatic driver muta-tions in the triple-negative MPN might also be revealed.

Although the identification of the somatic driver mutations in JAK2, CALR, and MPL has provided us with a set of biomarkers greatly facilitating the diagnosis of MPN, the finding of constitutively activated JAK-STAT signaling resulting from each of these driver mutations has posed a relevant target for therapy.[2] Consequently, JAK2 inhib-itors have been developed and 2 compounds, ruxolitinib and fedratinib, have entered clinical use.[35–38] Because these currently available JAK2 inhibitors, which bind to the ATP pocket of the JAK2 kinase domain, are not selective for the JAK2 V617F mutant form of the kinase, they are able to interfere with activated JAK2-STAT signaling not just in JAK2 mutant, but also in CALR or MPL mutant patients, as well as in triple-negative MPN. Of note, the recent findings on mutant CALR being exposed at the cell surface could provide a therapeutic target specific to the MPN clone, which may be addressable in the future.[28]

SOMATIC MUTATIONS IN GENES BROADLY AFFECTED IN MYELOID MALIGNANCIES

Several genes commonly mutated across myeloid malignancies were found to be affected by somatic mutations also in MPN[25,39] (see **Fig. 2**, **Table 2**). Overall, more than one-half of individuals suffering from MPN carry accompanying mutations in these myeloid cancer genes with increasing frequency at more advanced ages and most prominently in PMF. Epigenetic modifiers and factors involved in messenger RNA splicing are predominantly affected, whereas blast phase MPN shows character-istic additional mutations.[3]

Epigenetic Modifiers

The DNA methylation status of CpG islands modulating gene expression results from a complex interplay of methylating and demethylating events. DNMT3A represents a de novo methyltransferase prevalently mutated in AML, most commonly with the hotspot mutation R882H. DNMT3A mutations were also frequently found in MPN with 3% to 15% in patients with PMF and up to 9% in patients with PV and patients with ET.[40] A loss of DNMT3A function has been shown to occur early in MPN disease evolution, typically before the acquisition of JAK2 V617F and to induce a clonal advantage with overall expansion of the hematopoietic stem cell pool.[39,41] The dynamics of clonal evolution seem to relate to specific MPN phenotypes with PMF developing rather from JAK2 V617F mutant clones with preexisting DNMT3A mutations, whereas JAK2 V617F followed by late acquisition of genetic alterations in DNMT3A would favor the occurrence of PV or ET.[42]

DNA demethylation occurs via the generation of 5-hydroxymethylcytosine con-verted from 5-methylcytosine by TET2 found to be mutated in solid tumors and myeloid malignancies. Also in MPN, TET2 mutations are prevalent and found in 7% to 22% of patients without a clear prognostic effect.[43] Genetic alterations in TET2 mediate expansion of the hematopoietic stem cell pool.[44] Similarly to DNMT3A, mutational order impacts clinical phenotype with patients acquiring JAK2 V617F before a TET2 mutation presenting rather with PV or ET as compared to patients acquiring JAK2 V617F afterwards.[16] The observation that TET2 mutations are mutually exclusive with mutations in the 2 isoforms of isocitrate dehydrogenase IDH1 and IDH2 with largely overlapping DNA methylation and gene expression pat-terns, has revealed their redundant functional effects. IDH1/2 mutations, initially described in glioblastoma and AML, induce the accumulation of the oncometabolite

Table 2
Approximate frequencies of additional somatic mutations in MPN

Class	Mutated Gene	Frequency (%)			Molecular Function
		PV	ET	PMF	
Epigenetic regulation	DNMT3A	2–7	0–9	3–15	De novo DNA methylase
	TET2	19–22	5–16	10–18	DNA demethylase
	IDH1/2[a]	2	1	0–6	Isocitrate dehydrogenase generating 2-HG
	ASXL1[a]	3–12	1–11	13–37	Chromatin remodeling as Polycomb group protein
	EZH2[a]	0–3	1–3	1–9	PRC2 complex H3K27me3 methyltransferase
	SUZ12	2–3	<1	2	PRC2 complex component
Messenger RNA splicing	SRSF2[a]	3	2	8–18	Serine/arginine-rich splicing factor
	U2AF1	<1	1	6–16	Spliceosome component
	SF3B1	3	5	6–10	Splicing factor 3B protein complex subunit 1
	ZRSR2	5	3	4–10	Spliceosome component
Signaling	N/KRAS	0–1	<1	3–4	Small GTPase activating MAPK pathway signaling
	CBL	1	1	4–7	E3 ubiquitin-protein ligase regulating JAK2
	SH2B3 (LNK)	9	3	3–6	Adaptor regulating hematopoietic signaling incl. JAK2
	PTPN11	<1	0–2	0–2	Protein tyrosine phosphatase dephosphorylating RAS
Transcriptional regulation	RUNX1	0–2	0–2	3–4	Transcription factor involved in differentiation of hematopoietic stem cells
	NFE2	2–3	<1	0–3	Transcription factor involved in myelopoiesis
DNA repair	TP53	1	2–6	1	Transcription factor, cell cycle regulator
	PPM1D	1	2	1	Regulatory inhibitor of TP53

[a] High molecular risk (HMR) mutations.

α-ketoglutarate interfering with proper TET2 function.[45] Of note, IDH1/2 mutations, which are detected in 1% to 6% of patients with MPN, significantly impact prognosis in PMF, with a higher risk for secondary AML, earlier transformation, and lower overall survival. In addition, IDH1/2 mutations are enriched in blast phase MPN occurring in 19% to 31% of patients.[46]

The factors involved in histone methylation via polycomb repressive complex 2 are also mutated in MPN, as for example, EZH2 and ASXL1, which mediate adverse prognostic effects. Genetic alterations in EZH2, the enzymatic component of polycomb repressive complex 2 mediating methylation at H3K27, are detected particularly in patients with PMF at 1% to 9%.[47] Several studies demonstrated aggravating effects on bone marrow fibrosis and observed EZH2 mutations to associate with adverse prognosis and decreased overall survival.[48,49] ASXL1, which is involved in mediating polycomb repressive complex 2 function, is mutated in 13% to 37% of patients with PMF and 1% to 12% of patients with PV and patients with ET.[50] Analogous to its adverse prognostic effect in other myeloid malignancies, ASXL1 mutations are also unfavorable in MPN and associate with a poor outcome.[51]

In addition to somatic mutations in epigenetic regulators modifying the epigenetic landscape in MPN, JAK2 V617F itself has also been reported to mediate epigenetic functions. JAK2 V617F phosphorylates the protein arginine methyltransferase PRMT5, which is increasingly studied in different malignancies, including MPN.[52,53] Additional reports have described the potential of JAK2 V617F to localize to the nucleus impacting on histone H3 phosphorylation.[54]

Splicing Factors

Mutations in genes involved in messenger RNA splicing are frequent in myeloid malignancies, particularly in myelodysplastic syndromes (MDS). Splicing factors are also recurrently mutated in MPN with up to approximately 20% of patients with PMF harboring genetic alterations in SRSF2, U2AF1, SF3B1 or ZRSR2 leading to mis-splicing.[55] Although SF3B1 is typically seen in MDS/MPN with ringed sideroblasts and thrombocytosis and rather associates with a favorable prognosis in this setting,[56] SRSF2 confers an increased risk for leukemic transformation and shortened overall survival in patients with PMF.[57]

Signaling Molecules

Beyond the somatic driver mutations in JAK2, CALR, and MPL, additional signaling molecules may also be subject to mutational events implicated in MPN pathogenesis. RAS isoforms, including KRAS and NRAS, which are central drivers of MAPK pathway signaling, represent well-established oncogenes not only in solid tumors, but also in myeloid malignancies.[58] Although AML particularly and certain MDS/MPN overlap syndromes (eg, chronic myelomonocytic leukemia) recurrently show somatic RAS mutations, N/KRAS have also been found mutated in MPN,[3,25,39] for which a relevance of MAPK signaling has been established.[59] Recent studies evaluating the significance of RAS activation in myelofibrosis have shown somatic N/KRAS mutations in 6% of patients.[3] They were typically subclonal relative to other, clonal genetic alterations and associated with progressive disease and additional, high molecular risk mutations. N/KRAS mutations predicted increased risk for leukemic transformation and significantly shorter overall survival, which was improved in patients treated with the JAK2 inhibitor ruxolitinib.[60]

High Molecular Risk Mutations and Blast Phase Myeloproliferative Neoplasms

Concomitant mutations in myeloid cancer genes as discussed elsewhere in this article play significant roles in determining MPN phenotypes, progression, and outcome.[3] Although the sequence of mutation acquisition may determine the presentation of PMF versus PV/ET as shown for TET2 and DNMT3A, several studies have demonstrated adverse prognostic effects mediated by a greater overall number of mutations, which often increase upon progression.[39] Unfavorable outcomes have directly been related with mutations in ASXL1, IDH1/2, EZH2, and SRSF2, which are therefore designated as high molecular risk mutations and are increasingly implemented in modern, molecularly-based prognostication schemes.[55] In blast phase MPN, mutations in IDH1/2 and SRSF2 are enriched and occur at an increased frequency.[46,61] In contrast, JAK2 V617F is frequently lost upon transformation to blast phase MPN, highlighting a clonal evolution from early subclones preceding JAK2 V617F or from independent JAK2 V617F negative clones.[62,63] Of note, genetic alterations in the tumor suppressor TP53 are seen in up to 35% of patients upon transformation. TP53 mutations often herald blast phase when acquired in advanced MPN and mostly affect both alleles via independent emergence of mutations or uniparental disomy at chromosome 17p.[61]

GERMLINE GENETIC FACTORS INVOLVED IN MYELOPROLIFERATIVE NEOPLASMS

Familial clustering of MPN with 5% of patients with MPN having an affected family member has suggested germline predisposition alleles, which increase the susceptibility to acquire somatic MPN driver mutations.[64] In 2009, several groups identified a so-called 46/1 or GGCC haplotype still representing the strongest germline predisposing factor for MPN today with 3- to 4-fold increased risk to develop sporadic or familial MPN.[65] The haplotype marked by several single nucleotide variants (as eg, rs10974944) encompasses the JAK2 gene itself and the somatic JAK2 V617F has typically been found in cis with the predisposition allele.[66] In addition, GWAS studies have identified germline susceptibility alleles also in TERT, MECOM, TET2, and SH2B3 (LNK) genes.[67] Although more prevalent risk alleles may promote the occurrence of sporadic or familial MPN, rarer germline factors would more strictly associate with familial cases as, for example, variants in RBBP6 involved in p53 function.[68] Importantly, analyses of multiple pedigrees demonstrated analogous clinical manifestations, genetic landscape, prognosis, and dynamics of progression for familial MPN as compared with sporadic cases.[69] In contrast, very rare germline variants with a high penetrance, which are involved in erythropoietin and thrombopoietin signaling, have been shown to mediate nonclonal, "MPN-like" diseases affecting only 1 myeloid lineage with a benign prognosis and no prospect of transformation. Such germline mutations in THPO, MPL, and JAK2 genes have been reported in hereditary thrombocytosis, whereas variants in EPOR, EPO, SH2B3, VHL, EGLN1, and EPAS1 (HIF2A) are known in hereditary erythrocytosis and germline mutations in CSF3R in hereditary neutrophilia. These hereditary MPN-like disorders have been reviewed in detail elsewhere.[68]

SOMATIC DRIVER MUTATIONS OF MYELOPROLIFERATIVE NEOPLASMS IN CLONAL HEMATOPOIESIS

Somatic driver mutations of MPN, including JAK2 V617F, are not restricted to MPN, but may occur in MDS, MDS/MPN overlap syndromes, and AML at lower frequencies.[70,71] Of note, the JAK2 V617F mutation has also been identified in clonal hematopoiesis of indeterminate potential (CHIP). This condition has gained increasing interest in recent years and delineates a hematopoietic clone arising from a hematopoietic stem cell with a somatic myeloid cancer gene mutation in a healthy individual with normal peripheral blood counts.[72] Although first insights came from X-chromosome inactivation studies showing an age-dependent skewing of hematopoiesis, modern sequencing methodologies have revealed clonal hematopoiesis characterized by somatic mutations in a greater than expected proportion of healthy persons. CHIP turns out to be prevalent and represents an age-dependent process, with 0.6% of individuals younger than 60 years, but up to 19.5% of individuals greater than 90 years of age presenting with clonal hematopoiesis. The most frequent are mutations in DNMT3A, TET2, ASXL1, SRSF2, and SF3B1 followed by JAK2 V617F.[73–76] Differential patterns have been described with DNMT3A and JAK2 V617F CHIP observed already in young adults with an increasing prevalence at older ages, whereas CHIP, characterized by splicing factor mutations as, for example, in SRSF2, rather present after the age of 70 years with a high risk for evolution to a myeloid malignancy.[77]

Why would JAK2 V617F CHIP matter? On the one hand, clonal hematopoiesis has been associated with an increased risk for vascular events, including coronary heart disease and ischemic stroke. This risk for vascular complications is particularly high for JAK2 V617F mutant CHIP and has been shown to increase with CHIP clone size.[78] It is likely that JAK2 V617F CHIP cooperates with classic vascular risk factors as hypertension, hyperlipidemia, diabetes, and smoking and may further promote vascular complications. Thus, JAK2 V617F CHIP may promote morbidity and mortality in so far healthy individuals in the absence of overt MPN. On the other hand, similar to CHIP with other myeloid cancer gene mutations, JAK2 V617F CHIP represents a pre-malignant stage with an increased risk of developing MPN. A study in more than 4000 healthy individuals reported higher platelet counts in JAK2 V617F versus wild-type CHIP, but still in the normal range, highlighting a propensity toward MPN development.[77] In a complementary approach, patients with JAK2 V617F mutant MPN with an availability of blood samples several years before MPN diagnosis were studied, which demonstrated JAK2 V617F CHIP in a majority of them.[79] Of note, the dynamics of clonal evolution were very variable between individuals ranging from an 0.36% to 6.20% annual increase of the JAK2 V617F allele burden, also among patients without co-mutations in common myeloid cancer genes. The 46/1 haplotype promoted the expansion of JAK2 V617F CHIP clones, but additional, as yet unknown factors are likely to contribute to this process. Given the prevalence and clinical consequences of JAK2 V617F CHIP, investigations into the biological processes driving clonal evolution and progression to overt MPN as well as vascular complications in pre-MPN and MPN phases are warranted.

CLINICAL SIGNIFICANCE OF GENETIC MARKERS IN MYELOPROLIFERATIVE NEOPLASMS

In the last 15 years, the insight into the genetics of MPN has been substantially extended and has started to immerse clinical practice at several levels including diagnosis, prognostication and therapeutic management.

Significance of Genetics for Diagnosis of Myeloproliferative Neoplasms

Although the World Health Organization implemented somatic JAK2 V617F, JAK2 exon 12, and MPL mutations promptly into its 2008 revision as a major diagnostic criterion for MPN, CALR mutations were added to the updated version in 2016 (**Table 3**). Thus, the somatic driver mutations, which constitutively activate JAK2-STAT signaling in MPN, serve as helpful biomarkers in approximately 98% of patients with PV and 85% to 90% of patients with ET and patients with PMF, representing a mainstay of MPN diagnosis. The prevalent co-mutations in myeloid cancer genes have also been implemented to provide support in diagnosing the more challenging cases of triple negative PMF. The 2016 World Health Organization guidelines recommend to test for ASXL1, EZH2, TET2, IDH1/2, SRSF2, and SF3B1 in triple-negative PMF to help determining a clonal nature.[4]

The Significance of Genetics for Prognostication in Myeloproliferative Neoplasms

Much has been learned from the sequencing efforts in myeloid malignancies as to differential effects of genetic alterations on the risk of transformation and overall outcome. In MPN, a set of high molecular risk mutations, including ASXL1, EZH2, IDH1/2, and SRSF2,[55] which confer adverse prognosis, as well as mutations enriched in blast phase MPN including IDH1/2 and TP53, have been delineated.[57] In contrast, mutations in CALR, particularly type 1, have been associated with favorable outcome in ET and PMF.[30] Although previous prognostication schemes for PMF, such as the International Prognostic Scoring System (IPSS), the Dynamic IPSS, and the Dynamic IPSS Plus have relied on clinical parameters and blood counts,[80] novel prognostic scoring systems are implementing the genetic make-up of MPN and are increasingly

Table 3
Diagnostic criteria for MPN implementing genetic markers according to the World Health Organization (2016)

	PV	ET	Myelofibrosis	
			Prefibrotic/Early	Overt/Fibrotic
Major criteria				
Blood (m/f)	Hemoglobin >165 g/L/ 160 g/L or Hematocrit >49%/48% or Red cell mass >25% above normal	Platelet count >450 × 10⁹/L	No specific requirement (cytoses or cytopenias possible)	No specific requirement (cytoses or cytopenias possible)
Marrow	Age-adjusted hypercellularity Trilineage growth (panmyelosis) including erythroid, granulocytic and megakaryocytic proliferation Pleomorphic, mature megakaryocytes	Proliferation of megakaryocytic lineage: increased, enlarged, megakaryocytes, hyperlobulated nuclei No increase in granulo/ erythropoiesis Rarely increase in reticulin fibers (grade 1)	Megakaryocytic proliferation/atypia No reticulin fibrosis greater than grade 1 Increased age-adjusted cellularity Granulocytic proliferation, often decreased erythropoiesis	Megakaryocytic proliferation and atypia Reticulin and/or collagen fibrosis of grade 2 or 3
Exclusion	No specific exclusions	Not PV, PMF, other myeloid neoplasm	Not CML, PV, ET, MDS, other myeloid neoplasms	
Genetics[a]	JAK2 V617F or exon 12 mutation	JAK2, CALR, or MPL mutation	JAK2, CALR, MPL mutation or Another clonal marker[b] or absence of reactive BM fibrosis	
Minor criteria				
Additional	Subnormal serum erythropoietin	Presence of a clonal marker or Absence of evidence of reactive cause	Anemia not owing to comorbidity Leukocytosis ≥11 × 10⁹/L Palpable splenomegaly LDH above reference	Anemia not owing to comorbidity Leukocytosis ≥11 × 10⁹/L Palpable splenomegaly LDH above reference Leukoerythroblastosis

(continued on next page)

Table 3
(continued)

| | PV | ET | Myelofibrosis | |
			Prefibrotic/Early	Overt/Fibrotic
Required	All 3 major criteria or First 2 major + minor criterion	All 4 major criteria or First 3 major + minor criterion	All 3 major + ≥1 minor criterion	All 3 major + ≥1 minor criterion

Abbreviations: BM, bone marrow; CML, chronic myeloid leukemia; LDH, lactate dehydrogenase; MDS, myelodysplastic syndromes.
[a] Genetic markers represent an integral part of diagnosis for all MPN subtypes according to the World Health Organization 2016 criteria.
[b] In absence of JAK2, CALR or MPL mutations genotyping of other mutations associated with myeloid malignancies, for example, in ASXL1, EZH2, TET2, IDH1/2, SRSF1, and SF3B1 to determine a clonal nature is recommended.

Table 4
Genetics-based prognostication schemes in myeloproliferative neoplasms

	GIPSS	Patients	MIPSS70	Patients	MYSEC	Patients
Genetic factors						
Driver mutations	CALR type 1/like mutation absent	1	CALR type 1/like mutation absent	1	CALR mutation absent	2
High-risk mutations	Somatic mutation in:		Somatic mutation in:		—	
	ASXL1	1	ASXL1	1		
	SRSF2	1	EZH2	1		
	U2AF1 Q157	1	SRSF2	1		
			IDH1/2	1		
			≥2 of the above "high molecular risk" mutations	2		
Conventional factors						
	Karyotype	2	Hemoglobin <100 g/L	1	Hemoglobin <110 g/L	2
	Very high risk: −7, i(17q), inv(3)/ 3q21, 12p−/12p11.2, 11q− 11q23, +21, other autosomal trisomies except +8/+9	1	WBC >25 × 10^9/L	2	Platelets <150 × 10^9/l	1
	Unfavorable: All other if not favorable (including normal, sole 13q−, +9, 20q−, +1, −Y)		Platelets <100 × 10^9/l	2	Peripheral blood blasts ≥3%	2
			Peripheral blood blasts ≥2%	1	Constitutional symptoms	1
			Fibrosis ≥ grade 2	1	Age at diagnosis 40–90 y	6–13.5
			Constitutional symptoms	1		
Risk category (points)	Low	0	Low	0–1	Low	0
	Intermediate-1	1	Intermediate	2–4	Intermediate-1	1
	Intermediate-2	2	High	≥5	Intermediate-2	2
	High	≥3			High	≥3

Abbreviations: GIPSS, genetically inspired prognostic scoring system; MIPSS, Mutation-Enhanced International Prognostic Score System; MYSEC, Myelofibrosis Secondary to Polycythemia Vera and Essential Thrombocythemia Prognostic Model; WBC, white blood cell count.

used. The Molecular IPSS70 adds genetic information on CALR and high molecular risk mutations, as well as on the number of mutations to the classical prognostic factors to assess the urgency of allogeneic hematopoietic stem cell transplantation in patients up to 70 years of age.[5] Rating the prognostic impact of genetics even higher, the genetically inspired IPSS purely relies on genetic information including a subset of high molecular risk mutations and mutations in CALR, as well as cytogenetic abnormalities to predict outcome.[6] The Myelofibrosis Secondary to Polycythemia Vera and Essential Thrombocythemia Prognostic Model specifically assesses prognosis for secondary, post-PV or post-ET myelofibrosis also implementing certain genetic factors[81] (**Table 4**). Promising further developments for prognostication are under way as exemplified by personalized prediction tools based on large-scale genomic data, which will be instrumental to individually assess the prognostic impact of a specific MPN patient's comprehensive genetic profile[3] (https://cancer.sanger.ac.uk/mpn-multistage).

Significance of Genetics for Myeloproliferative Neoplasm Therapy

Most importantly, the genetic characterization of MPN has initiated the era of targeted therapies for these entities, as several genetic lesions are actionable. The identification of JAK2 V617F as well as the observation that also CALR and MPL mutations induce constitutive activation of JAK-STAT signaling has led to the development of JAK2 inhibitors. Although the JAK1/2 inhibitor ruxolitinib represents now a clinical standard of care for the treatment of PMF and PV,[35–37] fedratinib, a JAK2/FLT3 inhibitor, has recently been approved.[38] The fact that current JAK2 inhibitors are not selective for mutant JAK2 turns out to be advantageous in the sense that activated JAK-STAT signaling in CARL and MPL mutant patients is also addressed. However, JAK2 inhibition selective for the MPN clone would be highly desirable to achieve more substantial disease-modifying activity with decreased mutant clone sizes and efforts toward refined JAK2 inhibitors are ongoing.[82] Adaptive changes of JAK2, MPL, or CALR mutant signaling are also extensively explored as co-targets including, for example, MEK-ERK or PI3K-AKT pathways.[59] The increasing insight into the biology of mutant CALR exposed at the cell surface holds potential as a target private to the mutant MPN clone, which could be addressable.[26] The genetic alterations in epigenetic and splicing factors could also provide interesting targets for therapeutic intervention, particularly in patients with JAK2 V617F–deficient founder clones or blast phase MPN with loss of JAK2 V617F. Although hypomethylating agents or histone deacetylase inhibition with beneficial effects in AML are also being studied in MPN,[83,84] PRMT5A or BRD4 inhibition represent innovative approaches to epigenetic targeting with promising preclinical results.[53,85] In addition to single-agent approaches, combination strategies with JAK2 inhibition are particularly explored aiming at increased efficacy of JAK2 inhibitor therapy. Important open questions relate to the significance of specific co-mutational profiles for response to targeted or conventional therapies.[86] Comprehensive genetic characterization of large treatment trials in MPN is desirable to evaluate which patient subgroups would benefit from specific therapeutic approaches.

SUMMARY

Our understanding of the genetics of MPN has expanded at a rapid pace with substantial impact on the way we diagnose, prognosticate and treat MPN. These developments are ongoing and will further refine our understanding of MPN pathogenesis for example, in regard to clonal hematopoiesis as a pre-MPN state, as well as our ability to develop genetically guided, individualized treatment concepts for patients with MPN.

CLINICS CARE POINTS

- JAK2, CALR, and MPL mutations are present in approximately 98% of patients with PV and 85% to 90% of patients with ET and patients with PMF and represent a mainstay for diagnosis of MPN according to World Health Organization criteria.

- In triple-negative MPN, evaluation for ASXL1, EZH2, TET2, IDH1/2, SRSF2, and SF3B1 mutations can assist to determine the clonal nature of the disease.

- Although CALR mutations associate with favorable prognosis in patients with ET and patients with PMF, the presence of high molecular risk mutations, including ASXL1, EZH2, IDH1,/2 and SRSF2, relate to an unfavorable prognosis in MPN.

- Genetic factors are increasingly implemented in modern prognostication schemes, including the genetically inspired IPSS, Molecular IPSS7, and Myelofibrosis Secondary to Polycythemia Vera and Essential Thrombocythemia Prognostic Model scores or novel personalized prediction tools (https://cancer.sanger.ac.uk/mpn-multistage).

- The constitutive activation of JAK-STAT signaling by somatic driver mutations in JAK2, CALR, and MPL provides a rational basis for JAK2 inhibitor therapy in patients with MPN.

- Novel targeted therapies, either as single agents or in combination with JAK2 inhibitors, are currently being developed to provide improved treatment concepts.

ACKNOWLEDGMENTS

The authors acknowledge research support to S.C. Meyer by the Swiss National Science Foundation (PBBEP3-144806, PCEFP3_181357), the Swiss Cancer League/ Swiss Cancer Research (KFS-3858-02-2016), the Swiss Bridge Foundation (PSB-4066-06-2016), the Cancer League Basel (KLbB-4784-02-2019), the Swiss Group for Clinical Cancer Research SAKK, the Foundation for the Fight against Cancer, the Nora van Meeuwen-Häfliger Foundation, the Foundation Peter-Anton and Anna-Katharina Miescher, and the Swiss Society of Hematology. Due to space restrictions, 1 or 2 publications may be referenced on behalf of several for certain key discoveries to which several groups have contributed. Figures were created with Biorender software (Biorender.com).

REFERENCES

1. Dameshek W. Editorial: some speculations on the myeloproliferative syndromes. Blood 1951;6(4):372–5.
2. Rampal R, Al-Shahrour F, Abdel-Wahab O, et al. Integrated genomic analysis illustrates the central role of JAK-STAT pathway activation in myeloproliferative neoplasm pathogenesis. Blood 2014;123(22):e123–33.
3. Grinfeld J, Nangalia J, Baxter EJ, et al. Classification and Personalized Prognosis in Myeloproliferative Neoplasms. N Engl J Med 2018;379(15):1416–30.
4. Arber DA, Orazi A, Hasserjian R, et al. The 2016 revision to the World Health Organization classification of myeloid neoplasms and acute leukemia. Blood. 2016;127(20):2391-2405. Blood 2016;128(3):462–3.
5. Guglielmelli P, Lasho TL, Rotunno G, et al. MIPSS70: mutation-enhanced international prognostic score system for transplantation-age patients with primary myelofibrosis. J Clin Oncol 2018;36:310–8.
6. Tefferi A, Guglielmelli P, Nicolosi M, et al. GIPSS: genetically inspired prognostic scoring system for primary myelofibrosis. Leukemia 2018;32(7):1631–42.

7. Levine RL, Wadleigh M, Cools J, et al. Activating mutation in the tyrosine kinase JAK2 in polycythemia vera, essential thrombocythemia, and myeloid metaplasia with myelofibrosis. Cancer Cell 2005;7(4):387–97.

8. Kralovics R, Passamonti F, Buser AS, et al. A gain-of-function mutation ofJAK2in myeloproliferative disorders. N Engl J Med 2005;352(17):1779–90.

9. Baxter EJ, Scott LM, Campbell PJ, et al. Acquired mutation of the tyrosine kinase JAK2 in human myeloproliferative disorders. Lancet 2005;365(9464):1054–61.

10. James C, Ugo V, Le Couédic J-P, et al. A unique clonal JAK2 mutation leading to constitutive signalling causes polycythaemia vera. Nature 2005;434(7037): 1144–8.

11. Ungureanu D, Wu J, Pekkala T, et al. The pseudokinase domain of JAK2 is a dual-specificity protein kinase that negatively regulates cytokine signaling. Nat Struct Mol Biol 2011;18(9):971–6.

12. Meyer SC, Levine RL. Molecular pathways: molecular basis for sensitivity and resistance to JAK kinase inhibitors. Clin Cancer Res 2014;20(8):2051–9.

13. Mullally A, Lane SW, Ball B, et al. Physiological Jak2V617F expression causes a lethal myeloproliferative neoplasm with differential effects on hematopoietic stem and progenitor cells. Cancer Cell 2010;17(6):584–96.

14. Vannucchi AM, Antonioli E, Guglielmelli P, et al. Clinical profile of homozygous JAK2 617V>F mutation in patients with polycythemia vera or essential thrombo-cythemia. Blood 2007;110(3):840–6.

15. Godfrey AL, Chen E, Pagano F, et al. JAK2V617F homozygosity arises commonly and recurrently in PV and ET, but PV is characterized by expansion of a dominant homozygous subclone. Blood 2012;120(13):2704–7.

16. Ortmann CA, Kent DG, Nangalia J, et al. Effect of mutation order on myeloprolif-erative neoplasms. N Engl J Med 2015;372(7):601–12.

17. Scott LM, Tong W, Levine RL, et al. JAK2 exon 12 mutations in polycythemia vera and idiopathic erythrocytosis. N Engl J Med 2007;356(5):459–68.

18. Passamonti F, Elena C, Schnittger S, et al. Molecular and clinical features of the myeloproliferative neoplasm associated with JAK2 exon 12 mutations. Blood 2011;117(10):2813–6.

19. Grisouard J, Li S, Kubovcakova L, et al. JAK2 exon 12 mutant mice display iso-lated erythrocytosis and changes in iron metabolism favoring increased erythro-poiesis. Blood 2016;128(6):839–51.

20. Pikman Y, Lee BH, Mercher T, et al. MPLW515L is a novel somatic activating mu-tation in myelofibrosis with myeloid metaplasia. PLoS Med 2006;3(7):e270.

21. Pardanani AD, Levine RL, Lasho T, et al. MPL515 mutations in myeloproliferative and other myeloid disorders: a study of 1182 patients. Blood 2006;108(10): 3472–6.

22. Oh ST, Simonds EF, Jones C, et al. Novel mutations in the inhibitory adaptor pro-tein LNK drive JAK-STAT signaling in patients with myeloproliferative neoplasms. Blood 2010;116(6):988–92.

23. Grand FH, Hidalgo-Curtis CE, Ernst T, et al. Frequent CBL mutations associated with 11q acquired uniparental disomy in myeloproliferative neoplasms. Blood 2009;113(24):6182–92.

24. Klampfl T, Gisslinger H, Harutyunyan AS, et al. Somatic mutations of calreticulin in myeloproliferative neoplasms. N Engl J Med 2013;369(25):2379–90.

25. Nangalia J, Massie CE, Baxter EJ, et al. Somatic CALR mutations in myeloprolif-erative neoplasms with nonmutated JAK2. N Engl J Med 2013;369(25):2391–405.

26. Elf S, Abdelfattah NS, Chen E, et al. Mutant calreticulin requires both its mutant c-terminus and the thrombopoietin receptor for oncogenic transformation. Cancer Discov 2016;6(4):368–81.
27. Chachoua I, Pecquet C, El-Khoury M, et al. Thrombopoietin receptor activation by myeloproliferative neoplasm associated calreticulin mutants. Blood 2016; 127(10):1325–35.
28. Marty C, Pecquet C, Nivarthi H, et al. Calreticulin mutants in mice induce an MPL-dependent thrombocytosis with frequent progression to myelofibrosis. Blood 2016;127(10):1317–24.
29. Rumi E, Pietra D, Ferretti V, et al. JAK2 or CALR mutation status defines subtypes of essential thrombocythemia with substantially different clinical course and outcomes. Blood 2014;123(10):1544–51.
30. Tefferi A, Lasho TL, Finke CM, et al. CALR vs JAK2 vs MPL-mutated or triple-negative myelofibrosis: clinical, cytogenetic and molecular comparisons. Leukemia 2014;28(7):1472–7.
31. Tefferi A, Lasho TL, Finke C, et al. Type 1 vs type 2 calreticulin mutations in primary myelofibrosis: differences in phenotype and prognostic impact. Leukemia 2014;28(7):1568–70.
32. Cabagnols X, Favale F, Pasquier F, et al. Presence of atypical thrombopoietin receptor (MPL) mutations in triple-negative essential thrombocythemia patients. Blood 2016;127(3):333–42.
33. Milosevic Feenstra JD, Nivarthi H, Gisslinger H, et al. Whole-exome sequencing identifies novel MPL and JAK2 mutations in triple-negative myeloproliferative neoplasms. Blood 2016;127(3):325–32.
34. Bercovich D, Ganmore I, Scott LM, et al. Mutations of JAK2 in acute lymphoblastic leukaemias associated with Down's syndrome. Lancet 2008;372(9648): 1484–92.
35. Harrison C, Kiladjian J-J, Al-Ali HK, et al. JAK Inhibition with Ruxolitinib versus Best Available Therapy for Myelofibrosis. N Engl J Med 2012;366(9):787–98.
36. Verstovsek S, Mesa RA, Gotlib J, et al. A double-blind, placebo-controlled trial of ruxolitinib for myelofibrosis. N Engl J Med 2012;366(9):799–807.
37. Vannucchi AM, Kiladjian JJ, Griesshammer M, et al. Ruxolitinib versus standard therapy for the treatment of polycythemia vera. N Engl J Med 2015;372(5): 426–35.
38. Harrison CN, Schaap N, Vannucchi AM, et al. Janus kinase-2 inhibitor fedratinib in patients with myelofibrosis previously treated with ruxolitinib (JAKARTA-2): a single-arm, open-label, non-randomised, phase 2, multicentre study. Lancet Haematol 2017;4(7):e317–24.
39. Lundberg P, Karow A, Nienhold R, et al. Clonal evolution and clinical correlates of somatic mutations in myeloproliferative neoplasms. Blood 2014;123(14):2220–8.
40. Abdel-Wahab O, Pardanani A, Rampal R, et al. DNMT3A mutational analysis in primary myelofibrosis, chronic myelomonocytic leukemia and advanced phases of myeloproliferative neoplasms. Leukemia 2011;25(7):1219–20.
41. Yang L, Rau R, Goodell MA. DNMT3A in haematological malignancies. Nat Rev Cancer 2015;15(3):152–65.
42. Nangalia J, Nice FL, Wedge DC, et al. DNMT3A mutations occur early or late in patients with myeloproliferative neoplasms and mutation order influences phenotype. Haematologica 2015;100(11):e438–42.
43. Tefferi A, Pardanani A, Lim K-H, et al. TET2 mutations and their clinical correlates in polycythemia vera, essential thrombocythemia and myelofibrosis. Leukemia 2009;23(5):905–11.

44. Moran-Crusio K, Reavie L, Shih A, et al. Tet2 loss leads to increased hematopoietic stem cell self-renewal and myeloid transformation. Cancer Cell 2011;20(1): 11–24.

45. Figueroa ME, Abdel-Wahab O, Lu C, et al. Leukemic IDH1 and IDH2 mutations result in a hypermethylation phenotype, disrupt TET2 function, and impair hematopoietic differentiation. Cancer Cell 2010;18(6):553–67.

46. Tefferi A, Lasho TL, Abdel-Wahab O, et al. IDH1 and IDH2 mutation studies in 1473 patients with chronic-, fibrotic- or blast-phase essential thrombocythemia, polycythemia vera or myelofibrosis. Leukemia 2010;24(7):1302–9.

47. Abdel-Wahab O, Pardanani A, Patel J, et al. Concomitant analysis of EZH2 and ASXL1 mutations in myelofibrosis, chronic myelomonocytic leukemia and blast-phase myeloproliferative neoplasms. Leukemia 2011;25(7):1200–2.

48. Shimizu T, Kubovcakova L, Nienhold R, et al. Loss of Ezh2 synergizes with JAK2-V617F in initiating myeloproliferative neoplasms and promoting myelofibrosis. J Exp Med 2016;213(8):1479–96.

49. Guglielmelli P, Biamonte F, Score J, et al. EZH2 mutational status predicts poor survival in myelofibrosis. Blood 2011;118(19):5227–34.

50. Abdel-Wahab O, Adli M, LaFave LM, et al. ASXL1 mutations promote myeloid transformation through loss of PRC2-mediated gene repression. Cancer Cell 2012;22(2):180–93.

51. Gelsi-Boyer V, Brecqueville M, Devillier R, et al. Mutations in ASXL1 are associated with poor prognosis across the spectrum of malignant myeloid diseases. J Hematol Oncol 2012;5:12.

52. Liu F, Zhao X, Perna F, et al. JAK2V617F-mediated phosphorylation of PRMT5 downregulates its methyltransferase activity and promotes myeloproliferation. Cancer Cell 2011;19(2):283–94.

53. Pastore F, Bhagwat N, Pastore A, et al. PRMT5 inhibition modulates E2F1 methylation and gene regulatory networks leading to therapeutic efficacy in JAK2V617F mutant MPN. Cancer Discov 2020. https://doi.org/10.1158/2159-8290.CD-20-0026.

54. Dawson MA, Bannister AJ, Göttgens B, et al. JAK2 phosphorylates histone H3Y41 and excludes HP1alpha from chromatin. Nature 2009;461(7265):819–22.

55. Vannucchi AM, Lasho TL, Guglielmelli P, et al. Mutations and prognosis in primary myelofibrosis. Leukemia 2013;27(9):1861–9.

56. Lasho TL, Finke CM, Hanson CA, et al. SF3B1 mutations in primary myelofibrosis: clinical, histopathology and genetic correlates among 155 patients. Leukemia 2012;26(5):1135–7.

57. Zhang S-J, Rampal R, Manshouri T, et al. Genetic analysis of patients with leukemic transformation of myeloproliferative neoplasms shows recurrent SRSF2 mutations that are associated with adverse outcome. Blood 2012; 119(19):4480–5.

58. Meyer SC, Levine RL. Translational implications of somatic genomics in acute myeloid leukaemia. Lancet Oncol 2014;15(9):e382–94.

59. Stivala S, Codilupi T, Brkic S, et al. Targeting compensatory MEK/ERK activation increases JAK inhibitor efficacy in myeloproliferative neoplasms. J Clin Invest 2019;129(4):1596–611.

60. Santos FPS, Getta B, Masarova L, et al. Prognostic impact of RAS-pathway mutations in patients with myelofibrosis. Leukemia 2020;34(3):799–810.

61. Rampal R, Ahn J, Abdel-Wahab O, et al. Genomic and functional analysis of leukemic transformation of myeloproliferative neoplasms. Proc Natl Acad Sci U S A 2014;111(50):E5401–10.

62. Campbell PJ, Baxter EJ, Beer PA, et al. Mutation of JAK2 in the myeloproliferative disorders: timing, clonality studies, cytogenetic associations, and role in leukemic transformation. Blood 2006;108(10):3548–55.

63. Theocharides A, Boissinot M, Girodon F, et al. Leukemic blasts in transformed JAK2-V617F-positive myeloproliferative disorders are frequently negative for the JAK2-V617F mutation. Blood 2007;110(1):375–9.

64. Rumi E, Passamonti F, Della Porta MG, et al. Familial chronic myeloproliferative disorders: clinical phenotype and evidence of disease anticipation. J Clin Oncol 2007;25(35):5630–5.

65. Jones AV, Chase A, Silver RT, et al. JAK2 haplotype is a major risk factor for the development of myeloproliferative neoplasms. Nat Genet 2009;41(4):446–9.

66. Kilpivaara O, Mukherjee S, Schram AM, et al. A germline JAK2 SNP is associated with predisposition to the development of JAK2(V617F)-positive myeloproliferative neoplasms. Nat Genet 2009;41(4):455–9.

67. Tapper W, Jones AV, Kralovics R, et al. Genetic variation at MECOM, TERT, JAK2 and HBS1L-MYB predisposes to myeloproliferative neoplasms. Nat Commun 2015;6:6691.

68. Bellanné-Chantelot C, Rabadan Moraes G, Schmaltz-Panneau B, et al. Germline genetic factors in the pathogenesis of myeloproliferative neoplasms. Blood Rev 2020;100710. https://doi.org/10.1016/j.blre.2020.100710.

69. Malak S, Labopin M, Saint-Martin C, et al. Long term follow up of 93 families with myeloproliferative neoplasms: life expectancy and implications of JAK2V617F in the occurrence of complications. Blood Cells Mol Dis 2012;49(3–4):170–6.

70. Bejar R, Stevenson K, Abdel-Wahab O, et al. Clinical effect of point mutations in myelodysplastic syndromes. N Engl J Med 2011;364(26):2496–506.

71. Lee JW, Kim YG, Soung YH, et al. The JAK2 V617F mutation in de novo acute myelogenous leukemias. Oncogene 2006;25(9):1434–6.

72. Bolton KL, Zehir A, Ptashkin RN, et al. The clinical management of clonal hematopoiesis: creation of a clonal hematopoiesis clinic. Hematol Oncol Clin North Am 2020;34(2):357–67.

73. Busque L, Patel JP, Figueroa ME, et al. Recurrent somatic TET2 mutations in normal elderly individuals with clonal hematopoiesis. Nat Genet 2012;44(11):1179–81.

74. Jaiswal S, Fontanillas P, Flannick J, et al. Age-related clonal hematopoiesis associated with adverse outcomes. N Engl J Med 2014;371(26):2488–98.

75. Genovese G, Kähler AK, Handsaker RE, et al. Clonal hematopoiesis and blood-cancer risk inferred from blood DNA sequence. N Engl J Med 2014;371(26):2477–87.

76. Xie M, Lu C, Wang J, et al. Age-related mutations associated with clonal hematopoietic expansion and malignancies. Nat Med 2014;20(12):1472–8.

77. McKerrell T, Park N, Moreno T, et al. Leukemia-associated somatic mutations drive distinct patterns of age-related clonal hemopoiesis. Cell Rep 2015;10(8):1239–45.

78. Jaiswal S, Natarajan P, Silver AJ, et al. Clonal Hematopoiesis and Risk of Atherosclerotic Cardiovascular Disease. N Engl J Med 2017;377(2):111–21.

79. McKerrell T, Park N, Chi J, et al. JAK2 V617F hematopoietic clones are present several years prior to MPN diagnosis and follow different expansion kinetics. Blood Adv 2017;1(14):968–71.

80. Gangat N, Caramazza D, Vaidya R, et al. DIPSS plus: a refined dynamic international prognostic scoring system for primary myelofibrosis that incorporates

prognostic information from karyotype, platelet count, and transfusion status. J Clin Oncol 2011;29(4):392–7.

81. Passamonti F, Giorgino T, Mora B, et al. A clinical-molecular prognostic model to predict survival in patients with post polycythemia vera and post essential thrombocythemia myelofibrosis. Leukemia 2017;31(12):2726–31.

82. Meyer SC, Keller MD, Chiu S, et al. CHZ868, a Type II JAK2 Inhibitor, Reverses Type I JAK Inhibitor Persistence and Demonstrates Efficacy in Myeloproliferative Neoplasms. Cancer Cell 2015;28(1):15–28.

83. Rampal RK, Mascarenhas JO, Kosiorek HE, et al. Safety and efficacy of combined ruxolitinib and decitabine in accelerated and blast-phase myeloproliferative neoplasms. Blood Adv 2018;2(24):3572–80.

84. Masarova L, Verstovsek S, Hidalgo-Lopez JE, et al. A phase 2 study of ruxolitinib in combination with azacitidine in patients with myelofibrosis. Blood 2018; 132(16):1664–74.

85. Kleppe M, Koche R, Zou L, et al. Dual targeting of oncogenic activation and inflammatory signaling increases therapeutic efficacy in myeloproliferative neoplasms. Cancer Cell 2018;33(4):785–7.

86. Guglielmelli P, Biamonte F, Rotunno G, et al. Impact of mutational status on outcomes in myelofibrosis patients treated with ruxolitinib in the COMFORT-II study. Blood 2014;123(14):2157–60.

Epigenetic Dysregulation of Myeloproliferative Neoplasms

Andrew Dunbar, MD[a,b], Young Park, MS[c], Ross Levine, MD[a,b,c,d],*

KEYWORDS

- Epigenetics of MPN • Myeloproliferative neoplasms • Myelofibrosis
- Fibrotic progression • Preclinical studies • Epigenetic pathways

KEY POINTS

- Mutations of epigenetic modifier proteins occur frequently in myeloproliferative neoplasms and influence clinical outcomes and treatment response.
- Mutations of epigenetic modifier proteins are enriched in myelofibrosis; however, the mechanisms of epigenetic dysregulation in disease progression remain poorly understood.
- Emerging epigenetic therapies provide promise for the treatment of myeloproliferative neoplasms, specifically myelofibrosis.

INTRODUCTION

Hematopoietic stem cells (HSCs) exist in a constant steady state, balancing self-renewal with proliferative gene expression programs in response to various cell-intrinsic and -extrinsic stimuli. Dynamic, reversable chromatin remodeling is essential for maintaining this steady state to ensure proper cell fate determination.[1] The dominant mechanisms by which this epigenetic remodeling occurs, either by post-translational modification of amino acid residues on histones or by methylation of DNA at cytosine residues, ensure that hematopoietic demands are met while maintaining the stem cell pool in response to stress.

It is perhaps not surprising then that mutations encoding the proteins involved in chromatin remodeling, such as those modulating DNA methylation, for example,

[a] Department of Medicine, Leukemia Service, Memorial Sloan Kettering Cancer Center, 1275 York Avenue, Box 20, New York, NY 10065, USA; [b] Center for Hematologic Malignancies, Memorial Sloan Kettering Cancer Center, 1275 York Avenue, Box 20, New York, NY 10065, USA; [c] Center for Epigenetics Research, Memorial Sloan Kettering Cancer Center, 1275 York Avenue, Box 20, New York, NY 10065, USA; [d] Human Oncology and Pathogenesis Program, Memorial Sloan Kettering Cancer Center, 1275 York Avenue, Box 20, New York, NY 10065, USA
* Corresponding author. Department of Medicine, Leukemia Service, Memorial Sloan Kettering Cancer Center, 1275 York Avenue, Box 20, New York, NY 10065.
E-mail address: leviner@mskcc.org

Hematol Oncol Clin N Am 35 (2021) 237–251
https://doi.org/10.1016/j.hoc.2021.01.001
0889-8588/21/© 2021 Elsevier Inc. All rights reserved.

ten-eleven translocation-2 (TET2), IDH, and DNA (cytosine-5)-methyltransferase 3 alpha (DNMT3A), as well as the histone modifiers enhancer of zeste homolog 2 (EZH2) and additional sex combs like 1 (ASXL1), are observed frequently across the spectrum of hematologic malignancies.[2] The aberrant DNA methylation and/or histone modification patterns occurring as a result of these mutations lead to transcriptional dysregulation, altered hematopoiesis, and, in many cases, enhanced competitive HSC fitness and mutant clonal expansion. Often, these clones do not evolve into overt hematologic disease but rather expand from a common ancestor to dominate the hematopoietic hierarchy leading to a so-called clonal hematopoiesis.[3] Interestingly, JAK2^{V617F}, a major myeloproliferative neoplasm (MPN) driver, is itself frequently observed in subclinical clonal hematopoiesis,[4] suggesting that mutant cells may lie dormant for years before manifesting as overt MPN. This finding further supports the notion that additional changes, including epigenetic alterations, are required for the initiation and progression of disease.

In MPNs, mutations of epigenetic modifying proteins co-occur frequently with the MPN driver mutations JAK2^{V617F}, MPL^{W515L}, and CALR. The presence of these mutations is thought to further enhance the fitness of an already hyperproliferative mutant clone expanded in response to constitutive JAK/STAT pathway activation. Recent data reveal that epigenetic dysfunction in MPNs also enhances aberrant proinflammatory cytokine signaling networks to promote a perturbed proinflammatory microenvironment favoring the mutant clone at the expense of normal hematopoiesis (and, in turn, fibrotic progression).[5] This might explain why epigenetic mutations are, in general, enriched to a much greater degree in myelofibrosis (MF) than in the other MPN subtypes polycythemia vera (PV) and essential thrombocythemia (ET).

Although considerable progress has been made over the last decade in our understanding of how epigenetic alterations cooperate with MPN driver mutations to promote disease progression, the specific ways by which chromatin alterations lead to fibrosis remain unclear. The order in which mutations are acquired (epigenetic mutation first, driver second, or vice versa) seems to influence this response. In addition, there is also increasing evidence that JAK2 itself has important epigenetic regulatory functions. Proinflammatory signaling pathways are also increasingly implicated in fibrotic progression. Excitingly, however, these insights have helped to pave the way for novel epigenetic therapies that increasingly show signs of promise for the treatment of this heterogeneous disease.

EPIGENETIC DYSFUNCTION FROM ABERRANT JAK/STAT SIGNALING

JAK2 functions as a receptor tyrosine kinase, transmitting signals from the cell surface by phosphorylating tyrosine residues on downstream effectors to stimulate gene regulatory programs important in cell division and differentiation.[6] Constitutive JAK/STAT signaling, occurring as a result of activating mutations of JAK2, CALR, or MPL, is a hallmark feature of MPNs. Emerging data, however, highlight the noncanonical role of JAK2 on the phosphorylation of important epigenetic mediators. Perhaps the most critical example is the epigenetic regulation of JAK2 in the post-translational modification of histones directly. In a seminal work, Dawson and colleagues[7] observed that JAK2 itself can localize to the nucleus to phosphorylate residues on histone H3 tyrosine 41 (H3Y41). The resultant alteration in chromatin structure disrupts binding of the chromatin repressor HP1a to DNA leading to up-regulation of several hematopoietic proto-oncogenes, including LMO2.

JAK2 has also been found to phosphorylate other proteins important for the epigenetic regulation of DNA. PRMT5 is a methyltransferase that functions to adds methyl groups to arginine residues on various intracellular proteins, including histones, and has an important role as a negative regulator of HSC division and differentiation.[8] Liu and colleagues[9] identified PRMT5 as a binding target of wild-type JAK2 that is phosphorylated in the setting of JAK2^{V617F}, leading to impaired PRMT5 methyltransferase activity, decreased global methylation, and enhanced HSC differentiation.[9] More recently, JAK2 was also found to phosphorylate TET2, an important epigenetic mediator of DNA methylation frequently mutated in myeloid disease. In patient samples, phosphorylation of TET2 by JAK2 promoted enhanced TET2 activity and, in turn, decreased global methylation levels.[10]

A perturbed methylation state seems to be common in MPNs, particularly MF, independent of any co-occurring mutation in an epigenetic modifying protein. Nischal and colleagues,[11] using targeted methylation assays to probe methylation profiles of neutrophils isolated from MPN patients, revealed an overall hypermethylation state in MPNs in comparison with healthy cells, with patients with primary MF showing a greater degree of global hypermethylation (as well as focal areas marked by hypomethylation) than patients with PV/ET. Similar findings were corroborated in a separate study; however, less of a differential methylation effect was observed across MPN subtypes.[12] Recent studies comparing the methylomes of individual cell types from patients with MF identified a distinct pattern of aberrant methylation changes in patients with ASXL1 mutations, particularly in areas marked by bivalent promoters[13] (eg, areas primed for differentiation and exquisitely sensitive to a myriad of histone marks), suggesting that ASXL1 might have an important role in regulating DNA methylation beyond its established role in polycomb-mediated histone modification.[14] Finally, a separate study using whole methylation profiling of patients with MF identified aberrant methylation patterns enriched at enhancer regions suggesting a role of altered cis-regulatory landscapes in MF.[15] In support of this finding, in a separate study by Kleppe and colleagues,[16] chromatin immunoprecipitation profiling of enhancer markers H3K4me1 and H3K27ac of megakaryocyte and erythroid progenitor cells from a hMPLW515L adoptive transfer model of fibrosis confirmed dramatic alterations in enhancer elements not observed in wild-type progenitors.[16] These changes were associated with greatly altered transcription, including enrichment in an HP1a signature and the upregulation of proinflammatory tumor necrosis factor α and nuclear factor κB (NF-κB) mediators, supporting an important role for these pathways in fibrotic development.

CO-OCCURRING EPIGENETIC MODIFYING MUTATIONS IN MYELOPROLIFERATIVE NEOPLASMS

Genetic discovery studies of patients with MPN have revealed the depth and breadth of somatic alterations across all MPN subtypes, reflecting the striking heterogeneity of this disease at the molecular level. Mutations involved in the epigenetic regulation of DNA are some of the most frequent co-occurring mutations in MPN and are associated with increased risk of progression to fibrosis and leukemia.[17] Other mutations frequently observed in MPNs, discussed elsewhere, include spliceosome modulators (eg, *SRSF2*, *SFB1*, *U2AF1*),[18] as well as transcription factors (eg, *RUNX1*, *CEBPA*, *TP53*), and the signaling molecules *NRAS/KRAS*, *CBL*, and *cKIT*, among others.

Epigenetic mutations are enriched to a greater degree in MF over other MPN subtypes (**Fig. 1**),[19–23] supporting the notion that progressive epigenetic dysregulation plays a critical role in fibrotic progression and development. Across multiple studies, mutations of *ASXL1*, *EZH2*, and isocitrate dehydrogenase 1/2 (*IDH1/2*), as well as the spliceosome modulator *SRSF2*, have all been shown to portend greater risk of fibrotic

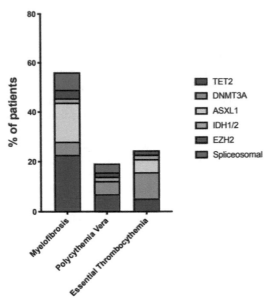

Fig. 1. Frequency of epigenetic modifying protein mutations across MPN subtypes.

and/or leukemic progression with associated impairment in overall survival.[19–23] Notably, the presence of 2 or more of these mutations co-occurring together seems to correlate with particularly poor outcomes. In 1 study, the median overall survival for those with 2 or more combined mutations was 2.6 years in comparison with 7 years for those with just 1 mutation, and 12.3 years for those with no mutations.[24] The presence of an *ASXL1* mutation seems to confer a particularly high risk, with significant enrichment in primary MF and in fibrosis evolved from an antecedent PV or ET.[20] Importantly, *ASXL1* mutations, and to a lesser extent *EZH2* mutations, were also associated with a decreased response to ruxolitinib inhibitor therapy,[25] a finding similarly observed in a more recent study also evaluating the alternative JAK2 inhibitor momelotinib.[26] These data suggest that *ASXL1*-mutant clones might be selected for in the setting of JAK inhibitor therapy; however, this process remains yet to be functionally dissected. Moreover, the presence of an *ASXL1* mutation (as well as *IDH1/2*) was shown in 1 study to be associated with worsened outcome and lower progression-free survival after allogeneic stem cell transplantation[27]; however, these findings were not corroborated in a more recent retrospective follow-up study,[28] possibly as a result of patient heterogeneity between the cohorts evaluated.

Importantly, the order in which mutations are acquired in MPN (ie, driver first, epigenetic modifying second, and vice versa) has also been shown to influence disease phenotype and clinical course. Certain mutations seem to be more likely to precede $JAK2^{V617F}$ than to follow. Lundberg and colleagues[29] and Grinfeld and colleagues,[22] for example, each demonstrated that *DNMT3A* mutations were more likely to occur before the acquisition of $JAK2^{V617F}$, whereas *IDH1/2* mutations were more likely to occur after $JAK2^{V617F}$.[30–32] Similarly, other data suggest that, in contrast with de novo acute myeloid leukemia (AML), *ASXL1* mutations occur as a late event (ie, following $JAK2^{V617F}$).[22,33] Importantly, *TET2* can be acquired both early or late, and the order in which *JAK2V617 F* versus *TET2* is acquired influences disease phenotype. Ortmann and colleagues[34] demonstrated that patients who acquired *TET2* first were older at time of diagnosis and exhibited expansion of their HSCs with a tendency toward an ET phenotype, whereas *JAK2*-first patients were younger at diagnosis, and displayed more proliferative HSCs with an erythroid predominance and an associated PV phenotype. This finding suggests that the mutational order might influence stem cell biology and disease progression in MPNs. Although this process remains unclear, the authors provide evidence to suggest that transcriptional changes occurring as a result of the first mutation can influence the mutant cell's response to the second.

Recent elegant work by Rodriguez-Meira and colleagues[33] combining DNA mutational and whole transcriptome analysis at the single-cell level has further highlighted the transcriptional heterogeneity observed between various mutant subclones within individual patients, including those with mutations in epigenetic-modifying proteins. In addition to confirming the non–cell autonomous effects of mutant MPN clones on gene expression patterns of surrounding wild-type HSCs, this study also revealed how mutations in epigenetic modifying proteins can alter the transcriptional landscape as the clone evolves. This result was evidenced in 1 patient in particular with multiple individual MPN clones at various stages of evolution, including one with combined $JAK2^{V617F}/EZH2$ mutations. Distinct transcriptomic signatures were observed in the $JAK2^{V617F}/EZH2$ clone alone not seen with single-mutant $JAK2^{V617F}$ cells, with enrichment in pathways involved in apoptosis, p53 signaling, hypoxia, and cell division. These data provide further clarity in regard to how the addition of epigenetic alterations might enhance clonal evolution over time.

PRECLINICAL MODELS OF EPIGENETIC MODIFYING PROTEINS IN MYELOPROLIFERATIVE NEOPLASMS

To further uncover the mechanisms of epigenetic modifying proteins in MPNs and the manner in which these mutations can cooperate with MPN driver mutations to augment disease, several groups have explored different mutational combinations using various $Jak2^{V617F}$ knockin mouse model systems. Here, we explore our current understanding of the specific mechanisms of action of epigenetic modifying proteins in the context of MPN.

Mutations in DNA Methylation Proteins: TET2 and DNMT3A

The methylation of cytosines in gene promoter regions is a highly dynamic process and essential for the maintenance of steady-state gene transcription in HSCs. In general, increased methylation of cytosines results in repression of gene transcription, whereas the loss of methyl groups enhances transcription. In MPN, 2 frequently mutated proteins involved in the methylation of DNA include those critical for the addition and removal of these methyl residues, specifically DNMT3A and TET2, respectively. Mutations of *DNMT3A* impair normal DNMT3A activity and the addition of methyl-groups (promoting a hypomethylation phenotype), whereas *TET2* mutations lead to loss of function and impairment in the removal of methyl groups (resulting in global hypermethylation).[2] Despite seemingly opposite effects on DNA methylation, both mutated *TET2* and *DNMT3A* models display a strikingly similar phenotype: enhanced HSC self-renewal, impaired myeloid differentiation, and clonal expansion on serial transplantation (**Fig. 2**).

The effect of *Tet2* loss in the context of MPN has been explored using combined $Jak2^{V617F}$ knockin and *Tet2* knockout mouse models.[35,36] Consistent with the enhanced HSC fitness observed with tet2 loss alone, double-mutant $Jak2^{V617F}/Tet2^{ko}$ mice display expansion of long-term HSC and multipotent progenitor populations with an enrichment in HSC gene signatures. In the model described by Kameda and

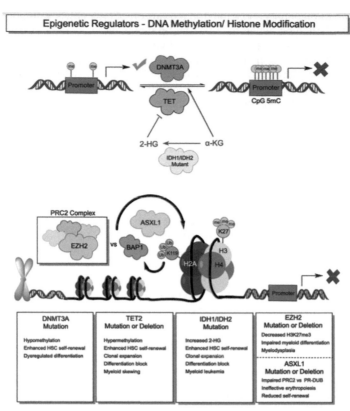

Fig. 2. (*Top*) schematic of role of DNMT3A and TET2 in the addition and removal of methyl-groups (lollipops) from DNA promoter regions respectively, and the role of IDH1/2 in oncome-tabolite 2-hydroxygluterate (2-HG) synthesis. (*Bottom*) schematic of role of EZH2/polycomb repressive 2 (PRC2) complex and ASXL1 in the placement of repressive methyl-marks on H3K27 to silence gene transcription.

colleagues,[35] this translated to enhanced leukocytosis and a more pronounced splenomegaly with an impaired overall survival of double-mutant mice in comparison with single-mutant mice. More recently, Shepherd and colleagues[37] analyzed the gene expression profiles of $Jak2^{V617F}$ versus double-mutant $Jak2^{V617F}/Tet2^{ko}$ cells at single-cell resolution. They observed that $Jak2^{V617F}$-mutant HSCs exhibit a hyper-proliferative state exiting quiescence at a greater rate with defective self-renewal, whereas $Tet2$-mutant HSCs displayed slower division with durable self-renewal. Combined mutation resulted in a combinatorial effect whereby dual-mutant HSCs shared both highly proliferative and durable self-renewal properties highlighting how 2 separate cell programs, division and stemness, might cooperate in a potent way to prop-agate disease.

To assess how $Dnmt3A$ mutations augment $Jak2^{V617F}$, Jacquelin and colleagues[38] used a $Jak2^{V617F}/Dnmt3A^{-/-}$ inducible Cas9 system in mice. Notably, the authors observed a biphasic disease course in double-mutant mice not observed with $Jak2^{V617F}$ alone, characterized by an early PV phenotype evolving to a myelofibrotic phase after 7 to 9 months with associated dense reticulin fibrosis in bone marrow and spleen, enhanced splenomegaly, and progressive bone marrow failure. Gene expression data combined with methylome profiling and chromatin accessibility analysis revealed, in addition to enhanced HSC identify signatures of double-mutant cells, an enrichment in proinflammatory signaling pathways including tumor necrosis factor α via NF-κB. These findings confirm *Dnmt3A* loss alone is sufficient to engender fibrotic transformation when co-occurring with *Jak2^{V617F}* and supports the notion that aberrant methylation may play an important role in the transcriptional dysregulation observed in MF.

Mutations in IDH1/2

Somatic alterations of *IDH1/2* represent a distinct subclass of epigenetic modifying protein mutations observed in myeloid disease, including MPNs. *IDH1/2* mutations occur with regular frequency in de novo AML, but are also observed in 2% to 5% of patients with chronic MPN.[21,30,31,39] Activating missense substitutions of *IDH1/2*, mostly commonly *IDH2^{R140Q}*, results in gain-of-function activity and excess production of the oncometabolite 2-hydroxyglutarate. Two-hydroxyglutarate has various intracellular effects, including the inhibition of TET enzymatic function, which results in a hypermethylation phenotype resembling in many ways that of TET2 loss of function.[40] It perhaps is not surprising that *IDH1/2* mutations are almost always mutually exclusive of *TET2* and that, like *TET2*, *IDH* mutant HSCs expand in vivo. A potent myeloid differentiation block is also characteristic of *IDH1/2* mutation, likely owing to more diverse effects of 2-hydroxyglutarate on cell state beyond the regulation of DNA methylation alone. Importantly, this differentiation block may explain why *IDH1/2* mutations are frequently present in de novo AML and are highly enriched at time of leukemic progression in MPNs (up to 20%–25% in some studies).[30–32]

When combined with *Jak2^{V617F}*, *Jak2^{V617F}/Idh2^{R140Q}* double-mutant mouse models display enhanced leukocytosis, hematocrit, and splenomegaly with differentiation block and increased immature progenitors consistent with the known effects of IDH2 mutation.[41] Of note, double-mutant cells were preferentially sensitive to the IDH2 inhibitor AG-221 and exhibited reductions in mutant allele burden in response to therapy—an effect that could be enhanced further when combined with ruxolitinib therapy—providing a rationale for combined directed JAK2/IDH2 inhibitor therapy for double mutant disease. Strikingly, however, leukemic progression was not observed, suggesting that still additional factors are required to induce a transformation event.

Mutations in Histone-Modifying Proteins: Additional Sex Combs Like 1 and Enhancer of Zeste Homolog 2

Post-translation modification of histones represents another critical regulator of chromatin structure and transcriptional state. Histones are subject to a wide array of post-translational changes including phosphorylation, acetylation, methylation, and ubiquitylation. These modifications alter the 3-dimensional structure of the histone octamer allowing for the folding and unfolding of DNA, as well as the subsequent induction or repression of gene transcription. The enzymes responsible for the deposition and removal of these various histone marks are numerous and act in a tightly coordinated fashion to mediate appropriate gene transcription. Like DNA methylation, aberrant modifications can alter this transcriptional balance to promote a clonal fitness advantage of mutant cells.

The histone modifier proteins ASXL1 and enhancer of zeste homolog 2 (EZH2), both named for their roles in homeotic gene regulation during *Drosophila* embryogenesis, are frequently mutated in MPNs[19–23] and are critical components of the polycomb group of protein complexes. Polycomb proteins, specifically the polycomb repressive 2 complex (consisting of core components EZH2, EED, and SUZ12), are highly conserved across species and are responsible for the addition of methyl groups to lysine residues on histone H3, specifically H3K27.[42] Placement of these repressive methyl "marks" promotes a closed chromatin state and the repression of gene transcription (see **Fig. 2**). Ablation of polycomb repressive 2 activity then dampens this repressive state, leading to the loss of the stem gene expression signatures necessary for HSC maintenance. Of note, EZH2 also has been shown to interact and recruit DNA methyltransferases to participate in DNA methylation, including DNMT3A,[43] highlighting the significant cross-talk that occurs between these 2 seemingly disparate epigenetic regulatory systems.

Conditional *Ezh2* knockout alleles have been explored in the context of *Jak2*^{V617F} knockin mouse models by 3 independent groups.[44–46] Remarkable concordance was observed across all 3 studies. Combined *Jak2*^{V617F} with *Ezh2* loss resulted in abnormal stem cell differentiation with impaired erythropoiesis and skewing and expansion of the megakaryocytic lineage. Loss of the repressive chromatin mark H3K27me3 leading to topological changes in chromatin structure was observed consistent with the known effects of EZH2. Importantly, as in *Jak2*^{V617F}/*Dnmt3A*$^{-/-}$ knockout mice, fibrotic progression was also observed, along with the upregulation of the proinflammatory genes *S100a8/a9*, *TGFB1*, and *Hmg2A*.[45,46] Enrichment in NF-κB expression signatures was also seen, once more highlighting the role of proinflammatory signaling, including NF-κB, in fibrotic progression.

Like EZH2, ASXL1 is a polycomb-associated protein important for the regulation of genes involved in stem cell maintenance; however, its role in myeloid progression remains incompletely understood. In addition to having activities to promote polycomb repressive 2–mediated gene repression,[47] ASXL1 also associates with BRCA1 associated protein 1 to form the canonical polycomb repressive deubiquitinase complex responsible for the removal of the repressive mark ubiquitin from histone H2A.[14] Thus, ASXL1 seems to have both silencing and enhancing effects on chromatin structure. ASXL1 mutations in myeloid diseases, including MPN, are frequently nonsense or frameshift mutations, which are hypothesized to lead to a truncated protein product. It is unclear, however, if truncated protein product persists and acts in a gain-of-function or dominant-negative fashion to suppress wild-type ASXL1 function, or if mutated protein is lost entirely (eg, by nonsense mediated decay) and thus functions as true loss of function. Both knockout and truncating knockin mouse models of *Asxl1* have been developed with varying effects on HSC fitness, serial transplantation, and disease phenotype,[48–52] but in general promotes a myelodysplastic-like syndrome with defective erythropoiesis and impaired repopulation capacity. Importantly, evidence suggests that the mechanisms driving polycomb dysfunction in the setting of perturbed *Asxl1* might vary based on the specific knockout versus truncated protein knockin system being evaluated, suggesting a more complicated, nuanced role for ASXL1 in the modulation of chromatin structure.

More recently, *Jak2*^{V617F}/*Asxl1*$^{f/f}$ knockout models have been evaluated to explore effects of combined mutation in MPNs.[53] In this study, the authors observed a spectrum of MPN phenotypes with a preponderance of MF or progression to fibrosis with enhanced leukocytosis and expanded megakaryocytic/erythroid progenitor populations. Notably, transformation to acute leukemia was also observed in a subset of mice. Transcriptional and chromatin analysis were not performed however, so it remains unclear the degree to which combined mutation alters histone modification and transcriptional changes. Regardless, these studies support the general high-risk phenotype of combined JAK2/ASXL1 mutation observed in humans. Further studies are required to more comprehensively identify the specific gene expression programs involved.

EMERGING EPIGENETIC MODIFYING THERAPIES FOR THE TREATMENT OF MYELOFIBROSIS

With our improved understanding of the role of epigenetic dysfunction in disease progression in MPNs, there has been an increasing movement to explore novel epigenetic modifying therapies. Here we explore these emerging therapies currently being evaluated for use in these diseases.

Hypomethylating Agent Therapy

As described elsewhere in this article, altered DNA methylation patterns are frequent in MPNs and in other myeloid diseases and likely contribute to the dysregulated transcriptional programs that promote mutant clonal expansion. Hypomethylating agent (HMA) therapy, either with decitabine or 5-azacytidine, inhibits DNA methyltransferase activity and the addition of methyl groups to DNA, resulting in a global decrease in genome methylation and, presumably, the restoration of key transcription programs influencing cell growth and differentiation.[54] Although HMA drugs have become a mainstay in the treatment of myelodysplastic syndromes and de novo AML for patients unfit for intensive induction, limited studies evaluating single-agent HMA for the treatment of chronic MF suggest only moderate effect.[55] Retrospective series, however, reveal some activity for HMA alone in the setting of accelerated- or blast-phase disease,[56] and a recent study evaluating combined HMA with ruxolitinib treatment for treatment-naïve chronic MF suggests a potential synergy between these 2 agents.[57] In this study, 72% of participants ultimately achieved objective improvements in spleen volume and/or symptom scores, and the combination was generally well-tolerated. Of those who exhibited a spleen response, 95% demonstrated persistent response at 4 years of follow-up, suggesting additive improvement beyond ruxolitinib alone (when compared with historical COMFORT-I/II data).[58] It should be noted, however, that the majority of responses were observed in the initial period on ruxolitinib, before the start of azacytidine, suggesting that ruxolitinib might be the major driver of response. Still, 28% of participants demonstrated clinical improvement after the addition of HMA suggesting that HMA might indeed have synergistic effects in the setting of JAK inhibition.

Bromodomain and Extraterminal Domain Inhibitor Therapy

The bromodomain and extraterminal domain (BET) protein family binds to acetylated histones to regulate a wide variety of genes implicated in cancer (ie, c-Myc, BCL-xL, and CDK4/6).[59] BET inhibitors impair the interaction of BET proteins to histones, leading to alterations in the chromatin state and subsequent gene transcription. As a result, BET proteins have become a promising therapeutic target across the spectrum of both liquid and solid tumors. In MPNs, Saenz and colleagues[60] observed that treatment of CD34+ cells from post-MPN AML patients with combined BET + JAK inhibition resulted in enhanced cell apoptosis and growth arrest over either single-agent therapy alone. Furthermore, recent important work by Kleppe and colleagues[16] demonstrated that BET inhibitor therapy attenuates NF-κB signaling and synergizes with ruxolitinib to abrogate fibrosis development in MPN animal models, and emerging data suggest that the presence of EZH2 or ASXL1 mutations might sensitize cells to BET inhibitor therapy.[44,52] Given these findings, BET inhibitor therapy with or without ruxolitinib is now currently under evaluation for the treatment of progressive MF. In a recent phase I/II clinical trial, treatment with the BET inhibitor CPI-0610 in combination with ruxolitinib resulted in a dramatic response in spleen volume reduction (67% of patients receiving combination therapy, as well as 35% of patients with CPI-0610 alone), and 52% of patients (including 38% of patients receiving CPI-0610 alone) reported a more than 50% improvement in total symptoms scores as well.[61,62] Notably, a decrease in bone marrow fibrosis was also observed in 33% of patients across all arms, suggesting potent disease-modifying activity. Based on these encouraging preliminary data, a phase III trial of CPI-0610 plus ruxolitinib for untreated MF is now currently underway.

LSD1 Inhibitor Therapy

LSD1 is emerging as a possible therapeutic target in MPNs. LSD1 carries enzymatic function to remove methyl groups on histone lysine residues at active promoters. LSD1 loss results in expansion of myeloid progenitor populations with impairment in terminal differentiation, including megakaryocyte maturation,[63] and has been found to be overexpressed in patients with MF.[64] Furthermore, LSD1 inhibition demonstrated significant disease modifying activity in various preclinical mouse models of MPNs.[65] These findings have led to early phase evaluation of LSD1 inhibition for the treatment of MF, including secondary MF. In a phase I/IIa trial of the LSD1 inhibitor bomedemstat, a more than 50% symptom improvement was observed in 30% of participants, with approximately 20% demonstrating a more than 35% decrease in spleen volume.[66] Improvements in bone marrow fibrosis have also been observed in a smaller percentage of patients.[67] Based on these findings, a current phase IIb expansion study remains on-going for high-risk MF (NCT03136185) and has been expanded further to other MPN subtypes, including ET, for those having failed 1 previous standard therapy (NCT04081220).

Isocitrate Dehydrogenase 1/2 Inhibitor Therapy

IDH1/2 inhibition is an attractive target for IDH-mutant MPNs, highlighting the potential role for combined mutation-directed precision therapy for specific MPN/post-MPN AML genotypes. Given the enrichment of IDH1/2 mutations in post-MPN AML specifically, there is a rationale for the use of IDH inhibitors for the treatment of IDH1/2-mutated blast-/accelerated-phase disease. As such, clinical trials for advanced IDH-mutant MPN, including post-MPL AML, are ongoing (NCT04281498), and recent retrospective data evaluating IDH1/2 inhibitor use in the post-MPN AML setting suggests some early promise.[68]

PRMT5 Inhibitor Therapy

Given the role of JAK2^{V617F} in the phosphorylation of the arginine methyltransferase PRMT5,[9] there is a rationale for targeted PRMT5 inhibition in MPNs. In support of this strategy, a recent study evaluating the PRMT5 inhibitor C220 demonstrated efficacy in preclinical animal models, including improvements in bone marrow fibrosis and overall decreases in the allele burden, possibly through the enhancement of apoptosis and cell cycle arrest through E2F transcriptional activity.[69] Given these findings, PRMT5 inhibitors are also now currently being planned alone or in combination with ruxolitinib therapy in clinical trials for the treatment of MF.

Histone Deacetylase Inhibitor Therapy

Histone deacetylases (HDACs) catalyze the removal of "active" acetyl groups from histones and thus act to silence gene transcription. HDAC inhibitors have been demonstrated to have a myriad of intracellular effects, including dampening the repression of genes critical for DNA damage and repair and cell cycle regulation, as well as enhancing protein degradation through acetylation of heat shock protein 90.[70] As a result, HDAC inhibitors have been evaluated as anticancer therapy in a variety of liquid and solid tumor malignancies and are currently approved for use in T-cell lymphomas and plasma cell disorders. In preclinical models of MPN, HDAC inhibition preferentially induces apoptosis in JAK2^{V617F}-mutant cells, including primary patient samples, possibly through the destabilization of mutant JAK2 as a result of enhanced shock protein 9 activity,[71–73] prompting the evaluation of HDAC inhibitors for clinical use in MPNs. However, given the general lack of specificity of current HDAC inhibitors for individual HDAC proteins, and the numerous (likely) pleotropic effects of these agents, response rates have varied,[74,75] and toxicity, primarily hematologic, is frequently observed and a major cause of treatment discontinuation. Notably, however, a recent study identified HDAC11 specifically as a key mediator of aberrant megakaryopoiesis in MPNs, and genetic deletion of *Hdac11* ameliorated fibrosis and prolonged survival in MPN animal models,[76] suggesting more selective targeting of individual HDACs might enhance therapeutic efficacy while limiting off-target effects.

SUMMARY

The enrichment of methylation/histone changes in MF compared with other MPN subtypes underscores the importance of epigenetic dysregulation in fibrotic progression. Emerging data highlight the role of aberrant proinflammatory signaling beyond JAK/STAT in influencing fibrosis development. Evolving state-of-the-art technologies allowing for the simultaneous detection of DNA mutation, gene expression, and chromatin state at the level of the single cell will provide granularity in ways never thought possible. Already, these techniques are allowing us to better dissect how mutant clones evolve and expand over time and how the acquirement of additional mutations, in particular epigenetic modifiers, enhance clonal dominance. An improved understanding of how mutant cells influence gene expression changes in healthy bystander cells to impair normal hematopoiesis and how aberrant cytokine production alters the bone marrow microenvironment to promote fibrotic progression will be critical for identifying even newer and more refined ways to treat this deadly disease.

CLINICS CARE POINT

- Extended mutational analysis in MPNs provide important prognostic information.

DISCLOSURE

The authors acknowledge the support of Memorial Sloan Kettering Cancer Center Support Grant NIH P30 CA008748. This work was supported by National Cancer Institute P01 CA108671 11 (R.L.L.) and the Janus Fund (O.S. and R.L.L.). R.L.L. is on the supervisory board of Qiagen and is a scientific advisor to Imago, Mission Bio, Zentalis, Ajax, Auron, Prelude, C4 Therapeutics and Isoplexis. He receives research support from and consulted for Celgene and Roche and has consulted for Incyte, Janssen, Astellas, Morphosys and Novartis. He has received honoraria from Roche, Lilly and Amgen for invited lectures and from Gilead for grant reviews.

REFERENCES

1. Rodrigues CSMA, A. Epigenetic Regulators as the Gatekeepers of Hematopoiesis. Trends in Genetics In press.

2. Shih AH, Abdel-Wahab O, Patel JP, et al. The role of mutations in epigenetic regulators in myeloid malignancies. Nat Rev Cancer 2012;12:599–612.

3. Bowman RL, Busque L, Levine RL. Clonal hematopoiesis and evolution to hematopoietic malignancies. Cell Stem Cell 2018;22:157–70.

4. Jaiswal S, Fontanillas P, Flannick J, et al. Age-related clonal hematopoiesis associated with adverse outcomes. N Engl J Med 2014;371:2488–98.

5. Kramann R, Schneider RK. The identification of fibrosis-driving myofibroblast precursors reveals new therapeutic avenues in myelofibrosis. Blood 2018;131: 2111–9.

6. Villarino AV, Kanno Y, O'Shea JJ. Mechanisms and consequences of Jak-STAT signaling in the immune system. Nat Immunol 2017;18:374–84.

7. Dawson MA, Bannister AJ, Gottgens B, et al. JAK2 phosphorylates histone H3Y41 and excludes HP1alpha from chromatin. Nature 2009;461:819–22.

8. Kim H, Ronai ZA. PRMT5 function and targeting in cancer. Cell Stress 2020;4: 199–215.

9. Liu F, Zhao X, Perna F, et al. JAK2V617F-mediated phosphorylation of PRMT5 downregulates its methyltransferase activity and promotes myeloproliferation. Cancer Cell 2011;19:283–94.

10. Jeong JJ, Gu X, Nie J, et al. Cytokine-regulated phosphorylation and activation of TET2 by JAK2 in hematopoiesis. Cancer Discov 2019;9:778–95.

11. Nischal S, Bhattacharyya S, Christopeit M, et al. Methylome profiling reveals distinct alterations in phenotypic and mutational subgroups of myeloproliferative neoplasms. Cancer Res 2013;73:1076–85.

12. Perez C, Pascual M, Martin-Subero JI, et al. Aberrant DNA methylation profile of chronic and transformed classic Philadelphia-negative myeloproliferative neoplasms. Haematologica 2013;98:1414–20.

13. Nielsen HM, Andersen CL, Westman M, et al. Epigenetic changes in myelofibrosis: distinct methylation changes in the myeloid compartments and in cases with ASXL1 mutations. Sci Rep 2017;7:6774.

14. Asada S, Fujino T, Goyama S, et al. The role of ASXL1 in hematopoiesis and myeloid malignancies. Cell Mol Life Sci 2019;76:2511–23.

15. Martinez-Calle N, Pascual M, Ordonez R, et al. Epigenomic profiling of myelofibrosis reveals widespread DNA methylation changes in enhancer elements and ZFP36L1 as a potential tumor suppressor gene that is epigenetically regulated. Haematologica 2019;104:1572–9.

16. Kleppe M, Koche R, Zou L, et al. Dual targeting of oncogenic activation and inflammatory signaling increases therapeutic efficacy in myeloproliferative neoplasms. Cancer Cell 2018;33:29–43 e7.

17. Skov V. Next generation sequencing in MPNs. Lessons from the past and prospects for use as predictors of prognosis and treatment responses. Cancers (Basel) 2020;12:2194.

18. Hautin M, Mornet C, Chauveau A, et al. Splicing anomalies in myeloproliferative neoplasms: paving the way for new therapeutic venues. Cancers (Basel) 2020; 12:2216.

19. Tefferi A, Lasho TL, Finke CM, et al. Targeted deep sequencing in primary myelofibrosis. Blood Adv 2016;1:105–11.

20. Vannucchi AM, Lasho TL, Guglielmelli P, et al. Mutations and prognosis in primary myelofibrosis. Leukemia 2013;27:1861–9.

21. Tefferi A, Lasho TL, Abdel-Wahab O, et al. IDH1 and IDH2 mutation studies in 1473 patients with chronic-, fibrotic- or blast-phase essential thrombocythemia, polycythemia vera or myelofibrosis. Leukemia 2010;24:1302–9.

22. Grinfeld J, Nangalia J, Baxter EJ, et al. Classification and personalized prognosis in myeloproliferative neoplasms. N Engl J Med 2018;379:1416–30.

23. Tefferi A, Lasho TL, Guglielmelli P, et al. Targeted deep sequencing in polycythemia vera and essential thrombocythemia. Blood Adv 2016;1:21–30.

24. Guglielmelli P, Lasho TL, Rotunno G, et al. The number of prognostically detrimental mutations and prognosis in primary myelofibrosis: an international study of 797 patients. Leukemia 2014;28:1804–10.

25. Patel KP, Newberry KJ, Luthra R, et al. Correlation of mutation profile and response in patients with myelofibrosis treated with ruxolitinib. Blood 2015;126:790–7.

26. Spiegel JY, McNamara C, Kennedy JA, et al. Impact of genomic alterations on outcomes in myelofibrosis patients undergoing JAK1/2 inhibitor therapy. Blood Adv 2017;1:1729–38.

27. Kroger N, Panagiota V, Badbaran A, et al. Impact of molecular genetics on outcome in myelofibrosis patients after allogeneic stem cell transplantation. Biol Blood Marrow Transplant 2017;23:1095–101.

28. Tamari R, Rapaport F, Zhang N, et al. Impact of high-molecular-risk mutations on transplantation outcomes in patients with myelofibrosis. Biol Blood Marrow Transplant 2019;25:1142–51.

29. Lundberg P, Karow A, Nienhold R, et al. Clonal evolution and clinical correlates of somatic mutations in myeloproliferative neoplasms. Blood 2014;123:2220–8.

30. Green A, Beer P. Somatic mutations of IDH1 and IDH2 in the leukemic transformation of myeloproliferative neoplasms. N Engl J Med 2010;362:369–70.

31. Pardanani A, Lasho TL, Finke CM, et al. IDH1 and IDH2 mutation analysis in chronic- and blast-phase myeloproliferative neoplasms. Leukemia 2010;24:1146–51.

32. Tefferi A, Jimma T, Sulai NH, et al. IDH mutations in primary myelofibrosis predict leukemic transformation and shortened survival: clinical evidence for leukemogenic collaboration with JAK2V617F. Leukemia 2012;26:475–80.

33. Rodriguez-Meira A, Buck G, Clark SA, et al. Unravelling intratumoral heterogeneity through high-sensitivity single-cell mutational analysis and parallel RNA sequencing. Mol Cell 2019;73:1292–305.e8.

34. Ortmann CA, Kent DG, Nangalia J, et al. Effect of mutation order on myeloproliferative neoplasms. N Engl J Med 2015;372:601–12.

35. Kameda T, Shide K, Yamaji T, et al. Loss of TET2 has dual roles in murine myeloproliferative neoplasms: disease sustainer and disease accelerator. Blood 2015;125:304–15.

36. Chen E, Schneider RK, Breyfogle LJ, et al. Distinct effects of concomitant Jak2V617F expression and Tet2 loss in mice promote disease progression in myeloproliferative neoplasms. Blood 2015;125:327–35.

37. Shepherd MS, Li J, Wilson NK, et al. Single-cell approaches identify the molecular network driving malignant hematopoietic stem cell self- renewal. Blood 2018;132:791–803.

38. Jacquelin S, Straube J, Cooper L, et al. Jak2V617F and Dnmt3a loss cooperate to induce myelofibrosis through activated enhancer-driven inflammation. Blood 2018;132:2707–21.

39. Brecqueville M, Rey J, Bertucci F, et al. Mutation analysis of ASXL1, CBL, DNMT3A, IDH1, IDH2, JAK2, MPL, NF1, SF3B1, SUZ12, and TET2 in myeloproliferative neoplasms. Genes Chromosomes Cancer 2012;51:743–55.

40. Montalban-Bravo G, DiNardo CD. The role of IDH mutations in acute myeloid leukemia. Future Oncol 2018;14:979–93.

41. McKenney AS, Lau AN, Somasundara AVH, et al. JAK2/IDH-mutant-driven myeloproliferative neoplasm is sensitive to combined targeted inhibition. J Clin Invest 2018;128:789–804.
42. Sparmann A, van Lohuizen M. Polycomb silencers control cell fate, development and cancer. Nat Rev Cancer 2006;6:846–56.
43. Vire E, Brenner C, Deplus R, et al. The Polycomb group protein EZH2 directly controls DNA methylation. Nature 2006;439:871–4.
44. Sashida G, Wang C, Tomioka T, et al. The loss of Ezh2 drives the pathogenesis of myelofibrosis and sensitizes tumor-initiating cells to bromodomain inhibition. J Exp Med 2016;213:1459–77.
45. Shimizu T, Kubovcakova L, Nienhold R, et al. Loss of Ezh2 synergizes with JAK2-V617F in initiating myeloproliferative neoplasms and promoting myelofibrosis. J Exp Med 2016;213:1479–96.
46. Yang Y, Akada H, Nath D, et al. Loss of Ezh2 cooperates with Jak2V617F in the development of myelofibrosis in a mouse model of myeloproliferative neoplasm. Blood 2016;127:3410–23.
47. Abdel-Wahab O, Adli M, LaFave LM, et al. ASXL1 mutations promote myeloid transformation through loss of PRC2-mediated gene repression. Cancer Cell 2012;22:180–93.
48. Abdel-Wahab O, Gao J, Adli M, et al. Deletion of Asxl1 results in myelodysplasia and severe developmental defects in vivo. J Exp Med 2013;210:2641–59.
49. Hsu YC, Chiu YC, Lin CC, et al. The distinct biological implications of Asxl1 mutation and its roles in leukemogenesis revealed by a knock-in mouse model. J Hematol Oncol 2017;10:139.
50. Nagase R, Inoue D, Pastore A, et al. Expression of mutant Asxl1 perturbs hematopoiesis and promotes susceptibility to leukemic transformation. J Exp Med 2018;215:1729–47.
51. Uni M, Masamoto Y, Sato T, et al. Modeling ASXL1 mutation revealed impaired hematopoiesis caused by derepression of p16Ink4a through aberrant PRC1-mediated histone modification. Leukemia 2019;33:191–204.
52. Yang H, Kurtenbach S, Guo Y, et al. Gain of function of ASXL1 truncating protein in the pathogenesis of myeloid malignancies. Blood 2018;131:328–41.
53. Guo Y, Zhou Y, Yamatomo S, et al. ASXL1 alteration cooperates with JAK2V617F to accelerate myelofibrosis. Leukemia 2019;33:1287–91.
54. Sato T, Issa JJ, Kropf P. DNA hypomethylating drugs in cancer therapy. Cold Spring Harb Perspect Med 2017;7:a026948.
55. Quintas-Cardama A, Tong W, Kantarjian H, et al. A phase II study of 5-azacitidine for patients with primary and post-essential thrombocythemia/polycythemia vera myelofibrosis. Leukemia 2008;22:965–70.
56. Dunbar AJ, Rampal RK, Levine R. Leukemia secondary to myeloproliferative neoplasms. Blood 2020;136:61–70.
57. Masarova L, Verstovsek S, Hidalgo-Lopez JE, et al. A phase 2 study of ruxolitinib in combination with azacitidine in patients with myelofibrosis. Blood 2018;132:1664–74.
58. Verstovsek S, Mesa RA, Gotlib J, et al. A double-blind, placebo-controlled trial of ruxolitinib for myelofibrosis. N Engl J Med 2012;366:799–807.
59. Stathis A, Bertoni F. BET proteins as targets for anticancer treatment. Cancer Discov 2018;8:24–36.
60. Saenz DT, Fiskus W, Manshouri T, et al. BET protein bromodomain inhibitor-based combinations are highly active against post-myeloproliferative neoplasm secondary AML cells. Leukemia 2017;31:678–87.

61. Mascarenhas J, Harrison C, Patriarca A, et al. CPI-0610, a bromodomain and extraterminal domain protein (BET) inhibitor, in combination with ruxolitinib, in JAK-inhibitor-naïve myelofibrosis patients: update of MANIFEST phase 2 study. Virtual: American Society of Hematology; 2020.

62. Talpaz MRR, Verstovsek S, Harrisonn C, et al. CPI-0610, a bromodomain and extraterminal domain protein (BET) inhibitor, as monotherapy in advanced myelofibrosis patients refractory/intolerant to JAK inhibitor: update from phase 2 MANIFEST study. Virtual: American Society of Hematology; 2020.

63. Sprussel A, Schulte JH, Weber S, et al. Lysine-specific demethylase 1 restricts hematopoietic progenitor proliferation and is essential for terminal differentiation. Leukemia 2012;26:2039–51.

64. Niebel D, Kirfel J, Janzen V, et al. Lysine-specific demethylase 1 (LSD1) in hematopoietic and lymphoid neoplasms. Blood 2014;124:151–2.

65. Jutzi JS, Kleppe M, Dias J, et al. LSD1 inhibition prolongs survival in mouse models of MPN by selectively targeting the disease clone. Hemasphere 2018;2:e54.

66. Yacoub APK, Bradley T, Gerds A, et al. A phase 2 study of the LSD1 inhibitor IMG7289 (bomedemstat) for the treatment of advanced myelofibrosis. Virtual: American Society of Hematology; 2020.

67. Pettit JGA, Yacoub A, Watts J, et al. A phase 2a study of the LSD1 inhibitor img-7289 (bomedemstat) for the treatment of myelofibrosis. Orlando, FL: American Society of Hematology; 2019.

68. Chifotides HT, Masarova L, Alfayez M, et al. Outcome of patients with IDH1/2-mutated post-myeloproliferative neoplasm AML in the era of IDH inhibitors. Blood Adv 2020;4:5336–42.

69. Pastore F, Bhagwat N, Pastore A, et al. PRMT5 inhibition modulates E2F1 methylation and gene-regulatory networks leading to therapeutic efficacy in JAK2(V617F)-Mutant MPN. Cancer Discov 2020;10:1742–57.

70. Falkenberg KJ, Johnstone RW. Histone deacetylases and their inhibitors in cancer, neurological diseases and immune disorders. Nat Rev Drug Discov 2014;13:673–91.

71. Wang Y, Fiskus W, Chong DG, et al. Cotreatment with panobinostat and JAK2 inhibitor TG101209 attenuates JAK2V617F levels and signaling and exerts synergistic cytotoxic effects against human myeloproliferative neoplastic cells. Blood 2009;114:5024–33.

72. Akada H, Akada S, Gajra A, et al. Efficacy of vorinostat in a murine model of polycythemia vera. Blood 2012;119:3779–89.

73. Evrot E, Ebel N, Romanet V, et al. JAK1/2 and Pan-deacetylase inhibitor combination therapy yields improved efficacy in preclinical mouse models of JAK2V617F-driven disease. Clin Cancer Res 2013;19:6230–41.

74. Bose P, Swaminathan M, Pemmaraju N, et al. A phase 2 study of pracinostat combined with ruxolitinib in patients with myelofibrosis. Leuk Lymphoma 2019;60:1767–74.

75. Mascarenhas J, Lu M, Li T, et al. A phase I study of panobinostat (LBH589) in patients with primary myelofibrosis (PMF) and post- polycythaemia vera/essential thrombocythaemia myelofibrosis (post-PV/ET MF). Br J Haematol 2013;161:68–75.

76. Yue L, Sharma V, Horvat NP, et al. HDAC11 deficiency disrupts oncogene-induced hematopoiesis in myeloproliferative neoplasms. Blood 2020;135:191–207.

Murine Modeling of Myeloproliferative Neoplasms

Karie Chen, MS, Alan H. Shih, MD, PhD*

KEYWORDS

- Myeloproliferative neoplasm • Mouse model • JAK2 • CALR • MPL • Epigenetics
- Preclinical trial

KEY POINTS

- MPN models closely mirror human disease, validate driver mutations in MPNs, and associate gene dysfunction with disease biology.
- MPN models confirm JAK2 pathway activation as central to MPN pathology with additional mutant genes in epigenetics, signaling, and cell-death that modify the disease phenotype.
- MPN models are used for preclinical testing of therapeutics that can then be advanced into clinical trials and for identification of new potential targets.

INTRODUCTION

Myeloproliferative neoplasms (MPNs), such as polycythemia vera (PV), essential thrombocythemia (ET), and primary myelofibrosis (MF), are hematologic disorders that have excess proliferation of myeloid blood elements with disease cells maintaining the ability to differentiate. Through dedicated sequencing of patient samples, disease-associated mutations in target genes have been identified and are used for diagnostic and prognostic determination.[1] In the case of MPNs, the associated genetic changes have pointed to specific pathways that underlie disease biology. Using mouse models of these genetic changes, investigators have gained understanding of pathophysiology and therapeutic potential.

MOUSE MODELING

Although primary samples and tissue culture are used to study disease alleles, they face limitations including the ability to investigate cellular differentiation and the microenvironment in a physiologic context. To enhance research capabilities, mouse models have been used throughout cancer research.[2] One technique in hematologic

Department of Medicine, Division of Hematology/Oncology, Icahn School of Medicine at Mount Sinai, One Gustave L. Levy Place, Box 1079, New York, NY 10029, USA
* Corresponding author.
E-mail address: alan.shih@mssm.edu

Hematol Oncol Clin N Am 35 (2021) 253–265
https://doi.org/10.1016/j.hoc.2020.11.007
0889-8588/21/© 2020 Elsevier Inc. All rights reserved.

malignancy studies is bone marrow transplantation (BMT) (**Fig. 1**A). Bone marrow cells are transduced using a retrovirus that delivers the target gene and then transplanted.[3] Multiple recipients can receive the same donor cells that can also be tracked. The disadvantage is viral vectors integrate randomly into the genome and expression of the target gene is nonphysiologic. Primary patient-derived cells (PDX) can also act as donor cells in BMT models (**Fig. 1**B). To avoid immune rejection, immune-compromised mice are used as recipients. Use of primary human cells has the clear advantage of being the best source of disease cells themselves but are hampered by variations between samples, difficulty in preserving primary cells, and the altered environment in immune-compromised mice. In a transgenic model, the target gene is integrated into the murine genome at a nonendogenous site (**Fig. 1**C).[4] This provides a consistent genetic model where regulation of the gene is under the same context. Knockin mouse models use targeted gene recombination or editing to express the mutant gene from the endogenous locus, under the control of the native promoter, and thus, more faithfully modeling physiologic expression levels (**Fig. 1**D).

JAK2

Efforts from different groups led to the identification of the cytokine signaling component Janus Kinase 2 (*JAK2*) as the most common mutation in MPNs. The first mouse models to study *JAK2V617 F* used BMT to demonstrate that this gene functions as a driver mutation.[5,6] Mice transplanted with *JAK2V617 F*-transduced bone marrow cells presented with a PV-like phenotype with increased hematocrit along with splenomegaly, leukocytosis, and neutrophilia. Over time they developed MF, mirroring the spent phase of PV with development of MF. Transgenic mouse models of *JAK2V617 F* also developed MPN phenotypes.[7-9] Because of the various promoters used to regulate gene expression and different integration sites, the level of *JAK2V617 F* expression differed across models. These models developed phenotypes ranging from thrombocytosis that resembled ET to erythrocytosis resembling PV with associated leukocytosis, suppressed *Epo* expression, splenomegaly, and evolution to MF.

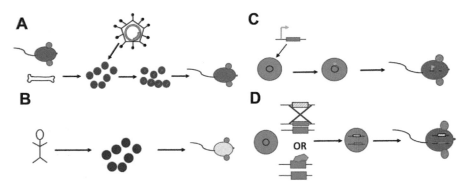

Fig. 1. Mouse models of MPN. (*A*) Retroviral-BMT model. Bone marrow cells are derived from a mouse and then transduced with a virus encoding a target gene. These cells are then reinjected into recipient mice. (*B*) Patient-derived cells model. Disease cells are derived from patient samples and then injected into immune-compromised mice. (*C*) Transgenic model. Embryonic stem (ES) cells are targeted with a transgene that integrates into the genome. Mice are then derived from these modified ES cells. (*D*) Knockin model. ES cells are targeted with either recombination methods or gene editing methods to modify a specific endogenous locus of the target gene. Mice are then derived from these modified ES cells.

Investigators also developed conditional knockin models with *JAK2V617 F*.[10–12] Again, these mice developed an MPN phenotype and had features similar to BMT and transgenic models. Use of human *JAK2V617 F* or murine *Jak2V617 F* was associated with variation in phenotype with heterozygous human *JAK2V617 F* developing more ET phenotypes and homozygous human or mouse *Jak2V617 F* developing more PV phenotypes. This suggests that the level of JAK2 activity may play a role in disease physiology and mirrors the human disease condition where *JAK2* mutations and homozygous mutant conditions are more common in PV than ET.[13] Mouse models have also been useful to understand more rare variants in *JAK2* mutations.[14] Transgenic mice that express human *JAK2-N542-E543del*, mirroring exon12 mutations, developed elevated hematocrits, splenomegaly, and other MPN features.[15]

Analysis of these conditional mice also showed defects in the stem-progenitor myeloid cell compartment. This defective hematopoietic stem cell (HSC) population correlates with observations that identified the *JAK2* mutation in patient HSCs.[16] There has been some disagreement among the models as to whether mutation in *JAK2* confers a competitive growth advantage in stem cells. Single cell analysis of the stem cells demonstrated decreased expression of important self-renewal regulators, such as *Bmi1*.[17] This agreed with other studies where transplanted mutant cells failed to outcompete wild-type cells in BMT experiments.[10] A knockin model that attempts to address this issue used a promoter that led to mutant *JAK2V617 F* expression only in a select number of HSCs in the bone marrow.[18] These mice over time evolved from an ET to PV phenotype and suggest that *JAK2V617 F* mutant HSCs can gain a growth advantage. The effect on stem cells is also supported by the observation of clonal hematopoiesis with *JAK2V617 F* mutation in which a mutant clone expands.[19]

MPL AND CALR

After the identification of *JAK2*, other components of the cytokine signaling pathway were deemed candidates in disease pathogenesis. Activated *Mpl* was identified early on as the gene responsible for transforming HSCs by the myeloproliferative leukemia virus.[20] Sequencing efforts led to the identification of mutations in the thrombopoietin receptor *MPL* in *JAK2V617F*-negative MPNs, specifically *MPLW515 L*.[21] The mutation was most commonly found in ET patients, and retroviral transduction models confirmed the oncogenic function of the mutant gene in ET-like disease.[21]

Using a more unbiased approach with next-generation sequencing, insertion and deletion mutations in calreticulin (*CALR*) were identified.[22] At first how *CALR* mutations lead to MPN was not obvious because *CALR* was not a known component of the cytokine signaling pathway. Using retroviral transduction BMT, transgenic, and knockin mouse models, expression of the *CALRdel52* mutation led to thrombocytosis and an ET-like phenotype with an increase in proliferation of megakaryocytes.[23–25] These results confirm *CALR* mutations as driver mutations in MPN. By using donor cells that were deleted for *c-mpl*, it was determined that MPL expression was essential for *CALR* mutation to induce disease. Furthermore, simple deletion of a C-terminal exon of murine *Calr* did not recapitulate the full extent of disease, suggesting that the specific human neopeptide generated by the frame-shift mutation had functional significance.[26,27] Knockin mice with type I *del52* mutant *Calr* developed ET-like disease with thrombocytosis particularly when the mutant gene was homozygous.[28] The data suggest that type I *CALRdel52* mutations may be associated with higher levels of signaling and thus more aggressive phenotypes. These data supported a model where a gain-of-function mutant CALR interacts with MPL and enhances signal transduction from the receptor.

PRECLINICAL TESTING

Besides functional genetic validation, mouse models have also been used to perform preclinical testing. MPN models generated by *JAK2V617 F* and *MPLW515 L* were first used to validate the utility of JAK2 inhibition and supported the development of ruxolitinib as targeted therapy.[29,30] The authors show that inhibition with these agents could decrease disease features, such as splenomegaly, bone marrow fibrosis, thrombocytosis, and leukocytosis. By using mice that encode deletion of *Stat5*, it was shown that when this pathway is disrupted, disease is largely attenuated.[31] Deletion of *Jak2* in an *MPLW515 L* retroviral model also greatly attenuated disease.[32] These models support efforts to target this pathway beyond ruxolitinib and the potential efficacy of more potent inhibition. For example, using a JAK2 inhibitor that binds to an alternative site, investigators were able to reverse resistance developed with ruxolitinib.[33]

These models have also been used to investigate additional therapeutic targets beyond JAK2. Interferon-α was validated as an effective therapy.[34] Targeting HSP90 and HSP27 heat shock protein and their chaperone effect on JAK2 were studied as potential treatments in MPNs.[35,36] The interaction of the JAK-STAT pathway and programmed death ligand-1 pathway has also been studied, forming the basis for potential studies with immunotherapy in MPNs.[37]

These models have been useful in testing combination therapies. In many studies with JAK2 inhibitors, the mutant MPN clone is not eliminated and the mutant allele burden persists in MPN models.[38] The combination of a histone deacetylase inhibitor, panobinostat was tested in combination with ruxolitinib.[39] This led to greater treatment response, and panobinostat itself has moved into clinical trials. MPN models have been used to test dual signaling blockade, specifically combining JAK2 with MEK inhibition.[40] This stemmed from the observation that although JAK2 inhibition was effective in inhibition MEK/ERK activation in vitro, it was less effective in vivo, implying an alternative activation pathway observed in this model. Dual JAK and MEK inhibition led to greater efficacy in this study.

These MPN models have been used to investigate pathways that may be implicated in MF including vitamin D and transforming growth factor-β.[41,42] Inhibition of AURKA has also been proposed to be effective in treating MF through its effects on megakaryocyte differentiation.[43] Using *JAK2V617 F* and *MPLW515 L* models, treatment with AURKA inhibitor was able to reduce disease burden, increase megakaryocyte maturation, and reduce pathogenic cytokines. This finding has been translated to clinical trials studying AURKA inhibition in MF.[44] Epigenetic therapy, such as bromodomain inhibition, has been studied alone and in combination to target fibrosis in MPN models.[45,46] MPN mice treated with JQ1, a BET inhibitor, alone or in combination with ruxolitinib showed signs of decreased fibrosis, prolonged survival, lowered cytokine levels, and reduced self-renewal capacity of disease cells. BET inhibitor clinical trials are in active investigation for MF.[47]

MPN models have also been used to investigate additional disease biology. Mouse models were used to understand pathology of cytokine production from stromal cells.[48] These models have been used to study the bone marrow microenvironment and how MPN disease modifies stromal cells and the HSC niche.[49,50] Mouse models have been used to study mechanisms of clotting defects that relates to thrombosis risk. These models have described differential adhesion in mutant cells.[51] They have shown how platelet aggregation is defective in the setting of MPN and increases the risk of bleeding.[52] *Jak2v617f* mutation in endothelial cells were shown to potentially contribute to thrombosis through P-selectin expression.[53] Intrinsic defects in *Jak2v617f* mutant megakaryocytes and platelets may contribute to thrombosis through responses to activating signals.[54] Mouse models of MPNs were also used to study how neutrophil extracellular traps lead to thrombosis.[55]

EPIGENETIC MUTATIONS

Although murine MPN models have shown that mutation of a single gene is sufficient to induce disease, sequencing of patient samples has identified additional mutations that co-occur with those in *JAK2*, *MPL*, and *CALR* in greater than 50% of patients.[56] Most of these genes fall within the class of epigenetic regulators, such as *TET2*, *ASXL1*, *DNMT3A*, *IDH1/2*, and *EZH2*. Mutation in these genes has been shown to affect processes including DNA and histone methylation. They are not specific to MPNs but instead are found across the spectrum of myeloid malignancies including myelodysplastic syndrome (MDS) and acute myeloid leukemia (AML). Typically, a single mutation in one of these genes is insufficient to induce overt myeloid disease. Often they affect HSC function, such as providing a competitive growth advantage or skewing their differentiation potential. To study this class of genes, investigators have crossed mice to generate compound mutant mice to assess mutational cooperativity.

TET2 acts as a 5-hydroxymethylase that leads to cytosine DNA demethylation. Combining *Tet2* and *Jak2* mutations, HSCs gain competitive growth advantage and have increased self-renewal, allowing disease to propagate in serial transplant experiments.[57,58] Specifically, these mice developed greater leukocytosis, splenomegaly, and disease stem cell expansion. TET2 has also been shown to be a potential mediator of *JAK2V617 F* activity, because specific tyrosines in TET2 are phosphorylation targets of JAK2.[59] Erythroid precursor cells isolated from MPN mouse models were used to define specific genes that may be affected by activated TET2. Thus, haploinsufficiency of *TET2* may influence *JAK2V617 F* activity.

EZH2 acts as member of polycomb repressive (PRC2) complex that leads to histone methylation and gene silencing. *Ezh2* loss in hematopoietic cells led to a variety of hematopoietic disorders including MDS, MDS/MPN overlap, and thrombocytosis.[60] Combining *Ezh2* with *Jak2* mutations generates a more aggressive disease with high platelet and neutrophil counts and advanced MF.[61,62] The addition of *Ezh2* mutation also affected MPN HSC activity because limiting dilution assays demonstrated that double mutant HSCs showed greater potency. Altered expression of genes regulated by *Ezh2* as marked by H3K27 methylation, such as *Hmga2*, and increased expression of transforming growth factor-β1 may also contribute to megakaryocyte pathology and MF. This tumor suppressive role has implications on the potential use of EZH2 inhibitors in myeloid diseases.

Modeling of *JAK2* mutation in combination with other additional mutations likewise generated models of more advanced disease. *JAK2V617 F* and *Asxl1* mutation generated a more aggressive model with increased MF and increased risk of progression to leukemia.[63] This agrees with clinical findings that *Asxl1* mutation is associated with worse prognosis in MF.[64] *JAK2V617 F* in combination with *Dnmt3a* deletion blocks erythroid development and also induces fibrosis. Disruption of PRC2 complexes affecting differentiation and increased inflammatory markers were determined to be part of the disease mechanism.[65] Mutations in *IDH1/2* occur rarely in MPN. These mutations are known to be gain-of-function that disrupt the activity of epigenetic regulators. When *JAK2V617 F* mutation is combined with *Idh2R140Q* in a mouse model, disease cells showed more aggressive phenotypes with blast-like cells.[66]

Another class of genes mutated in MPNs encode factors involved in RNA splicing including *SRSF2*, *U2AF1*, *ZRSR2*, and *SF3B1*. These mutations are rare in MPNs, and mouse models demonstrate a range of effects.[67–71] Pathways affected by aberrant RNA splicing have been identified including those regulating myeloid development and HSC, such as those involving *EZH2* and *RUNX1*.

SIGNALING, TRANSCRIPTION FACTOR, AND OTHER MUTATIONS

Mutations in signal transduction components other than *JAK2* and *MPL* have also been identified in patients with MPN. These include *LNK*, *CBL*, *PTPN11*, *NRAS/ KRAS*, and *PPM1D*.[56] *LNK* is an adaptor protein that can negatively regulate JAK2 signaling.[72] When disrupted in mouse models, *Lnk* mutant mice develop an MPN-like phenotype with increased in stem-progenitor cells, platelet counts, and megakaryocytes.[73–75] *CBL* is an ubiquitin ligase that regulates the stability and activity of signaling proteins including receptor tyrosine kinases and JAK2. Mouse models of *CBL* mutation lead to increased JAK-STAT signaling and enhances HSC renewal.[76,77] *PTPN11* is a tyrosine phosphatase that regulates Ras/MAPK signaling. *Ptpn11* mutant mice develop stem-progenitor cells with hyperactive signaling and leukocytosis with hepatosplenomegaly.[78,79] Activated *NRAS/KRAS* models develop a myeloproliferative disorder phenotype with elevated leukocytes, inflammation, anemia, and hepatosplenomegaly.[80,81] *PPM1D* is a downstream target of *TP53* that acts as a phosphatase, regulating the DNA damage response. *Ppm1d* mutant mice demonstrated relative resistance to chemotherapy, which is consistent with the observation that these mutations are more common in therapy-related myeloid neoplasms.[82]

The transcription factor *NFE2* is also mutated in a small proportion of patients with MPN ($\sim$2%) with mutations typically resulting in truncated proteins.[56] *NFE2* regulates myeloid differentiation, and murine BMT models develop increased counts in platelets, erythrocytes, and neutrophils with overexpression of wild-type protein.[83] In mice with compound mutations combining *JAK2V617 F* and *NFE2* mutation, a more advance MPN develops.[84]

Mutations in *TP53* occur in 2% to 4% of patients with MPN but are much more frequent in post-MPN AML. Mouse models combining *JAK2V617 F* with *Tp53* loss led to an aggressive AML that demonstrated megakaryocyte-erythroid progenitor dysfunction.[85] Cell of origin studies from mouse bone marrow suggest that stem-progenitor cells from various stages of differentiation can direct the type of disease that develops, with leukemic potential arising from the erythroid cell lineage in the setting of *JAK2* and *Tp53* mutation.[86]

Deletion in the long arm of chromosome 20 (20q) causing loss of heterozygosity has been observed in MPN, suggesting the presence of one or more tumor suppressor genes in this region.[87] No definitive target gene has been identified but candidate genes have been proposed by analyzing common and minimally deleted segments.[88] Using mouse models that have deleted specific genes in this region, candidate genes have been tested including *Ptpn1*, *Stk4*, and *Mbyl2* with varying degrees of MPN phenotype.[89–92] It is also possible that more than one gene in this 20q region may be responsible for the observed MPN association.

OTHER MYELOPROLIFERATIVE NEOPLASM DISEASE MODELS

Sequencing efforts have identified mutation profiles of other less common MPN diagnoses including chronic neutrophilic leukemia and atypical chronic myelogenous leukemia. Using a retroviral-BMT model, mutant *CSF3RT618I* was expressed in murine hematopoietic cells.[93] These mice developed an MPN disease that mirrored chronic neutrophilic leukemia with increased granulocytes and hepatosplenomegaly. The model was also useful in preclinical testing by demonstrating that ruxolitinib is an effective therapy by inhibiting JAK1/2 signaling downstream of the receptor.

Chronic myelomonocytic leukemia (CMML) is classified as a mixed MDS/MPN disease with features of both disease phenotypes. Mouse models with mutations found in MPN, such as CBL, TET2, and NRAS, can resemble CMML.[94–97] Enhanced PDX approaches have also been developed by altering recipient mice. By engineering the bone marrow microenvironment of mice to produce human cytokines that support HSCs (granulocyte-macrophage colony–stimulating factor, interleukin-3, stem cell factor), primary CMML samples have been more consistently engrafted into these NSGS immune-compromised mice.[98] These PDX models were then used to test treatment with pacritinib, a kinase inhibitor targeting JAK2 and being studied for MPN trials.

Human bone marrow–derived mesenchymal stromal cells have been used to generate ossicle-like niches in immunocompromised mice.[99] These then become sites to engraft a variety of primary human disease cells with greater efficiency. Intratibial injection of MF cells into NSGS mice has also been successful to model individual patient disease and was able to identify existing subclones that were at risk of evolving into acute leukemia and identify potential therapeutic targets.[100]

SUMMARY

Mouse models of MPNs have been guided by the identification of recurrently mutated genes. These models have confirmed activation of JAK2 pathway signaling as central to disease biology. They also show that disease is influenced by mutations in other disease-modifying genes in epigenetics, signal transduction, cellular differentiation, splicing, or cell-death. Although these mutations converge on similar pathways, the disease phenotypes are clearly different as seen in patients and mouse models. The levels to which the pathway is activated has an important influence on phenotypic outcomes. The specific cell types affected, the signaling node on which the mutation acts, and the modifying mutations all affect outcomes. Questions remain on what drives the rate of progression, particularly evolution to MF and acute leukemia transformation. More careful dissection of these models may lead to greater insights into these processes. What has been remarkable is how closely these murine models have mirrored human biology. Treatments that show promise in preclinical models have advanced to clinical trials. With improved mouse models and more in-depth analysis, much more can be learned regarding disease biology and contribute to improved treatments for MPN.

CLINICS CARE POINTS

- Preclinical testing in mouse models confirms activation of the JAK pathway in MPNs and the efficacy of JAK2 inhibitors such as ruxolitinib.
- The strength of JAK pathway signaling and specific cell type affected may determine the phenotype (whether PV, ET, or MF) that results from driver mutations.
- More than half of all MPN patients may have other mutations or chromosomal abnormalities in addition to JAK2, MPL, and CALR. As observed in modeling, particular mutations such as ASXL1 may portend more aggressive disease and worse prognosis.
- Based on modeling studies, additional targets are being invested in clinical trials to treat MPNs, including TGF-β, BET, MEK, and additional JAK inhibitors.

DISCLOSURE

K. Chen has nothing to disclose. A.H. Shih is supported by NCI grant K08CA181507.

REFERENCES

1. Rampal R, Levine RL. A primer on genomic and epigenomic alterations in the myeloproliferative neoplasms. Best Pract Res Clin Haematol 2014;27(2):83–93.
2. Kersten K, de Visser KE, van Miltenburg MH, et al. Genetically engineered mouse models in oncology research and cancer medicine. EMBO Mol Med 2017;9(2):137–53.
3. Nguyen TK, Morse SJ, Fleischman AG. Transduction-transplantation mouse model of myeloproliferative neoplasm. J Vis Exp 2016;118:54624.
4. Lampreht Tratar U, Horvat S, Cemazar M. Transgenic mouse models in cancer research. Front Oncol 2018;8:268.
5. Wernig G, Mercher T, Okabe R, et al. Expression of Jak2V617F causes a polycythemia vera-like disease with associated myelofibrosis in a murine bone marrow transplant model. Blood 2006;107(11):4274–81.
6. Lacout C, Pisani DF, Tulliez M, et al. JAK2V617F expression in murine hematopoietic cells leads to MPD mimicking human PV with secondary myelofibrosis. Blood 2006;108(5):1652–60.
7. Xing S, Wanting TH, Zhao W, et al. Transgenic expression of JAK2V617F causes myeloproliferative disorders in mice. Blood 2008;111(10):5109–17.
8. Tiedt R, Hao-Shen H, Sobas MA, et al. Ratio of mutant JAK2-V617F to wild-type Jak2 determines the MPD phenotypes in transgenic mice. Blood 2008;111(8): 3931–40.
9. Shide K, Shimoda HK, Kumano T, et al. Development of ET, primary myelofibrosis and PV in mice expressing JAK2 V617F. Leukemia 2008;22(1):87–95.
10. Mullally A, Lane SW, Ball B, et al. Physiological Jak2V617F expression causes a lethal myeloproliferative neoplasm with differential effects on hematopoietic stem and progenitor cells. Cancer Cell 2010;17(6):584–96.
11. Akada H, Yan D, Zou H, et al. Conditional expression of heterozygous or homozygous Jak2V617F from its endogenous promoter induces a polycythemia vera-like disease. Blood 2010;115(17):3589–97.
12. Marty C, Lacout C, Martin A, et al. Myeloproliferative neoplasm induced by constitutive expression of JAK2V617F in knock-in mice. Blood 2010;116(5): 783–7.
13. Godfrey AL, Chen E, Pagano F, et al. JAK2V617F homozygosity arises commonly and recurrently in PV and ET, but PV is characterized by expansion of a dominant homozygous subclone. Blood 2012;120(13):2704–7.
14. Scott LM, Tong W, Levine RL, et al. JAK2 exon 12 mutations in polycythemia vera and idiopathic erythrocytosis. N Engl J Med 2007;356(5):459–68.
15. Grisouard J, Li S, Kubovcakova L, et al. JAK2 exon 12 mutant mice display isolated erythrocytosis and changes in iron metabolism favoring increased erythropoiesis. Blood 2016;128(6):839–51.
16. Jamieson CH, Gotlib J, Durocher JA, et al. The JAK2 V617F mutation occurs in hematopoietic stem cells in polycythemia vera and predisposes toward erythroid differentiation. Proc Natl Acad Sci U S A 2006;103(16):6224–9.
17. Shepherd MS, Li J, Wilson NK, et al. Single-cell approaches identify the molecular network driving malignant hematopoietic stem cell self-renewal. Blood 2018;132(8):791–803.

18. Mansier O, Kilani B, Guitart AV, et al. Description of a knock-in mouse model of JAK2V617F MPN emerging from a minority of mutated hematopoietic stem cells. Blood 2019;134(26):2383–7.

19. Jaiswal S, Fontanillas P, Flannick J, et al. Age-related clonal hematopoiesis associated with adverse outcomes. N Engl J Med 2014;371(26):2488–98.

20. Souyri M, Vigon I, Penciolelli JF, et al. A putative truncated cytokine receptor gene transduced by the myeloproliferative leukemia virus immortalizes hematopoietic progenitors. Cell 1990;63(6):1137–47.

21. Pikman Y, Lee BH, Mercher T, et al. MPLW515L is a novel somatic activating mutation in myelofibrosis with myeloid metaplasia. PLoS Med 2006;3(7):e270.

22. Klampfl T, Gisslinger H, Harutyunyan AS, et al. Somatic mutations of calreticulin in myeloproliferative neoplasms. N Engl J Med 2013;369(25):2379–90.

23. Elf S, Abdelfattah NS, Chen E, et al. Mutant calreticulin requires both its mutant C-terminus and the thrombopoietin receptor for oncogenic transformation. Cancer Discov 2016;6(4):368–81.

24. Marty C, Pecquet C, Nivarthi H, et al. Calreticulin mutants in mice induce an MPL-dependent thrombocytosis with frequent progression to myelofibrosis. Blood 2016;127(10):1317–24.

25. Balligand T, Achouri Y, Pecquet C, et al. Knock-in of murine Calr del52 induces essential thrombocythemia with slow-rising dominance in mice and reveals key role of Calr exon 9 in cardiac development. Leukemia 2020;34(2):510–21.

26. Shide K, Kameda T, Kamiunten A, et al. Calreticulin haploinsufficiency augments stem cell activity and is required for onset of myeloproliferative neoplasms. Blood 2020;136(1):106–18.

27. Shide K, Kameda T, Kamiunten A, et al. Mice with Calr mutations homologous to human CALR mutations only exhibit mild thrombocytosis. Blood Cancer J 2019; 9(4):42.

28. Li J, Prins D, Park HJ, et al. Mutant calreticulin knockin mice develop thrombocytosis and myelofibrosis without a stem cell self-renewal advantage. Blood 2018;131(6):649–61.

29. Koppikar P, Abdel-Wahab O, Hedvat C, et al. Efficacy of the JAK2 inhibitor INCB16562 in a murine model of MPLW515L-induced thrombocytosis and myelofibrosis. Blood 2010;115(14):2919–27.

30. Quintas-Cardama A, Vaddi K, Liu P, et al. Preclinical characterization of the selective JAK1/2 inhibitor INCB018424: therapeutic implications for the treatment of myeloproliferative neoplasms. Blood 2010;115(15):3109–17.

31. Walz C, Ahmed W, Lazarides K, et al. Essential role for Stat5a/b in myeloproliferative neoplasms induced by BCR-ABL1 and JAK2(V617F) in mice. Blood 2012;119(15):3550–60.

32. Bhagwat N, Koppikar P, Keller M, et al. Improved targeting of JAK2 leads to increased therapeutic efficacy in myeloproliferative neoplasms. Blood 2014; 123(13):2075–83.

33. Meyer SC, Keller MD, Chiu S, et al. CHZ868, a type II JAK2 inhibitor, reverses type I JAK inhibitor persistence and demonstrates efficacy in myeloproliferative neoplasms. Cancer Cell 2015;28(1):15–28.

34. Mullally A, Bruedigam C, Poveromo L, et al. Depletion of Jak2V617F myeloproliferative neoplasm-propagating stem cells by interferon-alpha in a murine model of polycythemia vera. Blood 2013;121(18):3692–702.

35. Marubayashi S, Koppikar P, Taldone T, et al. HSP90 is a therapeutic target in JAK2-dependent myeloproliferative neoplasms in mice and humans. J Clin Invest 2010;120(10):3578–93.

36. Sevin M, Kubovcakova L, Pernet N, et al. HSP27 is a partner of JAK2-STAT5 and a potential therapeutic target in myelofibrosis. Nat Commun 2018;9(1):1431.

37. Prestipino A, Emhardt AJ, Aumann K, et al. Oncogenic JAK2(V617F) causes PD-L1 expression, mediating immune escape in myeloproliferative neoplasms. Sci Transl Med 2018;10(429):eaam7729.

38. Tyner JW, Bumm TG, Deininger J, et al. CYT387, a novel JAK2 inhibitor, induces hematologic responses and normalizes inflammatory cytokines in murine myeloproliferative neoplasms. Blood 2010;115(25):5232–40.

39. Evrot E, Ebel N, Romanet V, et al. JAK1/2 and Pan-deacetylase inhibitor combination therapy yields improved efficacy in preclinical mouse models of JAK2V617F-driven disease. Clin Cancer Res 2013;19(22):6230–41.

40. Stivala S, Codilupi T, Brkic S, et al. Targeting compensatory MEK/ERK activation increases JAK inhibitor efficacy in myeloproliferative neoplasms. J Clin Invest 2019;130:1596–611.

41. Wakahashi K, Minagawa K, Kawano Y, et al. Vitamin D receptor-mediated skewed differentiation of macrophages initiates myelofibrosis and subsequent osteosclerosis. Blood 2019;133(15):1619–29.

42. Yue L, Bartenstein M, Zhao W, et al. Efficacy of ALK5 inhibition in myelofibrosis. JCI Insight 2017;2(7):e90932.

43. Wen QJ, Yang Q, Goldenson B, et al. Targeting megakaryocytic-induced fibrosis in myeloproliferative neoplasms by AURKA inhibition. Nat Med 2015; 21(12):1473–80.

44. Gangat N, Marinaccio C, Swords R, et al. Aurora kinase a inhibition provides clinical benefit, normalizes megakaryocytes, and reduces bone marrow fibrosis in patients with myelofibrosis: a phase I trial. Clin Cancer Res 2019;25(16): 4898–906.

45. Sashida G, Wang C, Tomioka T, et al. The loss of Ezh2 drives the pathogenesis of myelofibrosis and sensitizes tumor-initiating cells to bromodomain inhibition. J Exp Med 2016;213(8):1459–77.

46. Kleppe M, Koche R, Zou L, et al. Dual targeting of oncogenic activation and inflammatory signaling increases therapeutic efficacy in myeloproliferative neoplasms. Cancer Cell 2018;33(1):29–43 e27.

47. Mascarenhas J, Kremyanskaya M, Hoffman R, et al. MANIFEST, a phase 2 study of CPI-0610, a bromodomain and extraterminal domain inhibitor (beti), as monotherapy or "add-on" to ruxolitinib, in patients with refractory or intolerant advanced myelofibrosis. Paper presented at: American Society of Hematology Annual Meeting 2019; Dec 7-10, 2019; Orlando, FL. Blood 2019; 134(Supplement 1):670.

48. Kleppe M, Kwak M, Koppikar P, et al. JAK-STAT pathway activation in malignant and nonmalignant cells contributes to MPN pathogenesis and therapeutic response. Cancer Discov 2015;5(3):316–31.

49. Oikonomidou PR, Casu C, Yang Z, et al. Polycythemia is associated with bone loss and reduced osteoblast activity in mice. Osteoporos Int 2016;27(4): 1559–68.

50. Zhan H, Ma Y, Lin CH, et al. JAK2(V617F)-mutant megakaryocytes contribute to hematopoietic stem/progenitor cell expansion in a model of murine myeloproliferation. Leukemia 2016;30(12):2332–41.

51. Edelmann B, Gupta N, Schnoeder TM, et al. JAK2-V617F promotes venous thrombosis through beta1/beta2 integrin activation. J Clin Invest 2018;128(10): 4359–71.

52. Lamrani L, Lacout C, Ollivier V, et al. Hemostatic disorders in a JAK2V617F-driven mouse model of myeloproliferative neoplasm. Blood 2014;124(7): 1136–45.

53. Guy A, Gourdou-Latyszenok V, Le Lay N, et al. Vascular endothelial cell expression of JAK2(V617F) is sufficient to promote a pro-thrombotic state due to increased P-selectin expression. Haematologica 2019;104(1):70–81.

54. Hobbs CM, Manning H, Bennett C, et al. JAK2V617F leads to intrinsic changes in platelet formation and reactivity in a knock-in mouse model of essential thrombocythemia. Blood 2013;122(23):3787–97.

55. Wolach O, Sellar RS, Martinod K, et al. Increased neutrophil extracellular trap formation promotes thrombosis in myeloproliferative neoplasms. Sci Transl Med 2018;10(436):eaan8292.

56. Grinfeld J, Nangalia J, Baxter EJ, et al. Classification and personalized prognosis in myeloproliferative neoplasms. N Engl J Med 2018;379(15):1416–30.

57. Kameda T, Shide K, Yamaji T, et al. Loss of TET2 has dual roles in murine myeloproliferative neoplasms: disease sustainer and disease accelerator. Blood 2015; 125(2):304–15.

58. Chen E, Schneider RK, Breyfogle LJ, et al. Distinct effects of concomitant Jak2V617F expression and Tet2 loss in mice promote disease progression in myeloproliferative neoplasms. Blood 2015;125(2):327–35.

59. Jeong JJ, Gu X, Nie J, et al. Cytokine-regulated phosphorylation and activation of TET2 by JAK2 in hematopoiesis. Cancer Discov 2019;9(6):778–95.

60. Mochizuki-Kashio M, Aoyama K, Sashida G, et al. Ezh2 loss in hematopoietic stem cells predisposes mice to develop heterogeneous malignancies in an Ezh1-dependent manner. Blood 2015;126(10):1172–83.

61. Shimizu T, Kubovcakova L, Nienhold R, et al. Loss of Ezh2 synergizes with JAK2-V617F in initiating myeloproliferative neoplasms and promoting myelofibrosis. J Exp Med 2016;213(8):1479–96.

62. Yang Y, Akada H, Nath D, et al. Loss of Ezh2 cooperates with Jak2V617F in the development of myelofibrosis in a mouse model of myeloproliferative neoplasm. Blood 2016;127(26):3410–23.

63. Guo Y, Zhou Y, Yamatomo S, et al. ASXL1 alteration cooperates with JAK2V617F to accelerate myelofibrosis. Leukemia 2019;33(5):1287–91.

64. Vannucchi AM, Lasho TL, Guglielmelli P, et al. Mutations and prognosis in primary myelofibrosis. Leukemia 2013;27(9):1861–9.

65. Jacquelin S, Straube J, Cooper L, et al. Jak2V617F and Dnmt3a loss cooperate to induce myelofibrosis through activated enhancer-driven inflammation. Blood 2018;132(26):2707–21.

66. McKenney AS, Lau AN, Somasundara AVH, et al. JAK2/IDH-mutant-driven myeloproliferative neoplasm is sensitive to combined targeted inhibition. J Clin Invest 2018;128(2):789–804.

67. Lee SC, North K, Kim E, et al. Synthetic lethal and convergent biological effects of cancer-associated spliceosomal gene mutations. Cancer Cell 2018;34(2): 225–241 e228.

68. Mupo A, Seiler M, Sathiaseelan V, et al. Hemopoietic-specific Sf3b1-K700E knock-in mice display the splicing defect seen in human MDS but develop anemia without ring sideroblasts. Leukemia 2017;31(3):720–7.

69. Fei DL, Zhen T, Durham B, et al. Impaired hematopoiesis and leukemia development in mice with a conditional knock-in allele of a mutant splicing factor gene U2af1. Proc Natl Acad Sci U S A 2018;115(44):E10437–46.

70. Kim E, Ilagan JO, Liang Y, et al. SRSF2 mutations contribute to myelodysplasia by mutant-specific effects on exon recognition. Cancer Cell 2015;27(5):617–30.

71. Smeets MF, Tan SY, Xu JJ, et al. Srsf2(P95H) initiates myeloid bias and myelodysplastic/myeloproliferative syndrome from hemopoietic stem cells. Blood 2018;132(6):608–21.

72. Tong W, Zhang J, Lodish HF. Lnk inhibits erythropoiesis and Epo-dependent JAK2 activation and downstream signaling pathways. Blood 2005;105(12): 4604–12.

73. Buza-Vidas N, Antonchuk J, Qian H, et al. Cytokines regulate postnatal hematopoietic stem cell expansion: opposing roles of thrombopoietin and LNK. Genes Dev 2006;20(15):2018–23.

74. Bersenev A, Wu C, Balcerek J, et al. Lnk controls mouse hematopoietic stem cell self-renewal and quiescence through direct interactions with JAK2. J Clin Invest 2008;118(8):2832–44.

75. Takizawa H, Eto K, Yoshikawa A, et al. Growth and maturation of megakaryocytes is regulated by Lnk/Sh2b3 adaptor protein through crosstalk between cytokine- and integrin-mediated signals. Exp Hematol 2008;36(7):897–906.

76. Lv K, Jiang J, Donaghy R, et al. CBL family E3 ubiquitin ligases control JAK2 ubiquitination and stability in hematopoietic stem cells and myeloid malignancies. Genes Dev 2017;31(10):1007–23.

77. Sanada M, Suzuki T, Shih LY, et al. Gain-of-function of mutated C-CBL tumour suppressor in myeloid neoplasms. Nature 2009;460(7257):904–8.

78. Chan G, Kalaitzidis D, Usenko T, et al. Leukemogenic Ptpn11 causes fatal myeloproliferative disorder via cell-autonomous effects on multiple stages of hematopoiesis. Blood 2009;113(18):4414–24.

79. Xu D, Wang S, Yu WM, et al. A germline gain-of-function mutation in Ptpn11 (Shp-2) phosphatase induces myeloproliferative disease by aberrant activation of hematopoietic stem cells. Blood 2010;116(18):3611–21.

80. Li Q, Haigis KM, McDaniel A, et al. Hematopoiesis and leukemogenesis in mice expressing oncogenic NrasG12D from the endogenous locus. Blood 2011; 117(6):2022–32.

81. Hamarsheh S, Osswald L, Saller BS, et al. Oncogenic Kras(G12D) causes myeloproliferation via NLRP3 inflammasome activation. Nat Commun 2020;11(1): 1659.

82. Hsu JI, Dayaram T, Tovy A, et al. PPM1D mutations drive clonal hematopoiesis in response to cytotoxic chemotherapy. Cell Stem Cell 2018;23(5):700–713 e706.

83. Kaufmann KB, Grunder A, Hadlich T, et al. A novel murine model of myeloproliferative disorders generated by overexpression of the transcription factor NF-E2. J Exp Med 2012;209(1):35–50.

84. Jutzi JS, Bogeska R, Nikoloski G, et al. MPN patients harbor recurrent truncating mutations in transcription factor NF-E2. J Exp Med 2013;210(5):1003–19.

85. Rampal R, Ahn J, Abdel-Wahab O, et al. Genomic and functional analysis of leukemic transformation of myeloproliferative neoplasms. Proc Natl Acad Sci U S A 2014;111(50):E5401–10.

86. Tsuruta-Kishino T, Koya J, Kataoka K, et al. Loss of p53 induces leukemic transformation in a murine model of Jak2 V617F-driven polycythemia vera. Oncogene 2017;36(23):3300–11.

87. Bench AJ, Nacheva EP, Hood TL, et al. Chromosome 20 deletions in myeloid malignancies: reduction of the common deleted region, generation of a PAC/BAC contig and identification of candidate genes. UK Cancer Cytogenetics Group (UKCCG). Oncogene 2000;19(34):3902–13.

88. Huh J, Tiu RV, Gondek LP, et al. Characterization of chromosome arm 20q abnormalities in myeloid malignancies using genome-wide single nucleotide polymorphism array analysis. Genes Chromosomes Cancer 2010;49(4):390–9.

89. Jobe F, Patel B, Kuzmanovic T, et al. Deletion of Ptpn1 induces myeloproliferative neoplasm. Leukemia 2017;31(5):1229–34.

90. Stoner SA, Yan M, Liu KTH, et al. Hippo kinase loss contributes to del(20q) hematologic malignancies through chronic innate immune activation. Blood 2019; 134(20):1730–44.

91. Clarke M, Dumon S, Ward C, et al. MYBL2 haploinsufficiency increases susceptibility to age-related haematopoietic neoplasia. Leukemia 2013;27(3):661–70.

92. Heinrichs S, Conover LF, Bueso-Ramos CE, et al. MYBL2 is a sub-haploinsufficient tumor suppressor gene in myeloid malignancy. Elife 2013;2: e00825.

93. Fleischman AG, Maxson JE, Luty SB, et al. The CSF3R T618I mutation causes a lethal neutrophilic neoplasia in mice that is responsive to therapeutic JAK inhibition. Blood 2013;122(22):3628–31.

94. Jin X, Qin T, Zhao M, et al. Oncogenic N-Ras and Tet2 haploinsufficiency collaborate to dysregulate hematopoietic stem and progenitor cells. Blood Adv 2018; 2(11):1259–71.

95. Kunimoto H, Meydan C, Nazir A, et al. Cooperative epigenetic remodeling by TET2 Loss and NRAS mutation drives myeloid transformation and MEK inhibitor sensitivity. Cancer Cell 2018;33(1):44–59 e48.

96. Nakata Y, Ueda T, Nagamachi A, et al. Acquired expression of Cbl(Q367P) in mice induces dysplastic myelopoiesis mimicking chronic myelomonocytic leukemia. Blood 2017;129(15):2148–60.

97. Wang J, Liu Y, Li Z, et al. Endogenous oncogenic Nras mutation promotes aberrant GM-CSF signaling in granulocytic/monocytic precursors in a murine model of chronic myelomonocytic leukemia. Blood 2010;116(26):5991–6002.

98. Yoshimi A, Balasis ME, Vedder A, et al. Robust patient-derived xenografts of MDS/MPN overlap syndromes capture the unique characteristics of CMML and JMML. Blood 2017;130(4):397–407.

99. Reinisch A, Hernandez DC, Schallmoser K, et al. Generation and use of a humanized bone-marrow-ossicle niche for hematopoietic xenotransplantation into mice. Nat Protoc 2017;12(10):2169–88.

100. Celik H, Krug E, Zhang CR, et al. A Humanized animal model Predicts Clonal evolution and therapeutic vulnerabilities in myeloproliferative neoplasms. bioRxiv; 2020. https://doi.org/10.1101/2020.11.12.378810v1.

Important Pathologic Considerations for Establishing the Diagnosis of Myelofibrosis

Mohamed E. Salama, MD

KEYWORDS

• Myelofibrosis • Histopathology • Fibrosis • Osteosclerosis • Grading

KEY POINTS

- The 2017 World Health Organization diagnostic criteria for primary myelofibrosis emphasized the relevance of histopathology and introduced scoring schemas for reticulin - collagen fibrosis and osteosclerosis.
- Despite this notable progress, histopathologic evaluation of myelofibrosis suffers some level of inconsistency related to interobserver variability and preanalytical variables. Central pathologic review for multicenter clinical trials is well established as an important quality control measure to mitigate inconsistencies in interpretation.
- Next-generation sequencing provides diagnostic and prognostic implications and can serve as a guide for selection of myelofibrosis (MF) patients for participation in clinical trials.
- There is increasing evidence that the clinical features and outcomes of PMF and post–polycythemia vera–MF and post–thrombocythemia-MF differ, providing a rationale for their identification.
- Secondary nonneoplastic causes of MF might be associated with a more favorable prognosis than PMF, emphasizing the need for establishing an accurate diagnosis in order to pursue appropriate prognostication and risk-adapted therapy.

INTRODUCTION

Primary myelofibrosis is a clonal stem cell disorder that is recognized as a distinct entity within the broader World Health Organization (WHO) myeloproliferative neoplasms (MPN) category, which also encompasses polycythemia vera (PV) and essential thrombocythemia (ET). Primary myelofibrosis is further subclassified into "prefibrotic" (pre-PMF) and overtly fibrotic primary myelofibrosis (PMF).[1] To render a diagnosis of

Department of Laboratory Medicine and Pathology, Division of Hematopathology, Mayo Clinic School of Medicine, Mayo Clinic, 200 First Street Southwest, Rochester, MN 55905, USA
E-mail address: Salama.Mohamed@mayo.edu

Hematol Oncol Clin N Am 35 (2021) 267–278
https://doi.org/10.1016/j.hoc.2020.11.002
0889-8588/21/© 2020 Elsevier Inc. All rights reserved.

pre-PMF or PMF, one must satisfy all major criteria and at least 1 minor criterion according to 2107 WHO revision for classification of hematopoietic neoplasms.[2] Overt myelofibrosis may also occur during the clinical course of a subset of ET and PV patients, which are diagnosed as post-ET and post-PV myelofibrosis (MF), in accordance with the International Working Group for MPN Research and Treatment (IWG-MRT) criteria (**Table 1**).

WHO emphasizes the role of morphology and histotopography of megakaryocytes (MK) in the classification of MPN. As such, histologic examination of peripheral blood smear and adequate bone marrow (BM) biopsy is indispensable for making the diagnosis of myelofibrotic disorders. In this review, the author highlights important pitfalls and pathology diagnostic considerations.

Discussion

Diagnosis of myelofibrosis

A classic picture of peripheral blood smears from a patient with PMF will show leukoerythroblastosis with dacrocytes (tear droperthrocytes) and anisopoikilocytosis. Leukoerythroblastosis is a manifestation of extramedullary hematopoiesis and is characterized by the presence of erythroid precursors, myeloid left shift with notable blasts, and teardrop cells in the peripheral blood. The number of circulating CD34[+] blasts are generally higher in PMF compared with other MPN; however, blasts appear in large numbers in the peripheral blood in PMF patients only in later stages of the disease. It is important to keep in mind that the etiologic causes of a leukoerythroblastic blood picture are diverse and have been described in hematologic disorders, including hemolytic and megaloblastic anemias, infections, metastatic cancers, and other hematologic malignancies.[3] In contrast to PMF, the peripheral blood smear in pre-PMF might not display overt leukoerythroblastosis.[2]

The BM histopathology examination entails microscopic evaluation of cellularity, lineage proliferation or reduction, and atypical morphology, along with quantification of blasts, fibrosis level, and osteosclerosis. Typically, the BM biopsy of PMF shows clear-cut reticulin fibrosis (ie, fibrosis grades 2 and 3). The BM is often hypercellular with increased MKs and granulocytic proliferation. However, cellular variability is not

Table 1
The International Working Group for Myelofibrosis Research and Treatment criteria for diagnosis of postessential thrombocythemia and postpolycythemia vera myelofibrosis

	Post-ET MF	Post-PV MF
Required criteria	Documented previous diagnosis of ET according to WHO criteria Bone marrow fibrosis grades 2–3 (on a 0–3 scale)	Documented previous diagnosis of PV according to WHO criteria Bone marrow fibrosis grades 2–3 (on 0–3 scale)
Additional criteria	Anemia and a <2 g/dL decrease in hemoglobin level Leukoerythroblastic peripheral blood picture Increasing splenomegaly Development of ≥1 constitutional symptoms Increased LDH	Anemia or sustained loss of requirement for phlebotomy Leukoerythroblastic peripheral blood picture Increasing splenomegaly Development of ≥1 constitutional symptoms

Diagnosis of both post-ET MF and post-PV MF must meet both required criteria and at least 2 additional criteria uncommon with normocellular or hypocellular areas of the biopsy. MK are conspicuously atypical and are arranged in tight clusters with juxtaposed cell surface without intervening hematopoietic marrow cells. MK typically will show variability based on the size of their cytoplasm. MK nuclei are bulbous ("cloudlike"), and hypolobated with dysmorphic and bizarre forms (**Fig. 1**). Denuded and bare nuclei with condensed chromatin are common. The BM in pre-PMF typically shows hypercellularity, with increased granulocytes and atypical MKs but without a significant increase in reticulin and/or collagen fibers (ie, fibrosis grades 0 and 1). Erythropoiesis is often reduced. The identification of atypical MK morphology and histotopography is fundamental for the recognition of pre-PMF. MKs form dense clusters and are frequently adjacent to the BM vascular sinuses and bone trabeculae. In addition, MKs will show variability in size and shape and will include hyperchromatic, bulbous, cloudlike, or balloon-shaped nuclei. Small forms are common and often require immunohistochemical staining with megakaryocytic markers, such as CD61 for visualization.

One notable improvement in revised 2017 WHO classification is the ability to distinguish pre-PMF from true ET. This distinction is important given that pre-PMF has a different predicted survival and progression rate as compared with ET. In contrast to pre-PMF, the MKs in ET are characteristically large with hyperlobulated nuclei ("staghornlike") and are arranged in loose clusters. Despite this notable progress, significant limitations and pitfalls exist and are discussed herein.

Pitfalls in grading of fibrosis, collagen deposition and osteosclerosis

MF is a collectively descriptive term that is used to label fibrotic changes affecting the BM in patients with PMF, post-PV, and post-ET MF as well as other nonneoplastic conditions. Patients with PMF, post-PV MF, and post-ET MF often have clinical similarities as well as indistinguishable histomorphologic BM findings particularly with marked fibrotic changes. However, distinct cytogenetic abnormalities and histomorphologic characteristics related to the underlying disease can provide support for their discrimination. The hallmark of all MF entities is increased density of reticulin fibers, along with increasing amount of collagen deposition and progressive osteosclerosis. It is important to stress the importance of assessing both reticulin and collagen deposition, as both are required to construct a comprehensive assessment of stromal fibrosis composition and extent.[4] Typically, reticulin fibers are visualized using silver

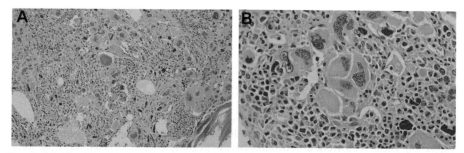

Fig. 1. (A) The histologic section from BM biopsy shows characteristic MF clues, including cell layering, increased MK, and dilated sinuses with intrasinusoidal hematopoietic cells (hematoxylin and eosin [H&E] stain, original magnification ×200). (B) This high-power magnification shows MK with hypolobated and bulbous nuclei arranged in tight cluster with no intervening hematopoietic cells (H&E stain, original magnification ×500).

impregnation methods, such as Gomori stain; however, collagen deposition is assessed using Masson trichrome staining of core biopsy sections.

The harmonized BM reticulin fibrosis grading system adopted by the WHO (**Fig. 2**, **Table 2**) enabled a high degree of reproducibility between pathologists.[2,4,5] However, the system suffers from some level of inconsistency related to the heterogeneity of fibrosis within a BM biopsy section and variations related to staining or other preanalytical variables, such as fixation and decalcification techniques. Reports that address these limitations are scarce. A recent consensus study for THE evaluation of reticulin fibrosis noted the frequent heterogeneity of fibrosis patterns and recommended the final score to be determined based on the highest grade present in at least 30% of the BM area. This approach improved reproducibility of fibrosis scoring from 76.2% to 83% between hematopathologists.[2,4]

Pitfalls to watch for in the assessment of reticulin fibrosis include assurance of adequate core biopsy size (1.5-cm core length), avoiding areas with significant crush artifacts, and insuring appropriate section thickness. Thick sections can lead to overestimation of fiber density. A staining of another section is warranted in cases with observed overstaining or weak staining. Clues to overstaining are distinct framing of adipocytes or dark precipitation, and inadequate weak staining can be inferred by the lack of internal perivascular control staining.[4]

The 2017 WHO grading system for MF did incorporate a scoring schema for collagen fibrosis and osteosclerosis.[2] This modification is a significant addition to the grading of MF, as it showed an overall hematopathologist agreement of 88.4%

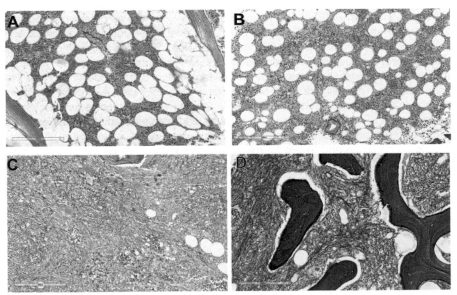

Fig. 2. Reticulin-stained sections showing MF scoring with reactive internal control as noted by blood vessel wall staining and dispersed linear fibers without crossover indicating MF-0 score (A). Loose meshwork of reticulin fibers with conspicuous crossover, MF-1 (B). Reticulin fiber density is markedly increased with diffuse and extensive intersection. Focal areas of thick fibers representing collagen depositions along with focal osteosclerosis could be recognized in these cases. MF-2 (C). There is increased reticulin fiber density with diffuse and extensive intersection, but with notable course and thick bundle of collagen along with significant osteosclerosis, MF-3 (D). (Silver stain, original magnification ×200).

Table 2
World Health Organization 2008 criteria for semiquantitative bone marrow fibrosis grading

MF-0	Scattered linear reticulin with no intersections (crossovers) corresponding to normal bone marrow
MF-1	Loose network of reticulin with many intersections, especially in perivascular areas
MF-2	Diffuse and dense increase in reticulin with extensive intersections, occasionally with focal bundles of thick fibers mostly consistent with collagen and/or focal osteosclerosis
MF-3	Diffuse and dense increase in reticulin with extensive intersections and coarse bundles of thick fibers mostly consistent with collagen, usually associated with osteosclerosis

Fiber density should be assessed in hematopoietic (cellular) areas.
Adapted from Thiele J, Kvasnicka HM, Tefferi A et al. Primary myelofibrosis In: Swerdlow SH, Campo E, Harris NL, et al (eds). WHO Classifications of Tumours of Haematopoietic and Lymphoid Tissues 4th edn. IARC Press: Lyon, France, 2008, pp 44–47.

and 92.6%, respectively.[4] Collagen deposition scoring takes into account either a local or an extensive deposition of collagen fibers in the BM space because of the employment of the 4-grade system (**Fig. 3**).[2–4] Scoring of osteosclerosis is also based on a 4-grade system reflecting the level of formation of new bone and trabecular thickness (**Fig. 4**).[2–4] Significant collagen deposition and osteosclerosis are associated with greater degree reticulin fibrosis, which remains the most significant biologic factor in

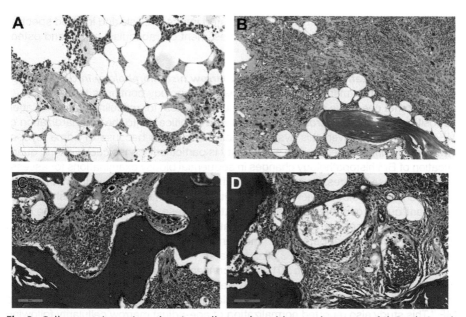

Fig. 3. Collagen stain sections showing collagen deposition scoring system. (*A*) Grade 0: only positive staining is depicted in the wall of the blood vessel, indicating adequate internal control. (*B*) Grade 1: Note only focal central collagen deposition without connecting meshwork. (*C*) Grade 1: More prominent central and paratrabecular deposition of collagen with focal bridging fibrosis. (*D*) Grade 3: There is diffuse effacement by collagen bundles replacing most BM hematopoietic space (Masson trichrome stain, original magnification ×200).

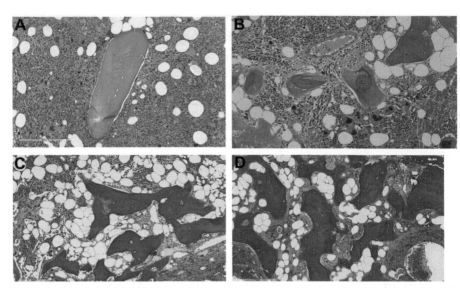

Fig. 4. Histologic sections depicting trabecular changes and osteosclerosis scoring in MF. (*A*) Grade 0: Normal trabecular bone architecture with smooth and defined trabecular border. (*B*) Grade 1: Note the new bone formation with focal buddings and spikes. (*C*) Grade 2: There is diffuse irregularity of bone trabecule with notable increased trabecular thickness and focal bridging connections. (*D*) Grade 3: There is diffuse and extensive new bone formation with effacement of BM hematopoietic space (H&E stain, original magnification ×200).

grading. The potential use of computer-assisted image analysis and infrared spectroscopic imaging as tools for quantitative assessment of trabecular volume and osteosclerosis grading has been reported.[6,7]

Assessment of treatment impact by bone marrow histomorphology in clinical trials
Assessment of treatment impact by BM histomorphology continues to represent an area of unmet need. The simplified WHO scoring system for reticulin fibrosis, collagen deposition, and osteosclerosis has contributed significantly to the standardization of MF evaluation; however, this system remains subjective because of some level of interobserver inconsistency. This subjectivity is particularly conspicuous during quantification of BM histopathology changes in sequential biopsy examinations for assessment of disease progression or treatment efficacy as a surrogate endpoint in clinical trials. Central pathology review for multicenter clinical trials is well established as an important quality control measure to mitigate for these inconsistencies.[8,9] The challenge was confirmed by the fair overall rate of agreement (low kappa statistic of 0.27) between the local pathologist and central pathology review MF grade assignment in 261 MPN patients from 3 clinical trials.[8]

Successful application of the 2017 WHO consensus-based adjudication in a central pathology review confirmed the long-term effect of ruxolitinib therapy as a disease-modifying agent to reverse or markedly delay BM fibrosis progression in advanced MF.[9] This study also reported normalization of age-adjust marrow cellularity following therapy in most cases in association with an improvement or stabilization of marrow fibrosis at 24-, 48-, and 60-month follow-up timepoints.[9] It is worth pointing out that assessment of marrow cellularity in the setting of marrow fibrosis remains an area that lacks consensus definition particularly with regards to accounting for the fibrotic areas.

Interestingly, fibrosis grade concordance between pathologists on 728 BM biopsies from clinical trials of fedratinib (SAR302503) was reported to be significantly lower for biopsies taken after therapy compared with those at baseline,[5] a finding further speaking to the need for more objective approaches. Whole-slide imaging coupled with image analysis has been proposed as a sensitive adjunct to morphology for detecting changes in the level of marrow fibrosis in clinical trials.[6,10] In addition, a stereology-based method has proven to provide A high level of reproducibility and can create a nonbiased random sampling to measure heterogeneity of marrow fibrosis.[11]

Clinical relevance of other testing beyond bone marrow histomorphology

A great level of agreement between pathologists was reported on the diagnosis of PMF compared with ET or PV.[12] However, it is worth highlighting that using histopathology alone to diagnose an MPN has limitations and that the availability of clinical data and other testing results to improve the accuracy of diagnostic interpretation of histomorphology cannot be emphasized.[13] Driver mutations involving JAK2V617F, *CALR*, and *MPL* are regarded as clonal markers that support PMF diagnosis. In the absence of these mutations, the presence of other clonal markers consistent with MF or the absence of reactive BM fibrosis meets this major criterion for MF diagnosis. The initial evaluation of the PMF patient typically begins with molecular testing for JAK2V617F mutation. If JAK2V617F testing is negative, then reflex testing for *CALR* and *MPL* mutations is contemplated. Immunostaining using antibody specifically recognizing the C-terminal peptide derived from all the frameshift mutations of *CALR* is commercially available, serve as a rapid test, and is a sensitive surrogate for the molecular assay (**Fig. 5**).[14] All 3 driver mutations are negative in approximately 10% of cases, so-called triple-negative (TN) cases. Detection of other common myeloid malignancy mutations in TN cases using large-scale next-generation sequencing (NGS) can help establish the clonal nature of the disease particularly when nonclonal causes of MF are being considered. In addition to establishing the diagnosis, NGS can contribute to molecular risk stratification, and management decisions, including clinical trial selection for patients when they are being evaluated for

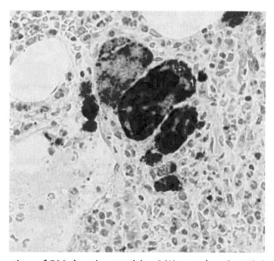

Fig. 5. Histologic section of BM showing positive MK cytoplasmic staining reactive to calreticulin antibody (CALR IHC stain, original magnification ×600).

MF. Similarly, karyotyping and fluorescence in situ hybridization testing can be helpful in discriminating PMF from myelodysplastic syndrome (MDS) with marrow fibrosis as well as providing some prognostic information.

Recent discoveries and characterization of driver mutations in JAK2, CALR, and MPL along with other somatic mutations have significantly improved the understanding of PMF pathogenesis and molecular prognostication relevance.[15] For example, detection of somatic mutations in ASXL1, EZH2, SRSF2, or IDH1/2, as well as the a lack of driver mutations in TN cases, denotes high-molecular-risk disease with a worse outcome and higher risk for transformation to acute leukemia.[16]

Prognosis and disease progression

BM from PMF patients usually contains foci of immature cells; however, myeloblasts typically account for less than 10% of the BM cellularity. Immunohistochemistry staining for CD34 and CD117 is useful for enumeration and localization of BM blasts in a fibrotic marrow. In patients with established PMF diagnosis, the identification of 10% to 19% blasts in the peripheral blood and/or BM and visualization of cluster formation and/or an abnormal endosteal location in the BM indicate an accelerated phase of the disease, whereas the finding of $\geq$20 blasts is diagnostic of blastic transformation. Transformation of PMF to acute leukemia occurs in 10% to 20% of cases within 10 years of diagnosis. Monocytosis is also reported to be a strong adverse predictor of inferior survival in PMF.[17]

Progression of BM fibrosis has prognostic implications. For example, it is well recognized that patients with PMF and post-PV or post-ET MF have a worse prognosis compared with patients with pre-PMF, PV, and ET.[18–21] The prognostication systems currently in use are based primarily on clinical characteristics; however, the Dynamic International Prognostic Scoring System also incorporates cytogenetics in the risk assessment. Two newly introduced risk-stratification systems for PMF include genetically inspired prognostic scoring system (GIPSS) and mutation- and karyotype-enhanced international prognostic scoring system (MIPSS70+). GIPSS represents a practical risk-assessment model based only on karyotype and a limited number of mutations and features 4 risk groups. MIPSS70+ (version 2.0) applies key clinical characteristics, cytogenetics, and mutations to stratify cases into 5 risk categories.[3] The MIPSS70: Mutation-Enhanced International Prognostic Score System for Transplantation-Age Patients with Primary Myelofibrosis does incorporate marrow fibrosis for assessing MF patient prognosis.

Differential diagnosis of myelofibrosis

A variety of other pathologic conditions could be associated with MF. As such, the appropriate caution must be exercised once MF is observed, particularly in TN PMF, and further investigation is warranted. In addition to BM morphology, other clinical findings (eg, splenomegaly), leukocyte count, karyotype, and molecular testing can serve as a guide to correct diagnosis.

Myeloid neoplasms associated with marrow fibrosis include acute myeloid leukemia (AML) with MF and myelodysplastic syndrome with myelofibrosis (MDS-MF). These conditions tend to have similar pathologic and laboratory characteristics and a misdiagnosis can occur because of overlapping morphology with PMF. Both panmyelosis with MF and acute megakaryoblastic leukemia with MF represent subtypes of AML that will show increased peripheral blood or BM blasts in a fibrotic background. CD34, CD41, and CD117 immunohistochemical stains are essential in these cases to highlight the increased (>20%) blast, which could be easily overlooked in the BM biopsy by morphology or a dry tap, limiting the ability to identify blasts in peripheral blood or BM aspirate smear either by morphology or by flow cytometry. Multilineage dysplasia and cytogenetic abnormalities commonly found in MDS patients, such as −5/del(5q), −7/del(7q), or +8, are critical to discriminate MDS-MF from PMF.[22] Other malignancies commonly associated with BM fibrosis include metastatic adenocarcinomas, Hodgkin lymphoma, mastocytosis, multiple myeloma, and hairy cell leukemia. In contrast to PMF, secondary MF associated with other malignancies lacks the characteristic MK tight clustering and nuclear dysplasia of PMF and often show higher degrees of reticulin fibrosis without expansion of the granulocytic lineage.[23,24]

Other reactive causes of MF that one must be consider while diagnosing MF include autoimmune conditions and infections (eg, tuberculosis, osteomyelitis, and visceral leishmaniasis). Autoimmune myelofibrosis (AIMF) is observed in association with systemic lupus erythematosus, systemic sclerosis, and Sjogren syndrome, but is also observed in patients who have autoantibodies without well-defined autoimmune disorders. AIMF has been proposed as a distinct entity that has a benign clinical course and responds well to steroids and/or other immunosuppressive therapy.[25] Peripheral cytopenias are the most common presentations in AIMF, and the BM is often hypercellular with erythroid and megakaryocytic hyperplasia noted in three-quarters of the cases. Granulocytic hyperplasia is noted in about one-third of cases. Although marrow fibrosis is often mild (1+ MF) in most cases, moderate (2+ MF) or marked (3+ MF) reticulin fibrosis is noted in 10% and 4% of the AIMF cases, respectively. In contrast to PMF, AIMF does not present with splenomegaly, eosinophilia, or basophilia. In addition, the absence of MK atypia or tight clustering, typically seen in PMF along with prominent lymphoid infiltrate in the BM, should be regarded as a clue to consider AIMF. Mild polytypic plasmacytosis and lymphoid aggregates are noted in the vast majority of cases, and a small subset of cases exhibits only interstitial lymphoid infiltrates. The lymphoid aggregates are typically well circumscribed, distributed in non-paratrabecular locations, and composed of small mature T cells.[25]

BM fibrosis also has been reported in a variety of other conditions, including a healing fracture site, osteopathies, and metabolic conditions (eg, hyperparathyroidism and Paget disease), as well as a result of the effects of medications (eg, eltrombopag, a thrombopoietin receptor agonist).[23,24,26,27]

Early-onset BM fibrosis should raise the possibility of nonneoplastic causes. Several studies reported BM fibrosis in the context of gray platelet syndrome (GPS) and other inherited platelet disorders (IPD) associated with variants in MPIG6B, Src family kinase member SRC, and VPS45. In the author's institution and in the literature, BM fibrosis noted in IPD is most associated with GPS. BM evaluation in these cases often shows normal MK number and histotopography (**Fig. 6**). Early recognition of IPD is critical for the care of these patients, given the progressive nature of MF and associated deterioration of peripheral counts often requiring transfusions.[28–30]

DISCERNING PRIMARY FROM SECONDARY POST–ESSENTIAL THROMBOCYTHEMIA AND POST–POLYCYTHEMIA VERA MYELOFIBROSIS

The diagnosis of post-ET MF and post-PV MF, together referred to here as secondary myelofibrosis (SMF), requires establishing moderate (MF 2+) or marked (MF 3+) fibrosis as documented in BM histopathological examination. Significant MF may obscure the BM histologic features of the underlying primary MPN to the degree that makes cases morphologically indistinguishable from PMF based on morphology alone. As such, adherence to IWG-MRT criteria (see **Table 1**) is required to make the diagnosis in these cases.

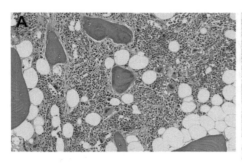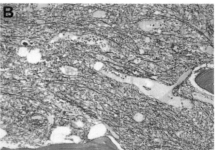

Fig. 6. Histologic section from a patient with IPD with MPIG6B nutation showing MK without atypia or histotopographic abnormalities (*A*) (H&E stain, original magnification ×200). Note the increased reticulin meshwork with frequent crossing indicating grade 2 MF (*B*) (reticulin stain, original magnification ×200).

Although PMF and SMF may receive the same treatment in clinical practice today, there is evidence that PMF and SMF patients differ in survival. For example, post-ET MF patients have a superior overall survival as compared with PMF and post-PV MF patients.[31] In addition, a distinct molecular risk profile was recently reported in PMF and SMF, whereby mutation involving *ASXL1*, *EZH2*, *SRSF2*, and *IDH* identifies PMF patients who are at risk for premature death or leukemic transformation, but only *SRSF2* mutations are reported to predict inferior survival in SMF patients.[16,32] In addition, a higher percent of complex karyotypic abnormalities were noted in SMF in contrast to PMF.[33] Recently, the MF secondary to the PV and ET prognostic model was introduced to effectively stratify patients at diagnosis into 4 distinct risk categories.[34–36] Taken together, these findings indicate that there are clinical and biological differences between PMF and SMF that influence outcomes, providing a rationale for separation of PMF from SMF.[33]

DISCLOSURE

The author has nothing to disclose.

REFERENCES

1. Arber DA, Orazi A, Hasserjian R, et al. The 2016 revision to the World Health Organization classification of myeloid neoplasms and acute leukemia. Blood 2016; 127(20):2391–405. Blood. 2016;128(3):462-463.
2. Swerdlow S, Campo E, Harris N, et al. WHO classification of tumours of haematopoietic and lymphoid tissues. Revised 4th edition. Lyon (France): IARC; 2017.
3. Clifford GO. The clinical significance of leukoerythroblastic anemia. Med Clin North Am 1966;50(3):779–90.
4. Kvasnicka HM, Beham-Schmid C, Bob R, et al. Problems and pitfalls in grading of bone marrow fibrosis, collagen deposition and osteosclerosis - a consensus-based study. Histopathology 2016;68(6):905–15.
5. Pozdnyakova O, Wu K, Patki A, et al. High concordance in grading reticulin fibrosis and cellularity in patients with myeloproliferative neoplasms. Mod Pathol 2014;27(11):1447–54.
6. Teman CJ, Wilson AR, Perkins SL, et al. Quantification of fibrosis and osteosclerosis in myeloproliferative neoplasms: a computer-assisted image study. Leuk Res 2010;34(7):871–6.

7. Mankar R, Bueso-Ramos CE, Yin CC, et al. Automated osteosclerosis grading of clinical biopsies using infrared spectroscopic imaging. Anal Chem 2020;92(1): 749–57.

8. Pozdnyakova O, Rodig S, Bhandarkar S, et al. The importance of central pathology review in international trials: a comparison of local vs. central bone marrow reticulin grading. Leukemia 2015;1:241–4.

9. Kvasnicka HM, Thiele J, Bueso-Ramos CE, et al. Long-term effects of ruxolitinib versus best available therapy on bone marrow fibrosis in patients with myelofibrosis. J Hematol Oncol 2018;11(1):42.

10. Zahr AA, Salama ME, Carreau N, et al. Bone marrow fibrosis in myelofibrosis: pathogenesis, prognosis and targeted strategies. Haematologica 2016;101(6): 660–71.

11. Eberhard DA, Potts SJ, Young GD, et al. Stereology and computer-based image analysis quantifies heterogeneity and improves reproducibility for grading reticulin in bone marrow. In: Eberhard DA, Potts SJ, Young GD, editors. Histopathology in pharmaceutical product development. 1st edition. NY, USA: Springer Publishing; 2014.

12. Garmezy B, Schaefer JK, Mercer J, et al. A provider's guide to primary myelofibrosis: pathophysiology, diagnosis, and management [published online ahead of print, 2020 Apr 7]. Blood Rev 2020;100691. https://doi.org/10.1016/j.blre. 2020.100691.

13. Gianelli U, Bossi A, Cortinovis I, et al. Reproducibility of the WHO histological criteria for the diagnosis of Philadelphia chromosome-negative myeloproliferative neoplasms. Mod Pathol 2014;27(6):814–22.

14. Bonifacio M, Montemezzi R, Parisi A, et al. CAL2 monoclonal antibody is a rapid and sensitive assay for the detection of calreticulin mutations in essential thrombocythemia patients. Ann Hematol 2019;98(10):2339–46.

15. Tefferi A. Novel mutations and their functional and clinical relevance in myeloproliferative neoplasms: JAK2, MPL, TET2, ASXL1, CBL, IDH and IKZF1. Leukemia 2010;24(6):1128–38.

16. Vannucchi AM, Lasho TL, Guglielmelli P, et al. Mutations and prognosis in primary myelofibrosis. Leukemia 2013;27(9):1861–9.

17. Tefferi A, Shah S, Mudireddy M, et al. Monocytosis is a powerful and independent predictor of inferior survival in primary myelofibrosis. Br J Haematol 2018;183(5): 835–8.

18. Gianelli U, Fiori S, Cattaneo D, et al. Prognostic significance of a comprehensive histologic evaluation of reticulin fibrosis, collagen deposition and osteosclerosis in primary myelofibrosis patients. Histopathology 2017;71(6):897–908.

19. Guglielmelli P, Pacilli A, Rotunno G, et al. Presentation and outcome of patients with 2016 WHO diagnosis of prefibrotic and overt primary myelofibrosis. Blood 2017;129:3227–36.

20. Guglielmelli P, Rotunno G, Pacilli A, et al. Prognostic impact of bone marrow fibrosis in primary myelofibrosis. A study of the AGIMM group on 490 patients. Am J Hematol 2016;91:918–22.

21. Guglielmelli P, Vannucchi AM. The prognostic impact of bone marrow fibrosis in primary myelofibrosis. Am J Hematol 2016;91:918–22.

22. Bae E, Park CJ, Cho YU, et al. Differential diagnosis of myelofibrosis based on WHO 2008 criteria: acute panmyelosis with myelofibrosis, acute megakaryoblastic leukemia with myelofibrosis, primary myelofibrosis and myelodysplastic syndrome with myelofibrosis. Int J Lab Hematol 2013;35(6):629–36.

23. Sharma P, Pali HP, Mishra PC, et al. Inability of immunomorphometric assessment of angiogenesis to distinguish primary versus secondary myelofibrosis. Anal Quant Cytol Histol 2011;33(4):236–44.

24. Kuter DJ, Bain B, Mufti G, et al. Bone marrow fibrosis: pathophysiology and clinical significance of increased bone marrow stromal fibres. Br J Haematol 2007; 139(3):351–402.

25. Vergara-Lluri ME, Piatek CI, Pullarkat V, et al. Autoimmune myelofibrosis: an update on morphologic features in 29 cases and review of the literature. Hum Pathol 2014;45(11):2183–91.

26. Ghanima W, Geyer JT, Lee CS, et al. Bone marrow fibrosis in 66 patients with immune thrombocytopenia treated with thrombopoietin-receptor agonists: a single-center, long-term follow-up. Haematologica 2014;99(5):937–44.

27. Brynes RK, Wong RS, Thein MM, et al. A 2-year, longitudinal, prospective study of the effects of eltrombopag on bone marrow in patients with chronic immune thrombocytopenia. Acta Haematol 2017;137(2):66–72.

28. Delario MR, Sheehan AM, Ataya R, et al. Clinical, Histopathologic, and genetic features of pediatric primary myelofibrosis–an entity different from adults. Am J Hematol 2012;87:461–4.

29. Saliba AN, Ferrer A, Gangat N, et al. Aetiology and outcomes of secondary myelofibrosis occurring in the context of inherited platelet disorders: a single institutional study of four patients [published online ahead of print, 2020 Jun 22]. Br J Haematol 2020. https://doi.org/10.1111/bjh.16897.

30. Hofmann I, Geer MJ, Vogtle T, et al. Congenital macrothrombocytopenia with focal myelofibrosis due to mutations in human G6b-B is rescued in humanized mice. Blood 2018;132:1399–412.

31. Masarova L, Bose P, Daver N, et al. Patients with post-essential thrombocythemia and post-polycythemia vera differ from patients with primary myelofibrosis. Leuk Res 2017;59:110–6.

32. Rotunno G, Pacilli A, Artusi V, et al. Epidemiology and clinical relevance of mutations in postpolycythemia vera and postessential thrombocythemia myelofibrosis: a study on 359 patients of the AGIMM group. Am J Hematol 2016;91(7):681–6.

33. Passamonti F, Mora B, Barraco D, et al. Post-ET and Post-PV myelofibrosis: updates on a distinct prognosis from primary myelofibrosis. Curr Hematol Malig Rep 2018;13(3):173–82.

34. Passamonti F, Giorgino T, Mora B, et al. A clinical-molecular prognostic model to predict survival in patients with post polycythemia vera and post essential thrombocythemia myelofibrosis. Leukemia 2017;31(12):2726–31.

35. Hernandez-Boluda JC, Pereira A, Correa JG, et al. Performance of the myelofibrosis secondary to PV and ET-prognostic model (MYSEC-PM) in a series of 262 patients from the Spanish Registry of Myelofibrosis. Leukemia 2018;32: 553–5.

36. Palandri F, Palumbo GA, Iurlo A, et al. Differences in presenting features, outcome and prognostic models in patients with primary myelofibrosis and post-polycythemia vera and/or post-essential thrombocythemia myelofibrosis treated with ruxolitinib. New perspective of the MYSEC-PM in a large multicenter study. Semin Hematol 2018;55(4):248–55.

Application of Single-Cell Approaches to Study Myeloproliferative Neoplasm Biology

Daniel Royston, MBChB, BMSc, DPhil, FRCPath[a],
Adam J. Mead, MA, BMBCh, FTCP, FRCPath, PhD[b],*,
Bethan Psaila, MA, MBBS, MRCP, FRCPath, PhD[b]

KEYWORDS

- Myeloproliferative neoplasm • Single-cell genomics • Digital pathology

KEY POINTS

- Myeloproliferative neoplasms (MPNs) are an excellent tractable disease model for the application of single-cell approaches to study human disease.
- Single-cell genetic analysis of MPNs has provided important insights into disease latency and the importance of the order of mutation acquisition during disease pathogenesis, of broader relevance for cancer biology.
- Single-cell transcriptomics has revealed aberrant megakaryocyte differentiation trajectories in persons with myeloproliferative neoplasms.
- Digital pathology analysis combined with deep learning allows objective analysis of megakaryocyte heterogeneity in persons with MPNs.

INTRODUCTION

Philadelphia-negative myeloproliferative neoplasms (MPNs) are an excellent tractable disease model of a number of aspects of human cancer biology, including genetic evolution, tissue-associated fibrosis, and cancer stem cells.[1,2] MPN is associated with long disease duration, well-characterized normal hematopoietic hierarchy, ability to purify cell populations by flow cytometry, and ease of accessibility of tissue derived from the malignant clone, facilitating the study of how this disease perturbs normal blood cell development through time. Accordingly, new technologies developed to study cancer biology have often been pioneered for the study of MPN. In this review,

[a] Nuffield Division of Clinical Laboratory Sciences, Radcliffe Department of Medicine and NIHR Biomedical Research Centre, University of Oxford, Headley Way, Oxford OX39DS, UK; [b] Medical Research Council (MRC) Molecular Haematology Unit, MRC Weatherall Institute of Molecular Medicine, NIHR Biomedical Research Centre, University of Oxford, Headley Way, Oxford OX3 9DS, UK
* Corresponding author.
E-mail address: adam.mead@imm.ox.ac.uk

Hematol Oncol Clin N Am 35 (2021) 279–293
https://doi.org/10.1016/j.hoc.2021.01.002
hemonc.theclinics.com

we discuss recent insights into MPN biology gained from the application of a number of new single-cell technologies to study human disease: single-cell genomics, single-cell transcriptomics and digital pathology (**Fig. 1**).

SINGLE-CELL GENOMICS

In the era of personalized medicine, genetic intratumoral heterogeneity (ITH) is increasingly recognized as a critical factor defining the behavior of a particular tumor in terms of clinical presentation, response to treatment, and risk of disease progression.[3] Although bulk next generation sequencing (NGS) techniques have undoubtedly provided extensive insights into genetic diversity of clones within any given tumor,[4,5] ultimately ITH can only be fully resolved using single-cell technologies.[6] For example, inferring clonal structures from bulk variant allele fractions is inherently confounded by the presence of loss of heterozygosity or convergent evolution in which the same genetic events might occur multiple times in the same tumor.[7,8] This makes it difficult to elucidate which mutations are present in the same clone, to accurately measure clonal diversity during therapy, to track disease evolution, or determine the order of mutations.

MPN has proven to be an important disease model providing an illustration of how single-cell genomics techniques can be applied to provide new insights into disease biology and how the technology might be moved toward application for precision medicine. Indeed, to a degree, single-cell genomics approaches are already in routine clinical use in myeloid diseases through application of cytogenetic analysis, including fluorescent in situ hybridization. The most common driver mutation in MPN occurs in exon 14 of the Janus kinase 2 (*JAK2*) gene, *JAK2V617F*, causing constitutive JAK-signal transducer and activator of transcription (JAK-STAT) signaling and driving the

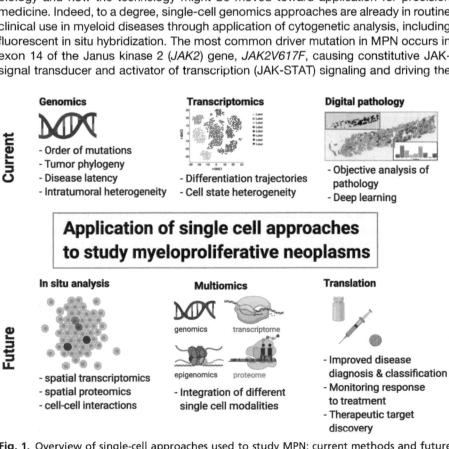

Fig. 1. Overview of single-cell approaches used to study MPN: current methods and future applications. Created with BioRender.com.

aberrant proliferation that is characteristic of MPN. Subsequently other mutations causing aberrant JAK-STAT signaling in MPN have been reported to occur in patients with MPN who are negative for the *JAK2V617F* mutation,[9–11] confirming that constitutive JAK-STAT signaling is the key pathway driving MPN phenotype.[12] The mutational landscape of MPN has been extensive studied, revealing that MPNs are genetically relatively simple compared with other tumors.[12,13] Together with other disease characteristics described in the introduction, this makes MPN an ideal tractable model for the application of single-cell genomics to understand the genetic evolution and clonal selection of mutant cells during disease development and progression. Consequently, single-cell assessment of genetic clonal evolution in MPN already has a rich history for the study of MPN over many years. Earlier studies benefited from the application of well-established clonogenic hematopoietic assays,[2] overcoming limitations of direct genetic analysis of single cells by providing an expanded cell population derived from a single cell for genetic analysis. For example, through the analysis of X-chromosome linked polymorphisms, including the study of single-cell–derived hematopoietic colonies, it has long been appreciated that MPNs are clonal diseases[14,15] that develop on acquisition of a disease-initiating mutation in a single multipotent hematopoietic stem cell (HSC).[1] This mutant HSC clone undergoes a poorly understood process of clonal expansion over time, with subsequent proliferation of mature cells of the myeloid lineages.[1] At the time that the *JAK2V617F* mutation was first described,[16] it was demonstrated that *JAK2V617F* selectively promoted the growth of single-cell–derived erythropoietin-independent colonies in patients with polycythemia vera (PV).[17] This approach was also used to characterize clonal diversity in patients with MPN with concurrent *JAK2V617F* mutation and a cytogenetic abnormality, demonstrating that these genetic events were present in the same clone in some patients but in separate clones in others.[18] Furthermore, combined analysis of *JAK2V617F* zygosity and loss of heterozygosity breakpoints using microsatellite markers in 6495 colonies revealed that *JAK2V617F* homozygous clones are recurrently acquired in patients with PV and patients with essential thrombocythemia (ET).[19] However, PV was typically associated with presence of a dominant homozygous subclone, unlike in ET. The study of single-cell–derived colonies in MPN has more recently provided novel insights into the importance of the order of acquisition of driver mutations. Analysis of colonies derived from single cells from patients with JAK2 and TET2 co-mutated MPN revealed differences in disease phenotype and response to targeted therapy that were dependent on the order of acquisition of these mutations.[20] The acquisition of *JAK2V617F* first, followed by *TET2* mutation, was more likely to result in a PV phenotype, typically in younger patients, but if *JAK2V617F* was acquired on a *TET2*-mutated background ("*TET2*-first"), an ET phenotype was more frequent. Similar observations also applied to DNMT3A and JAK2 mutations.[21] Together these studies nicely illustrate how the study of MPN can provide insights into pathways of genetic evolution of broader relevance for cancer biology.

Although analysis of hematopoietic colonies is a powerful approach, it is also associated with certain limitations and potential biases, as not all stem/progenitors are capable of growing colonies in vitro. Direct genetic analysis of single cells provides a potential solution, but is more challenging than analysis of material derived from colonies due to the very small amount of starting material and extensive amplification required.[22] Single-cell mutation analysis can be carried out by targeted NGS of known mutations, single-cell exome, or whole-genome sequencing.[23] A number of methods have been developed, each with advantages and also limitations in terms of the spectrum of mutations that can be analyzed and the sensitivity and specificity of mutation detection.[22,23]   Whole-genome   and   whole-exome   techniques   allow   the characterization of new genetic events, whereas targeted techniques rely on detection of known mutations within a given tumor. Targeted mutational analysis is a higher throughput and more cost-effective approach than whole-exome or genome sequencing of single cells with improved sensitivity and specificity of mutation detection and high-throughput commercially available droplet-based platforms.[24] Whole-genome single-cell techniques are typically associated with higher rates of allelic dropout, although new approaches to study low-input genomic DNA look set to change this.[6,25] To help address such technical problems, a number of bioinformatics tools to resolve the tumor phylogenetic trees have been developed.[26–28]

One of the first examples of single-cell exome sequencing in human cancer was a case of JAK2-mutation negative MPN, where 58 cells were sequenced, revealing monoclonal evolution of the disease in this patient and potential new candidate mutations driving clonal evolution.[29] The integration of single-cell genotyping with fluorescence-activated cell-sorting purification of specific cell populations allows mutations to be mapped to distinct phenotypically defined cell types, confirming that all mutations in MPN can be tracked back to the phenotypic HSC population.[30] Single-cell targeted mutation analysis in serial samples from patients with myelofibrosis has revealed the very high level of clonal dominance in the CD34+ compartment seen in almost all patients with myelofibrosis.[31] This study also elucidated pathways of clonal evolution during JAK2 inhibitor therapy, and demonstrated that complex clonal architecture correlates with risk of disease progression, particularly in association with the acquisition of RAS/RTK pathway mutations.[31]

New technologies now allow targeted mutational analysis of single cells to be done in a high-throughput manner using droplet-based approaches. For example, some of the first examples of direct single-cell sequencing using the Tapestri platform report the study of patients with MPN. In rare cases in which JAK2, CALR, and/or MPL mutations co-occur, this approach was used to determine that the mutations are present in independent clones.[32] In a landmark study, the Tapestri platform has also recently been used to analyze 740,526 cells from 123 patients with myeloid malignancies, including cases of MPN that have progressed to secondary acute myeloid leukemia (AML).[24] As might be expected, the number of mutations present and clonal diversity was higher in AML than MPN and also higher in MPN than in clonal hematopoiesis. In 4 of 6 patients with transformation of MPN to secondary AML, a new dominant subclone emerged that in some cases was present as a minor subclone during chronic phase. In this study, the investigators also describe an exciting new methodology to combine protein expression at the single-cell level with genotyping to link phenotype and genotype.

Perhaps the most remarkable recent finding, revealed through single-cell genomics approaches, relates to the origins and disease latency of MPN. These studies used state-of-the-art single-colony whole-genome sequencing lineage tracing approaches that rely on identification of background somatic mutations as a "molecular clock" to determine the timing of clonal expansion and disease development following acquisition of the JAK2V617F mutation.[33,34] With the caveat that both papers are available only as "preprints" and have not yet undergone peer review, it is striking that both studies reach a similar conclusion that the JAK2V617F mutation was reported to be acquired typically decades before disease development; remarkably, in many cases, the mutation was acquired in utero or in early childhood and yet only caused disease after many decades in adult life. In the study from the Cambridge group, 448,553 somatic mutations were identified and used to determine clonal dynamics in 843 hematopoietic colonies from 10 patients with MPN. This study estimated the median latency between JAK2V617F acquisition and disease onset to be 31 years, with remarkable interpatient variation in fitness advantage of the MPN clone.[33] The study by Van Egeren and colleagues[34] analyzed a smaller number of colonies from 2 patients, also concluding that there was a disease latency of decades between *JAK2V617F* acquisition and disease onset. This long latency is particularly striking in view of the observation that many persons with normal hematopoietic parameters have evidence of a small *JAK2V617F* clone.[35] This suggests that many persons acquire a *JAK2V617F* mutation and live with this mutation for decades, and perhaps in many cases lifelong, without ever developing disease. The challenge is now to understand the heterogeneity of clonal fitness advantage exerted by the *JAK2V617F* mutation in HSCs. It is likely that this will involve an interplay among germline genetics influencing HSC biology,[36] heterogeneity of the HSC of origin, and extrinsic factors such as "inflammaging."[37] To unravel this crucial aspect of MPN biology will no doubt require extensive use of single-cell methodologies that look set to be at the forefront of MPN research in coming years.

SINGLE-CELL TRANSCRIPTOMICS

Single-cell RNA-sequencing (scRNAseq) is the most widely applied assay in single-cell genomics, and is extensively used to provide a comprehensive and unbiased assessment of normal cellular and molecular tissue architecture and their perturbations in disease states. Over the past decade, experiments have massively expanded in their scale and implementation, due to technological advances resulting in high-throughput methods that are relatively easy to implement.[38,39] In parallel, there now exists a wealth of user-friendly and open-source computational pipelines for data analysis.[40] Transcriptional profiling of cells individually has several advantages over "bulk" analyses, including detection of rare cell types; determination of whether differences between samples are due to differences in the frequencies of cell types present or alternatively changes in individual cell phenotype; and exploration of combinatorial patterns of gene expression and differentiation trajectories.

A typical analytical pipeline includes organizing cells according to their transcriptional profiles into discrete groups, or "clusters" that correlate with cell type or state.[40] Although cells are captured as transcriptional "snapshots," their differentiation trajectories can be inferred computationally using trajectory analyses or ordering over "pseudotime," to identify key transition states and bifurcation points.[41–44] In addition, studying the ratio of spliced versus unspliced mRNA, or the "RNA velocity," can be used to predict the future direction of travel of individual cells along a computed trajectory.[45,46] scRNAseq can be readily combined with cell surface proteomics by incorporating barcoded antibodies,[47] and analytical techniques have been developed to infer cell-cell interactions using databases of receptor-ligand pairs.[48]

scRNAseq techniques have been widely used to study MPN, as these diseases provide an exemplar model of a cancer involving complex interactions among malignant cells, diverse immune cell types (clonal and nonclonal), and mesenchymal stromal cells. In chronic myeloid leukemia, stem cells were studied from patients before and after tyrosine kinase inhibitor treatment and from the same patient before and after transformation from chronic phase to blast crisis.[49] Studying cells individually provided the necessary resolution to detect the rare, highly quiescent, BCR-ABL + stem cells in those responding to tyrosine kinase inhibition, and to demonstrate that these cells were transcriptionally distinct from normal stem cells, suggesting possible new targets for therapy. In this study, scRNAseq was combined with a novel method enabling BCR-ABL positive and negative cells to be reliably distinguished with high sensitivity, revealing that BCR-ABL negative stem cells also showed an aberrant transcriptional signature with activation of inflammatory pathways, especially in those patients who failed to achieve an optimal response to treatment.[49]

scRNAseq has also been applied to study how mutations alter hematopoiesis in Philadelphia-negative MPN, both in mouse models and in primary patient samples. In studies of primary cells isolated from patients with MPN, high-throughput scRNA-seq has been applied to study how hematopoiesis is altered in patients with MPN.[50,51] In a study of approximately 40,000 cells from patients with mutCALR-driven MPN, scRNAseq using a widely used droplet-based 3′ scRNAseq platform (10x Genomics, Pleasanton, CA) with a new genotyping method involving targeted amplification of mutation transcripts was performed.[50] This method can easily be applied to profile 10 to 100s of 1000s of cells in parallel, and is sensitive for mutations that are highly expressed, such as mutCALR, for which approximately 90% cells were accurately genotyped, albeit less sensitive for low-expressed mutations (eg, 7.3% of JAK2V617F-mutant cells were genotyped) or those distant from the 3′ end, for example, SF3B1 (~24% sensitive).[50] This study showed that CALR mutations in patients with ET affect the entire hematopoietic hierarchy, with mutant cells detected in all stem and progenitor subsets, although a higher proportion of mutant cells in the megakaryocyte progenitor (MKP) compartment. Trajectory analyses indicated that hematopoiesis was biased toward myeloid and myeloid-megakaryocytic differentiation, with MKP showing increased cell cycling, and mutant cells had upregulation of genes involved in the unfolded protein response to an NF-kB signaling pathway.[50] A highly-sensitive method combining genomic DNA and complementary DNA genotyping in parallel with scRNAseq was also developed in MPN, enabling resolution of transcriptional signatures of genetic subclones in MPN and confirming that nonclonal stem/progenitors show aberrant, inflammatory gene expression signatures, highlighting the importance cell-extrinsic effects of MPN mutant clones.[30]

A recent study of a mouse model of mutant calreticulin (CALR)-driven ET reported similar findings. In this model, mutCALR resulted in an expansion of both HSCs and megakaryocyte progenitors, and the investigators identified an aberrant intermediary population termed "proliferative megakaryocyte progenitors (pMKP)" that fell on a distinct differentiation pathway to MKP in normal hematopoiesis in their analyses.[52] In addition, mutCALR HSC and MKP cell clusters showed significant dysregulation of genes involved in cholesterol biosynthesis as compared with wild-type cells,[52] in addition to cell cycle and unfolded protein response genes as previously been described in mutCALR patients with MPN.[50]

Profiling of more than 120,000 individual cells from a range of patients with primary and secondary myelofibrosis and both *JAK2V617F* and mutCALR-driven disease also demonstrated megakaryocyte-biased hematopoiesis, with an 11-fold increase in MKP detected in patients with myelofibrosis as compared with controls in all clinical and molecular subgroups.[51] Notably, the MKP in patients with myelofibrosis fell into 2 distinct transcriptional subgroups: a small subset with a transcriptional profile similar to MKP detected in age-matched healthy donors, and a larger population with global upregulation of inflammatory/profibrotic genes. This study also identified that megakaryocyte-associated genes, including a cell surface marker, G6B, as being widely upregulated in myelofibrosis stem/progenitor cells, suggesting a strategy for immunotherapeutic targeting of cells derived from the myelofibrosis clone.[51]

Single-cell analyses have also shed light on the changes to the nonhematopoietic stromal cell compartment in MPN. Creating a "map" of certain stromal cell populations in myelofibrosis mouse models highlighted mesenchymal progenitor cells as showing the strongest upregulation in expression of extracellular matrix proteins in fibrosis. This study highlighted the S100A8/S100A9 alarmin complex as a potential therapy target, demonstrating that its inhibition was able to ameliorate the disease phenotype in the mouse model.[53]

These insights highlight the power of single-cell "omic" techniques to accurately dissect cellular and molecular perturbations in MPN. Combined with emerging techniques to capture cell states and transcriptomes in unperturbed tissues, so-called "in situ sequencing" (see **Fig. 1**) single-cell approaches will prove to be a powerful approach for target discovery and in the future look set to play a key role in clinical diagnosis through more accurate disease classification and risk stratification.

DIGITAL PATHOLOGY

The bone marrow represents a complex, dynamic, and highly regulated tissue in which diverse cell populations lie in close proximity to an orchestrated network of extracellular (stromal) matrix, blood vasculature, and bone.[54] This complexity is compounded by physiologic changes in response to aging, stress, and environmental factors that manifest as shifting patterns of tissue cellularity, heterogeneity, and lineage maturation.[55] Such complex spatiotemporal relationships are increasingly recognized as important for disease initiation, progression, therapeutic response, and relapse in patients with various myeloid malignancies, including MPN.[56] Although advances in high-resolution single-cell genomic technologies are well established in the search for new treatment strategies, advanced diagnostics, and disease monitoring in MPN, complementary approaches to decipher the important interactions among neoplastic hemopoietic cells, stromal constituents, and immune cell populations of the marrow in MPN are required.[55,57] Recent developments in digital pathology, computer vision, and image analysis have the potential to address this imbalance and revolutionize the assessment of bone marrow tissues in MPN.

Key morphologic features relating to marrow cellularity, megakaryocyte pleomorphism/atypia, and fibrosis are firmly embedded in current MPN classification schemes.[58,59] However, inconsistencies in the interpretation of key morphologic features may lead to inaccurate diagnosis and disease classification, with multiple studies suggesting significant intraobserver and interobserver variability among pathologists.[60-63] Although this appears to be partly attributable to experience and training,[64] the subjective and qualitative nature of routine marrow biopsy reporting remains a fundamental limiting factor in any classification scheme incorporating morphology-based assessment of marrow tissue. The importance and value of more accurate and objective strategies for capturing the complexity of marrow tissue architecture in MPN extends beyond the potential for improving diagnosis and classification using current recommended criteria. As perturbations in the relationship between clonal and nonclonal hematopoietic cells and components of the marrow stem cell niche are gradually elucidated using sophisticated murine models of myeloid malignancies,[55,56,65-68] therapeutic strategies targeting the mediators of tumor cell survival, proliferation, and chemoresistance are beginning to emerge.[69-72] Translating these findings to human disease and validating novel therapies will require a concerted effort to move from the conventional, subjective, and laborious description of tissue morphologic features by pathologists to objective, quantitative, and automated descriptions of marrow constituents and their interactions.

Computational analysis of digitized images prepared from glass slide material has evolved over the past few decades and significantly accelerated in recent years with the development of sophisticated deep learning (DL) methods that emulate the structure and function of human neurons in the form of artificial neural networks.[73,74] DL methods have found ready application in the field of pathology, with image recognition convolutional neuronal networks (CNN) increasingly adopted for computer vision tasks in histopathology and cytology.[75–77] In contrast to common solid tumors, image analysis has seen relatively limited application to disorders of the bone marrow, with most studies describing strategies for cell identification, quantification, and the resolution of specific leukemic differential diagnoses including B-ALL and common B-cell lymphoma/leukemia subtypes.[78–83] These machine learning strategies have generally relied on morphology-based criteria to distinguish tumor cell subtypes rather than interrogate tumor cells with the intention of gaining novel insights into disease biology. However, recently machine learning has been used to correlate bone marrow aspirate morphologic features with somatic mutations in myelodysplastic syndrome, with specific morphologic profiles linked to unique clinical characteristics.[84]

Despite the central role of bone marrow biopsy assessment in the diagnosis and classification of MPNs, and the importance of the marrow microenvironment in disease biology (as outlined previously), few studies have attempted to apply advanced machine learning approaches to these disorders. In response, we recently demonstrated the utility of an automated image analysis pipeline that uses machine learning techniques to extract important cytomorphological and topographic features of individual megakaryocytes from digitized images of bone marrow biopsies.[85] This enabled the differentiation of reactive samples from common MPN subtypes (ET, PV, and primary myelofibrosis) and assisted in disease classification. Clustering of megakaryocytes using the machine-learned features from extracted megakaryocytes identified cellular subtypes beyond the sensitivity of detection by specialist hematopathologists and were seen to correlate with the underlying MPN driver mutation status. When combined with topographic assessment incorporating patterns of megakaryocyte clustering and cell distribution, the extracted features could be combined to produce a multidimensional representation of an individual sample well beyond conventional microscopic assessment. Moreover, the rapid automated analysis of samples allowed index cases of MPN or reactive marrow to be contextualized against libraries of previously analyzed samples (**Fig. 2**). This could be used to monitor or track morphologic features over time, corresponding to either stable disease or

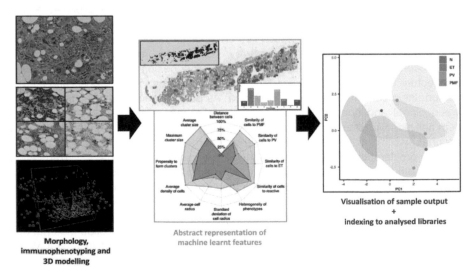

Morphology, immunophenotyping and 3D modelling

Abstract representation of machine learnt features

Visualisation of sample output
+
indexing to analysed libraries

Fig. 2. Illustration of how digital pathology approaches can be used to study cellular heterogeneity in MPN.

progression. This work highlights the potential of image analysis, driven by advanced machine learning approaches, to improve tissue diagnosis in MPN and correlate tissue-based morphologic features with standard mutational and clinical data collected during the routine investigation of patients with MPN. Importantly, the automated extraction of objective quantitative data from routinely prepared hematoxylin–eosin–stained slides is ideally suited to future integration with the results of whole-tissue immunolabeling studies, advanced single-cell genomic analysis, and the outputs from high-resolution multiplexed tissue imaging performed in the research setting.

An important consideration in the development of improved descriptions of tissue morphology and the marrow microenvironment using digital pathology and machine learning is the development of intuitive yet sufficiently detailed data visualization. The methods used will depend on the application and requirements of the end user, but it seems likely that for clinicians and researchers unfamiliar with the normal bone marrow tissue architecture and its heterogeneity, visual representation of the cellular target(s) of interest in the context of normal and/or previously analyzed disease tissue will aid interpretation and understanding. Successfully designed outputs should capture temporal changes in the course of disease or following treatment, but also have the potential to highlight relevant diagnostic and prognostic features with attention drawn to potential therapeutic targets.

Notwithstanding the potential clinical application of automated analysis of discrete single-cell populations, such as megakaryocytes in biopsies of MPN, a deeper understanding of the complex cellular interactions within the bone marrow of patients with myeloid malignancies requires a more comprehensive description of the spatiotemporal relationships that exist between the cellular and stromal components of the marrow. This will require integration of discrete cellular and extracellular morphologic features with lineage specific markers of differentiation and maturation using multiplexed immunolabeling approaches. Although several analytical platforms already use such approaches in the research setting, they are typically restricted to relatively small tissue fields (roughly equivalent to conventional microscopic high-power fields) from limited sample numbers.[86–88] Translating the insights of such studies to cohorts of routinely prepared clinical bone marrow samples will require the development of powerful and robust computational approaches that can be adapted to identify, quantitate, and integrate diverse cellular and extracellular targets at scale. An additional challenge will be building advanced 3-dimensional models of the bone marrow environment and establishing methods for their validation using cohorts of patient samples analyzed in 2 dimensions.

Although automated analytical pipelines using convolutional neural networks to detect and segment targets of interest in digital images offer the potential for rapid sample analysis, their generation is typically dependent on access to large numbers of tissue samples accompanied by detailed clinical, laboratory, and genomic data. In general, machine learning applications in pathology use supervised approaches in which functions are learned by mapping annotated tissue features into some qualitative or quantitative output.[77,89,90] This process is dependent on access to high-quality training data that are sufficiently labeled to allow the training phase to ultimately emulate the expert's input data. Strategies to reduce the burden of manual annotations by pathologists include transfer learning from preexisting CNNs and the development of human-in-the-loop annotation approaches that leverage human interactions to more rapidly train, test, and validate machine-learned functions.

Given the importance of accessing sufficient quantities of high-quality training and validation material, important practical considerations surround access to suitable tissue. Few centers can rely solely on locally retained tissue archives to build and validate models of discrete MPN subtypes that are sufficiently enriched with relatively rare samples corresponding to important clinical or genomic events, such as disease transformation or response to novel therapeutics. Access to trial sample cohorts and sharing of tissue libraries between collaborating clinical centers will likely optimize use of available diagnostic material and accelerate the development and validation of machine learning models of MPN.

In summary, machine learning approaches to image analysis have already received broad acceptance in several branches of solid tissue pathology and are widely accepted as a transformational technology with significant clinical and research potential. Realizing this potential in MPN will depend on the identification and extraction of important cell-cell and cell-stroma interactions that complement and enhance our understanding of the dynamics underlying the clonal expansion of single-cell precursors that ultimately drive the disease phenotype in individual patients. This will require close collaboration among hematologists, pathologists, bioinformaticians, biomedical engineers, and software engineers and the integration of multimodality approaches spanning novel single-cell and whole-tissue sample technologies.

SUMMARY

Single-cell technologies have over many years provided remarkable insights into MPN biology, making conceptual advances of broader relevance across cancer biology. Future technological developments in digital pathology, in situ sequencing, and single-cell multiomics approaches (see **Fig. 1**) will undoubtedly be applied over the coming years to tackle crucial questions in the field. One key question that will definitively require single-cell approaches is why different HSC clones carrying MPN driver mutations such as *JAK2V617F* show such heterogeneity in fitness advantage. This is crucial to understand if we are to develop treatment approaches that reverse the fitness advantage to induce molecular responses and ultimately alter the natural history of MPN. Another key challenge in the field is to translate these single-cell technological developments through to direct patient benefit. Although at the present time it may seem farfetched for single-cell methodologies to be applied routinely in clinical diagnostics, this will surely become a reality over the coming years with obvious utility for improved approaches to diagnose and classify disease as well as monitor response to treatment and predict risk of disease progression.

FINANCIAL SUPPORT AND SPONSORSHIP

None.

ACKNOWLEDGMENTS

All authors contributed equally to this work. A.J. Mead is funded by a Cancer Research UK Senior Clinical Fellowship. This work was supported by the National Institute for Health Research (NIHR) Oxford Biomedical Research Center (BRC). B.P. is supported by a CRUK Advanced Clinician Scientist Fellowship and Oxford BRC Senior Fellowship. The views expressed are those of the author(s) and not necessarily those of the NHS, the NIHR or the Department of Health.

DISCLOSURES

None.

REFERENCES

1. Mead AJ, Mullally A. Myeloproliferative neoplasm stem cells. Blood 2017;129(12): 1607–16.
2. Nangalia J, Mitchell E, Green AR. Clonal approaches to understanding the impact of mutations on hematologic disease development. Blood 2019;133(13): 1436–45.
3. McGranahan N, Swanton C. Biological and therapeutic impact of intratumor heterogeneity in cancer evolution. Cancer Cell 2015;27(1):15–26.
4. Martincorena I, Campbell PJ. Somatic mutation in cancer and normal cells. Science 2015;349(6255):1483–9.
5. Yates LR, Campbell PJ. Evolution of the cancer genome. Nat Rev Genet 2012; 13(11):795–806.
6. Wills QF, Mead AJ. Application of single-cell genomics in cancer: promise and challenges. Hum Mol Genet 2015;24(R1):R74–84.
7. Baslan T, Hicks J. Unravelling biology and shifting paradigms in cancer with single-cell sequencing. Nat Rev Cancer 2017;17(9):557–69.
8. Brierley CK, Mead AJ. Single-cell sequencing in hematology. Curr Opin Oncol 2020;32(2):139–45.
9. Klampfl T, Gisslinger H, Harutyunyan AS, et al. Somatic mutations of calreticulin in myeloproliferative neoplasms. N Engl J Med 2013;369(25):2379–90.
10. Nangalia J, Massie CE, Baxter EJ, et al. Somatic CALR mutations in myeloproliferative neoplasms with nonmutated JAK2. N Engl J Med 2013;369(25):2391–405.
11. Pardanani AD, Levine RL, Lasho T, et al. MPL515 mutations in myeloproliferative and other myeloid disorders: a study of 1182 patients. Blood 2006;108(10): 3472–6.
12. O'Sullivan J, Mead AJ. Heterogeneity in myeloproliferative neoplasms: causes and consequences. Adv Biol Regul 2019;71:55–68.
13. Lawrence MS, Stojanov P, Polak P, et al. Mutational heterogeneity in cancer and the search for new cancer-associated genes. Nature 2013;499(7457):214–8.
14. Adamson JW, Fialkow PJ, Murphy S, et al. Polycythemia vera: stem-cell and probable clonal origin of the disease. N Engl J Med 1976;295(17):913–6.
15. Gilliland DG, Blanchard KL, Levy J, et al. Clonality in myeloproliferative disorders: analysis by means of the polymerase chain reaction. Proc Natl Acad Sci U S A 1991;88(15):6848–52.
16. James C, Ugo V, Le Couedic JP, et al. A unique clonal JAK2 mutation leading to constitutive signalling causes polycythaemia vera. Nature 2005;434(7037): 1144–8.
17. Baxter EJ, Scott LM, Campbell PJ, et al. Acquired mutation of the tyrosine kinase JAK2 in human myeloproliferative disorders. Lancet 2005;365(9464):1054–61.
18. Beer PA, Jones AV, Bench AJ, et al. Clonal diversity in the myeloproliferative neoplasms: independent origins of genetically distinct clones. Br J Haematol 2009; 144(6):904–8.
19. Godfrey AL, Chen E, Pagano F, et al. JAK2V617F homozygosity arises commonly and recurrently in PV and ET, but PV is characterized by expansion of a dominant homozygous subclone. Blood 2012;120(13):2704–7.
20. Ortmann CA, Kent DG, Nangalia J, et al. Effect of mutation order on myeloproliferative neoplasms. N Engl J Med 2015;372(7):601–12.
21. Nangalia J, Nice FL, Wedge DC, et al. DNMT3A mutations occur early or late in patients with myeloproliferative neoplasms and mutation order influences phenotype. Haematologica 2015;100(11):e438–42.

22. Lim B, Lin Y, Navin N. Advancing cancer research and medicine with single-cell genomics. Cancer Cell 2020;37(4):456–70.
23. Povinelli BJ, Rodriguez-Meira A, Mead AJ. Single cell analysis of normal and leukemic hematopoiesis. Mol Aspects Med 2018;59:85–94.
24. Miles LA, Bowman RL, Merlinsky TR, et al. Single-cell mutation analysis of clonal evolution in myeloid malignancies. Nature 2020;587(7834):477–82.
25. Ellis P, Moore L, Sanders MA, et al. Reliable detection of somatic mutations in solid tissues by laser-capture microdissection and low-input DNA sequencing. Nat Protoc 2020. https://doi.org/10.1038/s41596-020-00437-6.
26. Roth A, McPherson A, Laks E, et al. Clonal genotype and population structure inference from single-cell tumor sequencing. Nat Methods 2016;13(7):573–6.
27. Ross EM, Markowetz F. OncoNEM: inferring tumor evolution from single-cell sequencing data. Genome Biol 2016;17:69.
28. Sohrab Salehi AS, Roth Andrew, Aparicio Samuel, et al. ddClone: joint statistical inference of clonal populations from single cell and bulk tumour sequencing data. Genome Biol 2017. https://doi.org/10.1186/s13059-017-1169-3.
29. Hou Y, Song L, Zhu P, et al. Single-cell exome sequencing and monoclonal evolution of a JAK2-negative myeloproliferative neoplasm. Cell 2012;148(5):873–85.
30. Rodriguez-Meira A, Buck G, Clark SA, et al. Unravelling intratumoral heterogeneity through high-sensitivity single-cell mutational analysis and parallel RNA sequencing. Mol Cell 2019;73(6):1292–1305 e1298.
31. Mylonas E, Yoshida K, Frick M, et al. Single-cell analysis based dissection of clonality in myelofibrosis. Nat Commun 2020;11(1):73.
32. Thompson ER, Nguyen T, Kankanige Y, et al. Clonal independence of JAK2 and CALR or MPL mutations in co-mutated myeloproliferative neoplasms demonstrated by single cell DNA sequencing. Haematologica 2020. https://doi.org/10.3324/haematol.2020.260448.
33. Williams N, Lee J, Moore L, et al. Phylogenetic reconstruction of myeloproliferative neoplasm reveals very early origins and lifelong evolution. bioRxiv 2020; 2020. 2011.2009.374710.
34. Van Egeren D, Escabi J, Nguyen M, et al. Reconstructing the lineage histories and differentiation trajectories of individual cancer cells in JAK2-mutant myeloproliferative neoplasms. bioRxiv 2020;2020. 2008.2024.265058.
35. Cordua S, Kjaer L, Skov V, et al. Prevalence and phenotypes of JAK2 V617F and calreticulin mutations in a Danish general population. Blood 2019;134(5):469–79.
36. Bao EL, Nandakumar SK, Liao X, et al. Inherited myeloproliferative neoplasm risk affects haematopoietic stem cells. Nature 2020;586(7831):769–75.
37. Karantanos T, Kaizer H, Chaturvedi S, et al. Inflammation exerts a nonrandom risk in the acquisition and progression of the MPN: insights from a Mendelian randomization study. EClinicalMedicine 2020;21:100324.
38. Stubbington MJT, Rozenblatt-Rosen O, Regev A, et al. Single-cell transcriptomics to explore the immune system in health and disease. Science 2017;358(6359): 58–63.
39. Aldridge S, Teichmann SA. Single cell transcriptomics comes of age. Nat Commun 2020;11(1):4307.
40. Stuart T, Satija R. Integrative single-cell analysis. Nat Rev Genet 2019;20(5): 257–72.
41. Wolf FA, Hamey FK, Plass M, et al. PAGA: graph abstraction reconciles clustering with trajectory inference through a topology preserving map of single cells. Genome Biol 2019;20(1):59.

42. Becht E, McInnes L, Healy J, et al. Dimensionality reduction for visualizing single-cell data using UMAP. Nat Biotechnol 2018. https://doi.org/10.1038/nbt.4314.

43. Coifman RR, Lafon S, Lee AB, et al. Geometric diffusions as a tool for harmonic analysis and structure definition of data: diffusion maps. Proc Natl Acad Sci U S A 2005;102(21):7426–31.

44. Trapnell C, Cacchiarelli D, Grimsby J, et al. The dynamics and regulators of cell fate decisions are revealed by pseudotemporal ordering of single cells. Nat Biotechnol 2014;32(4):381–6.

45. La Manno G, Soldatov R, Zeisel A, et al. RNA velocity of single cells. Nature 2018; 560(7719):494–8.

46. Bergen V, Lange M, Peidli S, et al. Generalizing RNA velocity to transient cell states through dynamical modeling. Nat Biotechnol 2020;38(12):1408–14.

47. Stoeckius M, Hafemeister C, Stephenson W, et al. Simultaneous epitope and tran-scriptome measurement in single cells. Nat Methods 2017;14(9):865–8.

48. Efremova M, Vento-Tormo M, Teichmann SA, et al. CellPhoneDB: inferring cell-cell communication from combined expression of multi-subunit ligand-receptor com-plexes. Nat Protoc 2020;15(4):1484–506.

49. Giustacchini A, Thongjuea S, Barkas N, et al. Single-cell transcriptomics un-covers distinct molecular signatures of stem cells in chronic myeloid leukemia. Nat Med 2017;23(6):692–702.

50. Nam AS, Kim KT, Chaligne R, et al. Somatic mutations and cell identity linked by genotyping of transcriptomes. Nature 2019;571(7765):355–60.

51. Psaila B, Wang G, Rodriguez-Meira A, et al. Single-cell analyses reveal megakaryocyte-biased hematopoiesis in myelofibrosis and identify mutant clone-specific targets. Mol Cell 2020;78(3):477–492 e478.

52. Prins D, Park HJ, Watcham S, et al. The stem/progenitor landscape is reshaped in a mouse model of essential thrombocythemia and causes excess megakaryocyte production. Sci Adv 2020;6(48):eabd3139.

53. Leimkuhler NB, Gleitz HFE, Ronghui L, et al. Heterogeneous bone-marrow stro-mal progenitors drive myelofibrosis via a druggable alarmin axis. Cell Stem Cell 2020. https://doi.org/10.1016/j.stem.2020.11.004.

54. Mendez-Ferrer S, Michurina TV, Ferraro F, et al. Mesenchymal and haemato-poietic stem cells form a unique bone marrow niche. Nature 2010;466(7308): 829–34.

55. Batsivari A, Haltalli MLR, Passaro D, et al. Dynamic responses of the haemato-poietic stem cell niche to diverse stresses. Nat Cell Biol 2020;22(1):7–17.

56. Mendez-Ferrer S, Bonnet D, Steensma DP, et al. Bone marrow niches in haema-tological malignancies. Nat Rev Cancer 2020;20(5):285–98.

57. Dufva O, Polonen P, Bruck O, et al. Immunogenomic landscape of hematological malignancies. Cancer Cell 2020;38(3):424–8.

58. Guglielmelli P, Pacilli A, Rotunno G, et al. Presentation and outcome of patients with 2016 WHO diagnosis of prefibrotic and overt primary myelofibrosis. Blood 2017;129(24):3227–36.

59. Arber DA, Orazi A, Hasserjian R, et al. The 2016 revision to the World Health Or-ganization classification of myeloid neoplasms and acute leukemia. Blood 2016; 127(20):2391–405.

60. Wilkins BS, Erber WN, Bareford D, et al. Bone marrow pathology in essential thrombocythemia: interobserver reliability and utility for identifying disease sub-types. Blood 2008;111(1):60–70.

61. Alvarez-Larran A, Ancochea A, Garcia M, et al. WHO-histological criteria for myeloproliferative neoplasms: reproducibility, diagnostic accuracy and

correlation with gene mutations and clinical outcomes. Br J Haematol 2014; 166(6):911–9.

62. Buhr T, Hebeda K, Kaloutsi V, et al. European Bone Marrow Working Group Trial on reproducibility of world health organization criteria to discriminate essential thrombocythemia from prefibrotic primary myelofibrosis. Haematologica 2012; 97(3):360–5.

63. Harrison CN, McMullin MF, Green AR, et al. Equivalence of BCSH and WHO diagnostic criteria for ET. Leukemia 2017;31(7):1660.

64. Barbui T, Thiele J, Gisslinger H, et al. The 2016 WHO classification and diagnostic criteria for myeloproliferative neoplasms: document summary and in-depth discussion. Blood Cancer J 2018;8(2):15.

65. Arranz L, Sanchez-Aguilera A, Martin-Perez D, et al. Neuropathy of haematopoictic stem cell niche is essential for myeloproliferative neoplasms. Nature 2014;512(7512):78–81.

66. Itkin T, Gur-Cohen S, Spencer JA, et al. Distinct bone marrow blood vessels differentially regulate haematopoiesis. Nature 2016;532(7599):323–8.

67. Gleitz HFE, Dugourd AJF, Leimkuhler NB, et al. Increased CXCL4 expression in hematopoietic cells links inflammation and progression of bone marrow fibrosis in MPN. Blood 2020;136(18):2051–64.

68. Christodoulou C, Spencer JA, Yeh SA, et al. Live-animal imaging of native haematopoietic stem and progenitor cells. Nature 2020;578(7794):278–83.

69. Cho BS, Kim HJ, Konopleva M. Targeting the CXCL12/CXCR4 axis in acute myeloid leukemia: from bench to bedside. Korean J Intern Med 2017;32(2): 248–57.

70. Drexler B, Passweg JR, Tzankov A, et al. The sympathomimetic agonist mirabegron did not lower JAK2-V617F allele burden, but restored nestin-positive cells and reduced reticulin fibrosis in patients with myeloproliferative neoplasms: results of phase II study SAKK 33/14. Haematologica 2019;104(4):710–6.

71. Ben-Batalla I, Schultze A, Wroblewski M, et al. Axl, a prognostic and therapeutic target in acute myeloid leukemia mediates paracrine crosstalk of leukemia cells with bone marrow stroma. Blood 2013;122(14):2443–52.

72. Nimmagadda SC, Frey S, Muller P, et al. SDF1alpha-induced chemotaxis of JAK2-V617F-positive cells is dependent on Bruton tyrosine kinase and its downstream targets PI3K/AKT, PLCgamma1 and RhoA. Haematologica 2019;104(7): e288–92.

73. LeCun Y, Bengio Y, Hinton G. Deep learning. Nature 2015;521(7553):436–44.

74. Janowczyk A, Madabhushi A. Deep learning for digital pathology image analysis: a comprehensive tutorial with selected use cases. J Pathol Inform 2016;7:29.

75. Litjens G, Sanchez CI, Timofeeva N, et al. Deep learning as a tool for increased accuracy and efficiency of histopathological diagnosis. Sci Rep 2016;6:26286.

76. Khosravi P, Kazemi E, Imielinski M, et al. Deep convolutional neural networks enable discrimination of heterogeneous digital pathology images. EBioMedicine 2018;27:317–28.

77. Rashidi HH, Tran NK, Betts EV, et al. Artificial intelligence and machine learning in pathology: the present landscape of supervised methods. Acad Pathol 2019;6. 2374289519873088.

78. Kimura K, Tabe Y, Ai T, et al. A novel automated image analysis system using deep convolutional neural networks can assist to differentiate MDS and AA. Sci Rep 2019;9(1):13385.

79. Singh A, Ohgami RS. Super-resolution digital pathology image processing of bone marrow aspirate and cytology smears and tissue sections. J Pathol Inform 2018;9:48.

80. Puigvi L, Merino A, Alferez S, et al. New quantitative features for the morphological differentiation of abnormal lymphoid cell images from peripheral blood. J Clin Pathol 2017;70(12):1038–48.

81. El Achi H, Khoury JD. Artificial intelligence and digital microscopy applications in diagnostic hematopathology. Cancers (Basel) 2020;12(4):797.

82. Alferez S, Merino A, Mujica LE, et al. Automatic classification of atypical lymphoid B cells using digital blood image processing. Int J Lab Hematol 2014;36(4):472–80.

83. Hagiya AS, Etman A, Siddiqi IN, et al. Digital image analysis agrees with visual estimates of adult bone marrow trephine biopsy cellularity. Int J Lab Hematol 2018;40(2):209–14.

84. Nagata Y, Zhao R, Awada H, et al. Machine learning demonstrates that somatic mutations imprint invariant morphologic features in myelodysplastic syndromes. Blood 2020;136(20):2249–62.

85. Sirinukunwattana K, Aberdeen A, Theissen H, et al. Artificial intelligence-based morphological fingerprinting of megakaryocytes: a new tool for assessing disease in MPN patients. Blood Adv 2020;4(14):3284–94.

86. Goltsev Y, Samusik N, Kennedy-Darling J, et al. Deep profiling of mouse splenic architecture with CODEX multiplexed imaging. Cell 2018;174(4):968–981 e915.

87. Gerdes MJ, Sevinsky CJ, Sood A, et al. Highly multiplexed single-cell analysis of formalin-fixed, paraffin-embedded cancer tissue. Proc Natl Acad Sci U S A 2013;110(29):11982–7.

88. Di Palma S, Bodenmiller B. Unraveling cell populations in tumors by single-cell mass cytometry. Curr Opin Biotechnol 2015;31:122–9.

89. Chang HY, Jung CK, Woo JI, et al. Artificial intelligence in pathology. J Pathol Transl Med 2019;53(1):1–12.

90. Serag A, Ion-Margineanu A, Qureshi H, et al. Translational AI and deep learning in diagnostic pathology. Front Med (Lausanne) 2019;6:185.

Unmet Need in Essential Thrombocythemia and Polycythemia Vera

Ashwin Kishtagari, MD, Aaron T. Gerds, MD, MS*

KEYWORDS

- Myeloproliferative neoplasms • MPN • ET • PV • Bomedemstat • IFN-α
- Idasanutlin • Givinostat

KEY POINTS

- Therapies that have demonstrated true disease modification are needed in PV and ET.
- Given the relatively favorable disease course for most patients with PV and ET, identifying disease-modifying treatments is difficult.
- Development of new measures of disease modification along with new therapies will be key to improving the long-term outcomes of patients.

INTRODUCTION

BCR-ABL1–negative myeloproliferative neoplasms (MPNs) comprise a group of clonal hematopoietic stem cell disorders characterized by aberrant proliferation of mature myeloid elements manifesting as erythrocytosis (polycythemia vera [PV]), thrombocytosis (essential thrombocytosis [ET]), leukocytosis and/or bone marrow fibrosis. Dysregulated JAK-STAT signaling resulting from the acquired mutations involving janus kinase 2 (*JAK2*), calreticulin (*CALR*), and myeloproliferative leukemia virus (*MPL*) with in the hematopoietic stem and progenitor cells is at the heart of MPN pathophysiology.[1] This leads to elevated inflammatory cytokines, which contribute to the wide spectrum of symptomatology experienced by patients with PV and patients with ET, including pruritis, fatigue, and splenomegaly. Patients with PV/ET have lifelong propensity for thrombohemorrhagic complications, and in some cases progression to myelofibrosis, and evolution to acute myeloid leukemia.

CURRENT STATE OF TREATMENT OF ESSENTIAL THROMBOCYTOSIS/POLYCYTHEMIA VERA

Despite the tremendous advances in understanding the pathophysiology of these diseases, there are currently no curative treatments for these diseases outside of

Leukemia & Myeloid Disorders Program, Cleveland Clinic Taussig Cancer Institute, 9500 Euclid Avenue, CA60, Cleveland, OH 44120, USA
* Corresponding author.
E-mail address: gerdsa@ccf.org

Hematol Oncol Clin N Am 35 (2021) 295–303
https://doi.org/10.1016/j.hoc.2021.01.003
0889-8588/21/© 2021 Elsevier Inc. All rights reserved.

allogeneic hematopoietic stem cell transplantation. Given the lifelong propensity for thrombohemorrhagic complications, most currently approved treatments focus on mitigation of these risks. Current therapeutic options for PV/ET include aspirin (ASA), therapeutic phlebotomy for controlling hematocrit, and cytoreductive drugs such as hydroxyurea. Therapeutic options for ET and PV are expanding, with many new agents in various stages of clinical trial evaluation. Large-scale genomic studies have identified the molecular underpinnings (*JAK2*, *MPL*, *CALR*) of the *BCR-ABL1*–negative MPNs, leading to the development of molecularly targeted therapies, which are currently in clinical trials. Ruxolitinib, a JAK1/2 inhibitor, is approved for the treatment of hydroxyurea-resistant PV. Despite its benefit in management of symptoms and blood counts, it does not appear to change the natural history of the disease.[2] The quest for disease-modifying treatments in PV/ET has propelled the exploration of several agents in various stages of drug development, such as murine double minute 2 (MDM2) inhibitors, histone-deacetylase (HDAC) inhibitors, and lysine-specific histone demethylase 1 (LSD1) inhibitors (**Fig. 1**). Even with these exciting advances occurring, there are still several outstanding issues in considering the care of patients with PV and ET, which we discuss.

SHOULD WE USE LOW-DOSE ASPIRIN IN ALL PATIENTS WITH ESSENTIAL THROMBOCYTOSIS AND POLYCYTHEMIA VERA?

The ECLAP study has long been held up as the standard for antiplatelet therapy in MPNs. This study was conducted in 518 patients with PV with randomization in a double-blinded fashion to low-dose ASA (100 mg daily) or placebo.[3] The use of aspirin resulted in a relative reduction (60%) of combined risk of nonfatal myocardial infarction, nonfatal stroke, pulmonary embolism, major venous thrombosis, or death from

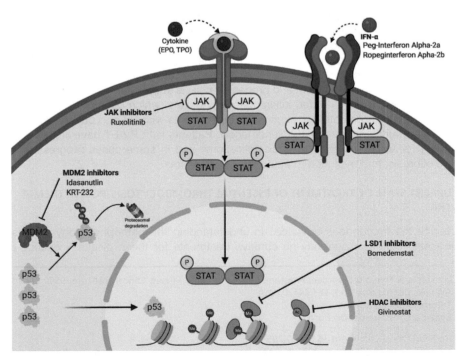

Fig. 1. Mechanism of action for IFN-α and emerging therapies in ET and PV.

cardiovascular causes (P = .03). The incidence of major bleeding was not significantly increased in the aspirin group as compared with placebo (P = .08). However, this study was conducted before the CYTO-PV study,[4] and hematocrit was not as tightly controlled as it is today. In fact, the median hematocrit was 48% and 47% for the ASA and placebo groups, respectively. It is unclear if better hematocrit control would affect the results of this study. Nonetheless, given the risk-to-benefit ratio demonstrated in the ECLAP study, low-dose ASA is still recommended in PV.[5,6]

Randomized, prospective studies evaluating ASA in ET have not been conducted, as noted in a Cochrane Review,[7] and the recommendation for the use of ASA in ET is largely extrapolated from the ECLAP study and retrospective analyses. In one retrospective analysis of patients with ET given either low-dose ASA as monotherapy versus observation alone, *JAK2* V617F-positive disease was associated with an increased risk of venous thrombosis in patients not receiving antiplatelet medication (incidence rate ratio [IRR] 4.0; 95% confidence interval [CI] 1.2–12.9; P = .02).[8] An additional retrospective analysis suggests that there is an increased risk of bleeding in patients with *CALR*-mutated disease who receive low-dose ASA as compared with those who did not (12.9 vs 1.8 episodes per 1000 patient-years, P = .03) and no reduction in thrombosis risk.[9] Based on this, low-dose ASA is recommended only for patients with high risk for thrombosis.[5,6]

IS THERE A TARGET PLATELET COUNT WHEN USING CYTOREDUCTION FOR ESSENTIAL THROMBOCYTOSIS?

The randomized CYTO-PV study set the standard for hematocrit control in PV.[4] Keeping the hematocrit less than 45%, as compared with less stringent range between 45% and 50%, resulted in a reduction in time until death from cardiovascular cause or major thrombotic event (hazard ratio [HR] 3.91; 95% CI 1.45–10.53; P = .007). Although the lower limit of the confidence interval includes possibility of marginal benefit (0.45-fold greater risk in the high hematocrit group), consensus guidelines have widely adopted the practice of keeping the hematocrit to less than 45% owing to a favorable risk-to-benefit ratio.[5,6] If you scour the guidelines, there is no equivalent evidence-based cytoreductive goal for platelet counts in ET.

At a minimum, it makes clinical sense to reduce the platelet count numbers in those who are at high risk for bleeding due to acquired von Willebrand syndrome as a result of extreme thrombocytosis. The paradox of an association between extreme thrombocytosis (platelet counts more than 1000 × 10^9/L) and bleeding has been known for some time.[10] In one retrospective analysis of 565 patients with ET, extreme thrombocytosis was associated with a 2.3-fold increase (95% CI 1.3–3.7, P = .003) in the risk of bleeding events in a multivariate analysis.[11] However, in low-risk young patients with ET, extreme thrombocytosis may not lead to an excess in bleeding events.[12] Further complicating the matter, acquired von Willebrand syndrome has been described in patients with ET without extreme thrombocytosis. A carefully taken bleeding history can help identify patients who may have excess bleeding and warrant a workup for a concurrent bleeding diathesis.

Extreme thrombocytosis aside, in the absence of a randomized controlled trial or rigorous retrospective study, there is no consensus on a goal platelet count when beginning cytoreduction to lower the platelet counts of patients with ET. In a prospective, randomized study of patients with high-risk ET (age >60 years and/or prior history of thrombosis), 56 patients received hydroxyurea and 58 were not given cytoreductive therapy.[13] With a median follow-up of 27 months, the incidence of thrombotic episodes was found to be significantly lower in patients treated with hydroxyurea

(3.6%) as compared with those who received no cytoreductive therapy (24%; difference of 20.4%, 95% CI 8.5%–32%; $P = .003$). As of note, 69% of the patients in either arm of the study were receiving antiplatelet therapy. In the treatment arm, the hydroxyurea dose was adjusted to a goal platelet count of 600×10^9/L or less based on a prior retrospective study.[14] For many patients, it takes little cytoreduction, such as hydroxyurea dosages of 500 to 1000 mg daily, to attain platelet counts in the normal range. However, for patients with counts more resistant to cytoreduction, the value of driving the counts into the normal range is unknown. This fact underscores both the need to approach platelet count goals on a case-by-case basis, and the need for new therapeutics that enact a deeper disease modification.

DO WE HAVE ANY MEDICATIONS THAT ARE TRULY DISEASE-MODIFYING?
Can Interferons Enact Disease Modification?

Interferon-alpha (IFN-α) and hydroxyurea are recommended cytoreductive treatments of symptomatic and high-risk patients with PV and ETs.[4,5] Over the past 3 decades, various forms of IFN-α have been successfully used to treat patients with MPNs, including PV and ET. IFN-α can control erythrocytosis and thrombocytosis, as well as reduce the risk of thrombotic complications, splenomegaly, and pruritis in most patients with PV or ET. IFN-α treatment has a disease-modifying potential by inducing complete hematologic-remissions, reversal of bone marrow fibrosis, and more recently evidenced by a reduction in mutation allele burden.[15] It induces this response via antiproliferative, anti-angiogenic, pro-apoptotic, immunomodulatory, and differentiating properties on hematopoietic progenitors and may preferentially target the malignant clone.[16]

Long-term efficacy and safety data show that IFN-α treatment accomplishes a high rate of complete hematologic response, minimized the occurrence of thromboembolic events, and remarkable rates of molecular responses.[17,18] Most of these responses are also durable, an appealing aspect of IFN-α treatment.

The efficacy of ropeginterferon alpha-2b, a monopegylated recombinant IFN-α, was evaluated in the noninferiority randomized phase III PROUD-PV trial and its extension study CONTINUATION-PV compared with best available therapy (80% of which was hydroxyurea) in 257 patients with PV. Ropeginterferon alpha-2b treatment was associated with well-controlled hematocrit (<45%) levels without requiring therapeutic phlebotomy and minimized the occurrence of thromboembolic events. Most importantly, disease progression was sporadic during 5-year results with ropeginterferon alpha-2b treatment. This indicates that the change in disease course may be related to deep and durable molecular responses achieved with this treatment.[19,20] Ropeginterferon alpha-2b is approved in the European Union as monotherapy for the treatment of patients with PV without symptomatic splenomegaly.

Other critical evidence of the potential for IFN-α treatment to alter the natural history of MPNs is that it is the only treatment that can provide a long-term complete hematologic response after discontinuation of the treatment. This is particularly evident in patients with a driver mutation VAF lower than 10% at the time of discontinuation.[21] This suggests that deeper driver mutation remission may be a biomarker surrogate for disease course modification. Recently published data show an association of germline genetic factors such as interferon lambda 4 (IFNL4) diplotype status and molecular remission with IFN-α therapy in patients with PV reflecting the differential effect of IFN-α treatment on JAK2 V617 F mutational burden.[22]

There is now evidence that IFN-α treatment in patients with PV will improve overall survival and alter the disease course by reversing the bone marrow fibrosis.[23] In this single-center retrospective study in 470 patients with PV, IFN-α (n = 93) demonstrated superior myelofibrosis-free survival and overall survival advantage over hydroxyurea (n = 189) or phlebotomy only (n = 133) treatments with a median follow-up of 10 years.[23] This constitutes other data supporting the disease-modifying potential of IFN-α.

A Case for Murine Double Minute 2 Inhibitors

The loss-of-function mutations in the *TP53* gene, located on chromosome 17p13.1, is seen in most cancers. Its protein product, p53, functions as an essential tumor suppressor, and is tightly regulated by several mechanisms, including posttranslational modifications and interaction with the negative regulator E3 ligase MDM2. *JAK2* V617 F increases MDM2 protein translation, resulting in upregulation of MDM2 levels in PV/ET CD34+ stem/progenitor cells, and nutlins, a class of drugs that inhibit MDM2 activity and in turn lead to increased p53 activity, are capable of depleting mutated PV/ET stem/progenitor cells.[24,25] This is strong rationale to treat patients with ET/PV with an MDM2 inhibitor.

The safety and efficacy of idasanutlin, a second-generation oral nutlin, was evaluated in a phase 1 trial, alone or in combination with IFN-α in patients with high-risk PV/ET for whom at least 1 prior line of therapy had failed.[26] Twelve patients (PV, n = 11; ET, n = 1) with *JAK2* V617 F-positive PV/ET were treated with idasanutlin at 100 and 150 mg daily, respectively, for 5 consecutive days of a 28-day cycle. The overall response rate after 6 cycles was 58% (7/12) with idasanutlin monotherapy. Median duration of response was 16.8 months (range, 3.5–26.7). Most importantly, the treatment was associated with a 43% mean reduction in the *JAK2* V617 F variant allele frequency signifying the disease-modifying potential of the treatment. These encouraging results prompted the international multicenter phase 2 study evaluating idasanutlin in patients with PV who were hydroxyurea-resistant/intolerant and phlebotomy-dependent (>1 phlebotomy in the 16-week period before screening). Idasanutlin was given orally once daily for 5 consecutive days of a 28-day cycle for up to 24 months. The primary endpoint at 32 weeks was the composite response of hematocrit control and spleen volume reduction greater than 35% by computed tomography/MRI in patients with splenomegaly and hematocrit alone in patients without splenomegaly; 27 patients were enrolled with median duration of treatment of 257 days (range, 5–677). The median number of treatment cycles was 8 (range, 1–22). At week 32, 16 patients were assessed for primary endpoint. Nine (56.3%) of the 16 patients have achieved hematocrit control and 8 (50%) of 16 patients achieved complete hematologic response. Idasanutlin treatment resulted in reduction in *JAK2* V617 F variant allele frequency, which was observed as early as after 3 cycles (median reduction, 39%; n = 19) and was sustained in patients receiving treatment. Interestingly, the reduction in the clonal burden was significantly greater in patients with complete hematologic response and hematocrit control, indicating the disease-modifying potential of the drug.[27,28] These enthusiastic results were dampened by the toxicities of the drug, a total of 3 serious adverse events were reported: atrial flutter, atrial fibrillation, and nausea/vomiting. The recurrent gastrointestinal toxicity (nausea/vomiting) was common and was not alleviated with antiemetic prophylaxis throughout the treatment and led to frequent treatment discontinuations.

KRT-232, another oral small molecule MDM2 inhibitor, is currently being evaluated for the treatment of patients with phlebotomy-dependent PV. A randomized, open-label, multicenter, phase 2a/2b study to determine the efficacy and safety of KRT-232 compared with ruxolitinib is currently accruing patients (NCT03669965).

Other Agents that May Lead to Disease Modification in Myeloproliferative Neoplasms

Givinostat is an orally bioavailable, potent inhibitor of class I and II histone-deacetylase (HDAC) that has demonstrated preclinical activity in selective targeting of the *JAK2* V617 F clone by attenuating JAK2/STAT5 signaling and inducing apoptosis.[29] Subsequently, several studies have shown that givinostat is clinically active either as monotherapy or in combination with hydroxyurea in patients with PV. The phase Ib/II proof-of-concept trial of givinostat in patients with PV was studied at the dosage of 100 mg twice daily. The objective response rate was 80.6% at the end of 3 cycles and 50% of patients reported symptomatic improvement (pruritus, headache) with givinostat treatment. Also, the givinostat treatment resulted in moderate reduction of *JAK2* V617 F allele burden after 3 and 6 cycles of treatment. Almost all patients experienced a grade 1/2 treatment-related adverse event (diarrhea, 51%; thrombocytopenia, 45%; increased serum creatinine, 37%).[30] Based on these results, a global registration phase III trial that will evaluate the efficacy of givinostat versus hydroxyurea in high-risk PV patients is under way.

Lysine-specific demethylase 1 (LSD1) is an epigenetic enzyme that can demethylate mono- and di-methylated lysine residues, specifically histone 3 and lysine 4 and 9 (H3K4 and H3K9), and plays a critical role in regulating gene transcription. LSD1 is essential for steady-state hematopoiesis as genetic knockdown or pharmacologic inhibition of LSD1 abrogates erythropoiesis, granulopoiesis, and thrombopoiesis in a reversible fashion. In addition, LSD1 is found to be overexpressed in patients with MPN.[31] Bomedemstat (IMG-7289), an irreversible LSD1 inhibitor, reduced splenomegaly and bone marrow fibrosis, and normalized blood counts in the *Jak2* V617 F murine model.[32] Most importantly, this treatment resulted in reduction in mutant allele burden and improved survival of treated mice. This encouraging result has led to the ongoing clinical evaluation of bomedemstat as a second-line agent in PV and ET (NCT04262141, NCT04254978).

Hematocrit control through therapeutic phlebotomy in PV is achieved by reducing the iron stores in the body available for erythropoiesis. However, iron deficiency can also lead to symptoms including fatigue, brittle nails, and pica syndrome. Iron deficiency also suppresses hepcidin levels, which, in turn, increases absorption of iron and enhances red blood cell production. The hepcidin-mimetic PTG-300 is aiming to control red cell counts, by degradation of the ferroportin receptor in iron-absorptive enterocytes and iron-recycling macrophages, thus inducing iron-restricted erythropoiesis. In the case of PV, the hematocrit could be controlled in the absence of therapeutic phlebotomy and iron deficiency. It is currently being evaluated in an ongoing phase II trial in patients requiring at least 3 phlebotomies in the preceding 24 weeks either with or without cytoreduction to maintain a hematocrit of less than 45% (ClinicalTrials.gov Identifier: NCT04057040). Of the first 13 patients enrolled (8 of whom have been treated for at least 3 months), all but 1 was phlebotomy-free on PTG-300.[33] Moreover, iron-related parameters suggested a steady improvement in iron deficiency. This provides an exciting new way of controlling red blood cell counts in PV, but it remains to be seen if there will be an associated reduction in symptom burden, thrombosis risk, or evidence of disease modification.

WHAT REALLY IS DISEASE-MODIFYING ANYWAY?

Most of the currently available treatment options for patients with PV/ET are mainly aimed at minimizing the risk of thrombosis and/or bleeding. So far, none of the approved treatments for PV/ET has shown clear evidence of disease-modifying potential. The ultimate goal of the novel treatments currently in various stages of drug development is disease modification; however, there is significant ambiguity in how to define this goal. Despite the tremendous success of JAK inhibitors in controlling the symptom burden, spleen size, and blood counts in patients with MPNs, as well as prolonging survival in MF, these treatments are not considered disease-modifying.[34] In the era of genomics, the standard approach is to measure disease modification with the reduction in the mutant allele burden of the driver mutation (*JAK2*, *CALR*, or *MPL*). Although it is intuitive, achieving molecular remission is not a validated endpoint in PV/ET, as its correlation with clinical outcomes, such has thrombotic events, disease progression, or overall survival, has not been established. Given that there are other pathways outside of JAK-STAT that are key in disease development, reduction of the driver mutant allele burden may prove not to be an effective surrogate endpoint for disease modification. Therefore, sustained exploration of the pathobiology and continued consensus on measurement of disease modification is needed for the future development of successful treatments.

SUMMARY

MPNs are a group of clonal hematopoietic stem cell disorders characterized by abnormal myeloproliferation leading to elevated blood counts, splenomegaly, systemic inflammation, and propensity to thrombosis. To date, none of the available therapies for PV/ET have been shown to improve survival or prevent transformation to myelofibrosis or acute leukemia, instead, therapies are primarily targeted at preventing thrombo-hemorrhagic complications and alleviating symptom burden. This is an urgent unmet clinical need in PV/ET. Although genetic driver mutation-specific targeted therapy is at the center of MPN drug development, recent evidence (eg, IFN-α, idasanutlin, givinostat, bomedemstat) highlights the importance of targeting other cellular pathways in MPN. There is now long-term evidence, albeit in a nonrandomized setting, that IFN-α treatment in patients with PV will improve overall survival and reverse bone marrow fibrosis in a fraction of treated patients, potentially altering the natural history of the disease. This emphasizes the importance of a broader approach to target novel pathways in MPN, with the goal of improving treatment outcomes.

CLINICS CARE POINTS

- Although low-dose aspirin is universal in PV to prevent thrombosis, it may not be needed for all patients with ET.
- There are no prospective, randomized data that have identified a platelet count target in ET, so platelet count goals are often individualized for each patient
- Retrospective data have suggested a potential myelofibrosis-free survival and overall survival advantage for interferon therapy over hydroxyurea therapy.
- In addition to controlling counts, new agents in development are aiming to alter the natural history of PV and ET.

DISCLOSURE

A.T. Gerds: Galecto (Advisory Board), PharmEssentia (Advisory Board), and Constellation (Advisory Board). A. Kishtagari: none.

REFERENCES

1. Spivak JL. Myeloproliferative neoplasms. N Engl J Med 2017;376(22):2168–81.
2. Kiladjian JJ, Zachee P, Hino M, et al. Long-term efficacy and safety of ruxolitinib versus best available therapy in polycythaemia vera (RESPONSE): 5-year follow up of a phase 3 study. Lancet Haematol 2020;7(3):e226–37.
3. Landolfi R, Marchioli R, Kutti J, et al. Efficacy and safety of low-dose aspirin in polycythemia vera. N Engl J Med 2004;350(2):114–24.
4. Marchioli R, Finazzi G, Specchia G, et al. Cardiovascular events and intensity of treatment in polycythemia vera. N Engl J Med 2013;368(1):22–33.
5. Network NCC. Myeloprolifertive neoplasms (version 1.2020). 2020. Available at: https://www.nccn.org/professionals/physician_gls/pdf/mpn.pdf. Accessed January 27, 2021.
6. Barbui T, Tefferi A, Vannucchi AM, et al. Philadelphia chromosome-negative classical myeloproliferative neoplasms: revised management recommendations from European LeukemiaNet. Leukemia 2018;32(5):1057–69.
7. Squizzato A, Romualdi E, Passamonti F, et al. Antiplatelet drugs for polycythaemia vera and essential thrombocythaemia. Cochrane Database Syst Rev 2013;(4):Cd006503.
8. Alvarez-Larrán A, Cervantes F, Pereira A, et al. Observation versus antiplatelet therapy as primary prophylaxis for thrombosis in low-risk essential thrombocythemia. Blood 2010;116(8):1205–10 [quiz: 1387].
9. Alvarez-Larrán A, Pereira A, Guglielmelli P, et al. Antiplatelet therapy versus observation in low-risk essential thrombocythemia with a CALR mutation. Haematologica 2016;101(8):926–31.
10. Epstein E, Goedel A. Hämorrhagische Thrombocythämie bei vasculärer Schrumpfmilz. Virchows Archiv 1934;292(2):233–48.
11. Palandri F, Polverelli N, Catani L, et al. Bleeding in essential thrombocythaemia: a retrospective analysis on 565 patients. Br J Haematol 2012;156(2):281–4.
12. Tefferi A, Gangat N, Wolanskyj AP. Management of extreme thrombocytosis in otherwise low-risk essential thrombocythemia; does number matter? Blood 2006;108(7):2493–4.
13. Cortelazzo S, Finazzi G, Ruggeri M, et al. Hydroxyurea for patients with essential thrombocythemia and a high risk of thrombosis. N Engl J Med 1995;332(17):1132–6.
14. Cortelazzo S, Viero P, Finazzi G, et al. Incidence and risk factors for thrombotic complications in a historical cohort of 100 patients with essential thrombocythemia. J Clin Oncol 1990;8(3):556–62.
15. Kiladjian JJ, Cassinat B, Chevret S, et al. Pegylated interferon-alfa-2a induces complete hematologic and molecular responses with low toxicity in polycythemia vera. Blood 2008;112(8):3065–72.
16. Mullally A, Bruedigam C, Poveromo L, et al. Depletion of Jak2V617F myeloproliferative neoplasm-propagating stem cells by interferon-α in a murine model of polycythemia vera. Blood 2013;121(18):3692–702.
17. Masarova L, Patel KP, Newberry KJ, et al. Pegylated interferon alfa-2a in patients with essential thrombocythaemia or polycythaemia vera: a post-hoc, median 83 month follow-up of an open-label, phase 2 trial. Lancet Haematol 2017;4(4):e165–75.
18. Yacoub A, Mascarenhas J, Kosiorek H, et al. Pegylated interferon alfa-2a for polycythemia vera or essential thrombocythemia resistant or intolerant to hydroxyurea. Blood 2019;134(18):1498–509.

19. Gisslinger H, Klade C, Georgiev P, et al. Ropeginterferon alfa-2b versus standard therapy for polycythaemia vera (PROUD-PV and CONTINUATION-PV): a randomised, non-inferiority, phase 3 trial and its extension study. Lancet Haematol 2020;7(3):e196–208.
20. Gisslinger H, Klade C, Georgiev P, et al. Long-term use of ropeginterferon alpha-2b in polycythemia vera: 5-year results from a randomized controlled study and its extension. Blood 2020;136(Supplement 1):33.
21. Daltro De Oliveira R, Soret-Dulphy J, Zhao L-P, et al. Interferon-alpha (IFN) therapy discontinuation is feasible in myeloproliferative neoplasm (MPN) patients with complete hematological remission. Blood 2020;136(Supplement 1):35–6.
22. Jäger R, Gisslinger H, Fuchs E, et al. Germline genetic factors influence outcome of interferon alpha therapy in polycythemia vera. Blood 2020. https://doi.org/10.1182/blood.2020005792.
23. Abu-Zeinah G, Krichevsky S, Cruz T, et al. Interferon in polycythemia vera (PV) yields improved myelofibrosis-free and overall survival. Blood 2020;136(Supplement 1):31–2.
24. Lu M, Wang X, Li Y, et al. Combination treatment in vitro with Nutlin, a small-molecule antagonist of MDM2, and pegylated interferon-α 2a specifically targets JAK2V617F-positive polycythemia vera cells. Blood 2012;120(15):3098–105.
25. Nakatake M, Monte-Mor B, Debili N, et al. JAK2(V617F) negatively regulates p53 stabilization by enhancing MDM2 via La expression in myeloproliferative neoplasms. Oncogene 2012;31(10):1323–33.
26. Mascarenhas J, Lu M, Kosiorek H, et al. Oral idasanutlin in patients with polycythemia vera. Blood 2019;134(6):525–33.
27. Passamonti F, Burbury K, El-Galaly TC, et al. Molecular response patterns in hydroxyurea (HU)-resistant or intolerant polycythemia vera (PV) during treatment with idasanutlin: results of an open-label, single-arm phase 2 study. Blood 2020;136(Supplement 1):38–40.
28. Mascarenhas J, Higgins B, Anders D, et al. Safety and efficacy of idasanutlin in patients (pts) with hydroxyurea (HU)-resistant/intolerant polycythemia vera (PV): results of an international Phase II study. Blood 2020;136(Supplement 1):29–31.
29. Chifotides HT, Bose P, Verstovsek S. Givinostat: an emerging treatment for polycythemia vera. Expert Opin Investig Drugs 2020;29(6):525–36.
30. Rambaldi A, Iurlo A, Vannucchi AM, et al. Safety and efficacy of the maximum tolerated dose of givinostat in polycythemia vera: a two-part Phase Ib/II study. Leukemia 2020;34(8):2234–7.
31. Niebel D, Kirfel J, Janzen V, et al. Lysine-specific demethylase 1 (LSD1) in hematopoietic and lymphoid neoplasms. Blood 2014;124(1):151–2.
32. Jutzi JS, Kleppe M, Dias J, et al. LSD1 inhibition prolongs survival in mouse models of MPN by selectively targeting the disease clone. Hemasphere 2018;2(3):e54.
33. Kremyanskaya M, Ginzburg Y, Kuykendall AT, et al. PTG-300 eliminates the need for therapeutic phlebotomy in both low and high-risk polycythemia vera patients. Blood 2020;136(Supplement 1):33–5.
34. Gerds AT. Beyond JAK-STAT: novel therapeutic targets in Ph-negative MPN. Hematology Am Soc Hematol Educ Program 2019;2019(1):407–14.

Thrombotic, Vascular, and Bleeding Complications of the Myeloproliferative Neoplasms

Andrew I. Schafer, MD

KEYWORDS

- Thrombosis • Vascular and microvascular disease • Bleeding
- Clonal hematopoiesis • Inflammation

KEY POINTS

- Thrombosis pathogenesis in the myeloproliferative neoplasms (MPNs) involves the synergistic effects of cell-intrinsic abnormalities of blood cells derived from the mutant MPN stem cell, endothelial cells, and a state of systemic inflammation.
- Venous, arterial, and microvascular thrombotic events are the most common causes of morbidity and mortality in the MPNs.
- Presentation of patients with unusual sites of thrombosis and vascular occlusion, such as splanchnic vein or cerebral vein thrombosis, microvascular disturbances such as erythromelalgia or neuro-ophthalmologic problems, and recurrent pregnancy loss, should raise clinical suspicion for an underlying MPN.
- Systemic bleeding complications in the MPNs are often caused by a form of acquired von Willebrand disease that develops as abnormal MPN platelets and neutrophils selectively remove the high-molecular-weight multimers of von Willebrand factor in the circulation by adsorbing them to their cell surfaces or by proteolysis.
- Phlebotomy to maintain hematocrits of less than 45% and cytoreductive therapy to target normalization of blood counts in patients who have had thrombotic or vascular complications are evidence-based mainstays of preventing their occurrence in patients with MPN, but antithrombotic agents are still used as for others without MPNs, with recent concerns about the indiscriminate use of aspirin.

INTRODUCTION

It has long been recognized that thrombosis, vascular events, and bleeding are the major causes of morbidity and mortality in patients with Philadelphia chromosome–negative myeloproliferative neoplasms (MPNs).[1] In a large, multinational cohort of patients with polycythemia vera (PV), the cause of death was thrombohemorrhagic events in 45%, compared with disease transformation in 13%.[2] Symptomatic patients with MPN may have exclusively thrombotic or exclusively bleeding complications during the course of their disease, but many have both. In 1899, Dr. Robert C. Cabot[3]

Weill Cornell Medicine, 1305 York Avenue, 8th Floor, Room Y-811, New York, NY 10021, USA
E-mail address: ais2007@med.cornell.edu

Hematol Oncol Clin N Am 35 (2021) 305–324
https://doi.org/10.1016/j.hoc.2020.11.006
0889-8588/21/© 2020 Elsevier Inc. All rights reserved.

described the case of a 46-year-old masseuse with polycythemia who had a history of spontaneous bruising and a transient ischemic attack. She presented with "very free hemorrhage, lasting half a day, and controlled only by packing the cavity with gauze … The bleeding seemed to make her feel better." She died of a cerebral hemorrhage.[3] Patients with PV are particularly prone to thrombosis, whereas patients with essential thrombocythemia (ET) and myelofibrosis (MF) tend to have more bleeding problems.

It is common for patients to present with thrombotic, vascular, or bleeding events that precede the diagnosis of MPN. In 9429 patients with MPNs and 35,820 matched control subjects from the Swedish Cancer Register, the hazard ratio (HR) for any thrombosis at 3 months after diagnosis was 4.0 in patients with MPN compared with controls. The HRs for thrombosis at 1 and 5 years after diagnosis of MPNs were 2.4 and 1.8, respectively. There was a nearly 10-fold increase in the rate of venous thrombosis specifically (HR, 9.7) 3 months after diagnosis, which decreased markedly at 1 and 5 years of follow-up, respectively, but remained significantly increased compared with control subjects.[4] The study clearly showed that most thrombotic events in patients with MPNs occur before or shortly after the diagnosis of MPN. Furthermore, the markedly decreased rate of venous thrombosis at 5 years after MPN diagnosis was sustained for at least 20 years. For arterial thrombosis, the greatest decrease is seen at 3 years after the MPN diagnosis, but then gradually increases by 20 years up to at least 50% of the rate seen at 3 months.

A systematic review and meta-analysis of 29 prospective and retrospective cohort studies showed that overall incidence of thrombosis at the time of diagnosis of an MPN (presumably occurring earlier) was 20.0%, including 6.2% for arterial events and 6.2% for venous thromboses.[5] Comparable findings were reported in a real-world study of a large, unselected group of patients with MPN seen at university and nonuniversity hospitals or office-based practices, reported by the MPN registry of the German Study Alliance Leukemia (SAL). Here, most thromboembolic events occurred either before or at the time of diagnosis of an MPN. In contrast, most bleeding complications in this population were noted after the MPN diagnosis.[6]

This finding raises the question of whether patients without known MPNs who present with apparently unprovoked thrombosis should be screened for an MPN as part of their hypercoagulability work-ups. It is reasonable to do so in individuals with sustained thrombocytosis, leukocytosis, and/or erythrocytosis following the thrombotic episode. However, transient blood count increases frequently occur as a reactive process immediately after the thrombotic event and do not warrant prompt evaluation for MPNs. Screening for an MPN after thrombosis in patients with unexplained splenomegaly is likewise reasonable. In those who present with thrombosis or a vascular event that is characteristic of MPNs, such as hepatic vein thrombosis, portal vein thrombosis, or erythromelalgia, evaluation for an underlying MPN is recommended. In the absence of any of these findings, evaluation of MPNs is not routinely indicated in patients who present with thrombosis.

GENOMIC PROFILE AND RISK OF THROMBOTIC AND VASCULAR COMPLICATIONS IN THE MPNs

The classic Philadelphia chromosome–negative MPNs are PV, ET, and primary myelofibrosis (PMF). Subsets of these disorders as they relate to progression of disease are prefibrotic myelofibrosis, post-PV myelofibrosis, and post-ET myelofibrosis. The major somatic driver mutations that have been identified to date for these MPNs are JAK2(V617F), JAK2 exon 12/13, calreticulin or CALR (mostly type 1 CALR del152 and type 2 CALR ins5), and MPL(W515). The prevalence of the JAK2(V617F) mutation is 95% in PV, 50% to 75% in ET, and 40% to 75% in PMF. *JAK2* exon 12 mutations are specific for PV. *CALR* mutations occur in 20% to 30% of patients with ET and PMF.[7] MPNs that do not have any of these driver mutations (approximately 10%) are termed triple negative, although many in this category do carry other rare mutations in these genes that are likely to be pathogenic. In addition to the driver mutations, patients with MPN can have other somatic mutations in cancer-associated genes. Such nondriver mutations occur in primarily in chromatin regulatory genes (eg, *ASXL1*, *EZH2*), epigenetic regulatory genes (eg, *TET2*, *DNMT3A*), or splicing machinery genes (eg, *SF3B1*), and can carry prognostic significance.

The mutational profile and order of mutation acquisition have major (but not exclusive) effects on MPN phenotype and patient outcomes, including the risk of thrombotic and vascular events. A *JAK2(V617F)* mutation is associated with an increased risk of thrombosis compared with patients with MPN with other driver mutations. Those who have a *JAK2(V617F)* allele frequency of greater than 75% are at particularly high risk of cardiovascular events and thrombosis, with each of these 2 complications carrying a relative risk of 7.1 ($P = .003$).[8] By contrast, patients with MPN who have a *CALR* mutation have a lower risk of thrombosis.[9] *CALR*-mutated and *JAK2(V617F)*-mutated CD34+ cells show different gene and microRNA expression profiles; in particular, patients with *CALR* mutation–positive ET are characterized by downregulation of several genes involved in thrombin signaling and platelet activation.[10]

In addition to the classic Philadelphia chromosome-negative MPNs, the 2016 revised World Health Organization (WHO) classification of MPNs[11] includes several other clonal hematopoietic disorders that have diagnostic somatic gene mutations: chronic myeloid leukemia (CML) with the *BCR-ABL* fusion gene; chronic neutrophilic leukemia with the *CSF3R* mutation; systemic mastocytosis with the *KIT*(D816V) mutation; and chronic hypereosinophilia with rearrangements of the *PDGFRA*, *PDGFRB*, and *FGFR1* genes. Some of these are also associated with thrombotic and vascular complications.

Chronic Myeloid Leukemia

In the pre–tyrosine kinase inhibitor (TKI) era, bleeding complications were found in some patients with CML, even in the absence of thrombocytopenia; however, thrombotic and vascular complications were rarely seen.[12] More recently the picture has changed. A recent meta-analysis and systematic review of 72 prospective studies including 9061 patients showed that the incidence rate of venous thromboembolism among patients with CML was 13% (95% confidence interval, 1%–36%), in contrast with incident rates of 5%, 3%, and 6% in patients with acute lymphoid leukemia, chronic lymphocytic leukemia, and acute myelogenous leukemia, respectively.[13] The potential confounding variable of treatment with TKIs that have been associated with vascular events in patients with CML was not addressed. Imatinib and the newer TKIs such as nilotinib, dasatinib, and ponatinib, to a greater or lesser extent clearly increase the risk of cardiovascular or atherothrombotic adverse events, particularly coronary, cerebrovascular, and peripheral arterial disease. Individual TKIs have different risk profiles, as well as different clinical manifestations and mechanisms of vascular toxicity.[14] Composite analysis of 531 patients treated with these frontline TKIs in different prospective CML trials found that, overall, 45% of patients developed cardiovascular adverse events and 9% had arteriothrombotic adverse events.[15]

Hypereosinophilia

Hypereosinophilia, whether it be clonal or nonclonal in cause, has been associated with various thrombotic and vascular complications, including deep vein thrombosis, pulmonary embolism, superficial venous thrombosis, portal vein thrombosis, cerebral arteriolar or venous thrombosis, and intracardiac mural thrombi. The frequency of thrombosis in hypereosinophilias has not been adequately determined but it is generally not common. When they do occur, most involve large-vessel, medium-vessel, or small-vessel arterial occlusions. A recently reported retrospective study of 63 consecutive patients with idiopathic hypereosinophilia or hypereosinophilic syndrome with concurrent venous thromboembolism, which excluded patients with provoking factors or any kind of underlying hypercoagulable states, found that independent risk factors included the level and duration of absolute eosinophilia.[16] The mechanism of thrombosis in these cases is probably multifactorial. Circulating eosinophils play a significant role in activation and regulation of coagulation, expressing tissue factor (TF) and TF-dependent thrombin generation.[17] The strong endogenous thrombin-generating capacity of eosinophils is also mediated by their procoagulant surfaces that are enriched in 12/15-lipoxygenase–derived phospholipids.[18] Eosinophil-derived mediators, including cationic proteins and reactive oxygen species, can also promote inflammation, fibrosis, and thrombosis by causing direct endothelial toxicity. The entity of eosinophilic vasculitis has been shown in 117 patients with hypereosinophilia who did not have asthma, antineutrophil cytoplasmic antibodies, or other causes of reactive eosinophilia. Histopathologic findings showed an eosinophil-rich, necrotizing form of vasculitis that affected not only arterial but also venous vessels.[19]

Systemic Mastocytosis

In contrast with the other MPNs discussed earlier, patients with systemic mastocytosis are at increased risk for only clinical bleeding, not thrombosis. The frequency of bleeding problems is very low but, when it does occur, it may be severe and even life threatening. In the French national database of 880 patients with well-characterized and well-followed systemic mastocytosis (CEREMAST), meeting WHO diagnostic criteria, 14 patients were identified as having a bleeding diathesis and none with venous thromboses.[20] Bleeding can be asymptomatic with only laboratory abnormalities in the prothrombin time (PT) and/or activated partial thromboplastin time (aPTT). In patients with overt bleeding, some had mucocutaneous bleeding, reflecting platelet-vascular abnormalities, and some had severe deep bleeding, indicating abnormalities in the coagulation system associated with prolonged PT and/or aPTT. Bleeding typically occurred at times of mast cell activation and degranulation flares, and was most severe in patients with aggressive disease who had multiorgan mast cell infiltration. Although it has been experimentally shown that mast cell granular contents are thrombogenic,[21] the almost exclusivity of clinical bleeding complications suggests that the balance between the antithrombotic properties of activated mast cells (containing heparin, tryptase, and tissue plasminogen activator) outweigh the effects of their proinflammatory/prothrombotic mediators (eg, histamine, tumor necrosis factor-α). In treating clinical bleeding in systemic mastocytosis, hemostatic management alone may be inadequate; simultaneous, aggressive treatment with mast cell mediator inhibitors and mast cell stabilizers may be required.[20]

VASCULAR DISEASE AND THROMBOSIS IN CLONAL HEMATOPOIESIS OF INDETERMINATE POTENTIAL

Clonal hematopoiesis of indeterminate potential (CHIP) refers to the acquisition of nonmalignant clonal mutations in genes that are associated mostly with hematologic neoplasms, including the MPNs, with variant frequencies of greater than or equal to 2% in the absence of any clinical evidence of a coexisting hematologic neoplasm. The risk of carrying CHIP increases dramatically with age, with a prevalence of greater than or equal to 50% in patients more than 85 years of age.[22] CHIP is now considered to be an inevitable consequence of normal aging. In population-based cohorts that had exome sequencing, the presence of CHIP was associated with an approximately 10-fold increased relative risk of developing a clinically overt hematologic malignancy, including MPN, within the subsequent 8 years.[23] Furthermore, it was unexpectedly found that the risk of future atherosclerotic coronary artery disease and ischemic stroke is more than doubled in carriers of CHIP.[24] Genes that are frequently mutated in CHIP may also be important mediators of inflammatory signals,[25] and inflammation (discussed later), which is an important contributor to the pathogenesis of MPNs, thrombosis, and atherosclerotic cardiovascular disease. In particular, JAK2 has been linked to inflammatory processes, serving as a signal transmitter downstream of major inflammatory cytokine receptors.[26]

NONGENOMIC RISKS OF THROMBOTIC AND VASCULAR COMPLICATIONS IN THE MYELOPROLIFERATIVE NEOPLASMS

Chronic inflammation is now recognized to be a critical participant in both the pathogenesis of MPNs and their thrombotic complications (**Fig. 1**). The progeny of *JAK2*-mutated MPN stem cells and the stromal cells within their bone marrow environment generate proinflammatory cytokines that promote mutant clonal evolution. Increased levels of interleukin (IL)-18, IL-6, IL-8, C-reactive protein, and other inflammatory mediators can be measured in circulating blood not only in patients with overt MPNs[27] but even in those with MPN driver mutation CHIP.[28,29] Some patients with progression

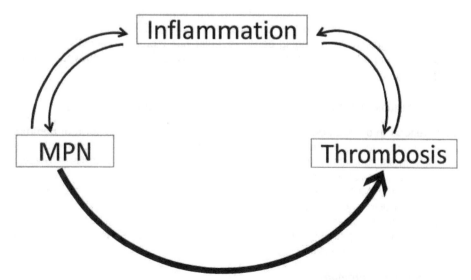

Fig. 1. The cycle of MPN, inflammation, and thrombosis. A simplified cartoon of thrombogenesis in the MPNs. The MPNs stimulate a microenvironmental and systemic inflammatory state. In turn, inflammation fuels MPN driver mutation–induced clonal expansion. There is also a reciprocal relationship between inflammation and thrombosis in MPN as well as patients without MPN. Thrombosis in general leads to an inflammatory state and inflammation, in turn, fuels thrombogenesis.

of disease have systemic symptoms (eg, night sweats, weight loss) that reflect their high level of systemic inflammation, but most patients with stable MPNs have only a subclinical systemic inflammatory state. A close functional interdependence between the processes of inflammation and thrombosis is now known to be operative in a wide spectrum of disorders, not only in the MPNs. Inflammation stimulates thrombosis and, in turn, thrombosis promotes inflammation (see **Fig. 1**), a generalizable pathophysiologic state that has been referred to as thromboinflammation.[30,31] Specifically in the MPNs, this sets up a potential vicious cycle wherein inflammation drives preferential proliferation of *JAK2(V617F)*-positive rather than wild-type clones, fueling more systemic inflammation that then leads to further mutant clonal evolution. The combined effects of an increasing population of *JAK2(V617F)*-positive circulating blood cells that have acquired prothrombotic and proadhesive phenotypes (discussed later), an activated coagulation system catalyzed by activated blood cells, and an increasing systemic proinflammatory state progressively heighten the risk of thrombotic and vascular complications in the MPNs.

Aging in general, even in the absence of MPNs, is a strong risk factor for both venous thrombosis and atherothrombosis.[32,33] Advanced age is well established as an independent risk factor for thrombosis in MPN risk stratification systems. Aging and systemic inflammation are not completely separate prothrombotic processes because advancing age is characterized by the gradual development of a state of chronic subclinical inflammation (so-called inflammaging) and by progressive immune system impairment.[34,35]

Other cardiovascular risk factors in addition to aging include obesity, smoking, diabetes mellitus, hypertension, hyperlipidemia, and the metabolic syndrome. Although their role in the development of atherothrombosis is well established, they are probably likewise risk factors for venous thrombosis. Several studies have shown that patients with atherosclerotic arterial disease are predisposed to venous thromboembolism and, conversely, patients with venous thromboembolism are at greater risk of arterial thrombotic complications than matched control individuals.[36] Therefore, aggressively managing cardiovascular risk factors in patients with MPN should be an important part of the armamentarium to prevent thrombotic and vascular complications.

VENOUS THROMBOEMBOLISM IN THE MYELOPROLIFERATIVE NEOPLASMS

Most venous thromboembolic complications in the MPNs take the form of common deep vein thrombosis of the lower extremities and/or pulmonary embolisms that are clinically indistinguishable from those seen in patients without MPNs. However, more unusual sites of venous thrombosis may occur in the MPNs that are by no means diagnostic of an MPN but are characteristic. These sites include superficial thrombophlebitis; jugular, subclavian, or axillary vein thrombosis of the upper extremities (Paget-Schroetter disease); renal vein thrombosis; central retinal or branch retinal vein thrombosis; splanchnic vein thrombosis (SVT); and cerebral venous and cavernous sinus thrombosis.

Splanchnic Vein Thrombosis

The splanchnic venous circulation involves predominantly the hepatic and portal veins, with extension to the mesenteric and splenic veins.

Hepatic vein thrombosis is also referred to as the Budd-Chiari syndrome. SVT[37] is often associated with hepatic cirrhosis, where the mechanism involves both local, anatomic factors as the nidus for thrombus formation and the systemic hemostatic abnormalities of liver failure. In noncirrhotic SVT, local intra-abdominal structural per-turbations such as malignant or benign tumors of the hepatobiliary system, ab-scesses, and abdominal surgery (eg, splenectomy, liver transplant, bariatric surgery) provoke adjacent clot development. Other local causes of SVT are contiguous inflam-matory disorders of the gastrointestinal tract, including inflammatory bowel disease, diverticulitis, and complicated hepatobiliary tract inflammation or infection. Systemic hypercoagulable states such as thrombophilias and hormonal changes (eg, oral con-traceptives, hormone replacement therapy, pregnancy) can be triggers for such events. Before the discovery of MPN driver mutations, at least one-third of patients presenting with SVT were classified as idiopathic. It is now known that almost all such cases are associated with MPNs or, rarely, another hematopoietic stem cell dis-order, paroxysmal nocturnal hemoglobinuria (PNH). In many such patients, an impor-tant clue that should raise suspicion of an underlying MPN is that circulating blood counts are inappropriately normal. With other causes of SVT that lead to portal hyper-tension, congestive splenomegaly, and hypersplenism, pancytopenia is expected. The low normal hemoglobin and hematocrit levels in patients with PV with hypersplen-ism has been referred to as masked PV.

The propensity for SVT in patients with MPN may be caused by several factors. These factors include the low blood flow velocity within the splanchnic venous system, which permits blood components to have prolonged contact with sinusoidal endothe-lial cells.[38,39] Vascular endothelial cells in MPNs have been shown to harbor the *JAK2(V617F)* mutation specifically in splanchnic veins,[40] and such JAK2-mutated endothelial cells promote a prothrombotic and proadherent phenotype[41] that has been attributed in part to overexpression of P-selectin.[42] SVT in PNH has been attrib-uted to bacterial and food antigens present in the gut-draining mesenteric and portal veins, which may locally activate complement, causing localized endothelial dam-age.[43] Similar mechanisms may be operative in SVT caused by MPNs. *JAK2(V617F)* mutation–positive patients with MPN have poor long-term outcomes despite anticoa-gulation,[44] although direct anticoagulants have been found to be safe and effective in patients with noncirrhotic portal vein thrombosis in general.[45]

Cerebral Venous and Cavernous Sinus Thrombosis

Cerebral venous thrombosis (CVT), a life-threatening condition, typically presents with headache, papilledema, and diplopia. The most common risk factors in adults are oral contraceptives, pregnancy, and thrombophilia. Even in the absence of other risk fac-tors, MPNs alone can be associated with these complications.[46] A significantly higher prevalence of coexisting thrombophilia has been found in patients with MPN with CVT compared with other patients with MPN. Furthermore, patients with MPNs and CVT have a higher risk of developing recurrent thromboses compared with those having other types of venous thromboses.[47,48] In addition to controlling the underlying MPN, anticoagulation is therefore required for an indefinite duration, even if coexisting hypercoagulable states such as oral contraceptives or pregnancy are no longer risks.

ARTERIAL THROMBOSIS AND ATHEROTHROMBOSIS IN THE MYELOPROLIFERATIVE NEOPLASMS

In contrast with venous thrombosis, most individuals with arterial thrombosis have un-derlying atherosclerotic cardiovascular disease (so-called atherothrombosis).[33,49] In these cases, the nidus for arterial thrombus tends to occur at sites of atherosclerotic plaque disruption. From the Swedish Canner Register, the 3-month HR for arterial thrombosis was increased 3-fold in patients with MPNs compared with age-matched and sex-matched controls from the general population, and the magnitude of this relative increased risk was comparable across MPN subtypes.[4] Similar findings were reported from the Danish National Patient Registry, adjusted for levels of comorbidity.[50] Patients with MPN are prone to the development of secondary cancers. Interestingly, after adjustments for confounders, multivariate analysis of a nested case-control study of patients with MPN showed that the occurrence of arterial thrombosis, but not venous thrombosis, was independently associated with an increased risk of subsequently diagnosed carcinomas (odds ratio, 1.97; confidence interval, 1.14–3.41), specifically noncutaneous malignancies.[51] The mechanisms underlying this observation remain unclear.

Acute myocardial infarction can be a presenting event in patients with MPN. The diagnosis of MPN should be considered in selected patients, especially those who have unexplained coronary ischemic events associated with persistent thrombocytosis and no cardiovascular risk factors. These individuals may have coronary artery thrombi, with or without spasm, but no underlying atherosclerotic changes in the coronary arteries.[52,53] The rates of ischemic cerebrovascular events in the MPNs are approximately 10-fold higher than in the general population.[54]

MICROVASCULAR COMPLICATIONS IN THE MYELOPROLIFERATIVE NEOPLASMS

Several microvascular disturbances have been described in the MPNs. Although infrequently seen, they can be disabling and distinctive, although they are not exclusive to the MPNs.

Erythromelalgia

Erythromelalgia typically presents as episodic burning and other forms of neuropathic pain with corresponding areas of erythema, warmth, and tenderness.[55] The symptoms and signs most commonly involve the lower extremities, usually asymmetrically, especially the plantar surfaces of the feet and toes. Less common sites are hands, fingers, and even face. Ambient heat, exercise, and limb dependence are provoking factors. Primary erythromelalgia is an autosomal dominant inherited disease caused by mutation in the SCN9A gene, which encodes for voltage-gated sodium channels. Secondary erythromelalgia is associated with many diseases but its most common cause is the MPNs. Histopathology by skin biopsy of an involved area, which is not routinely recommended, shows swelling of arteriolar endothelial cells, narrowing of the lumen by proliferating smooth muscle cells, and occlusion by platelet thrombi.[56] The presence of platelet thrombi in involved microvessels in patients with MPN, but their absence in involved areas in patients with primary erythromelalgia, may explain the lack of responsiveness to aspirin in the latter disorder.[57] The hypoxia caused by microvascular occlusions in erythromelalgia may also trigger a neuropathy through ischemic damage to cutaneous nociceptors, contributing to the sensorial manifestations.[58] In many cases, aspirin and, to a lesser extent, other nonsteroidal antiinflammatory drugs offer prompt improvement of symptoms but may require higher doses than are used for cardiovascular prevention. Coping strategies such as brief immersion of affected limbs in ice-cold water can provide transient relief. Optimal control of high blood counts may ameliorate the problem, but refractory cases pose a therapeutic challenge.[59]

Livedo Racemose and Livedo Reticularis

Livedo racemose and livedo reticularis are characterized by violaceous, netlike erythema of the skin. These disorders are caused by impairment of blood flow to cutaneous microvessels of the skin segments involved; the pattern of mottling relates to the vascular anatomy of normal skin. There continues to be debate about the differences between the 2 terms, with racemose generally preferred in the European and reticularis in the North American literature. The cutaneous manifestations are indistinguishable, but racemose tends to be more generalized, whereas reticularis is more localized to the legs. It is thought by some that livedo reticularis is a physiologic phenomenon caused by reactive cutaneous vasoconstriction (eg, to cold), whereas livedo racemose is always associated with a pathologic condition, such as antiphospholipid syndrome. If the two entities are not the identical disorder with merely different names, they likely represent a spectrum of cutaneous manifestations.[60] Livedo has been noted to be a rare microvascular complication of ET.[61,62]

Sneddon Syndrome

Sneddon syndrome[63] is an episodic or progressive disorder that is characterized by generalized livedo racemose and recurrent cerebrovascular events, sometimes leading to cognitive decline. Histopathology of skin and brain shows noninflammatory thrombotic vasculopathy involving medium-sized and small dermal and cerebral arteries. It is seen in patients with MPNs but it is more commonly linked to antiphospholipid syndrome.

Digital Ischemia

Large peripheral artery thromboses in the MPNs in the absence of underlying atherosclerosis is not well documented, but digital ischemia secondary to arteriolar thrombosis is well recognized. In these cases, the distal lower limb pulses are palpable and ankle-brachial pressure indices are normal. By angiography, normal large and medium-sized arteries are found to have minimal or no significant atherosclerotic changes. However, angiography can sometimes visualize small arterial vessel occlusions in the distal lower limb.[64] Patients can present this way and even undergo unsuccessful bypass surgery before thrombocytosis is noted and an MPN is diagnosed. The digital ischemia can appear de novo or follow manifestations of erythromelalgia. Without prompt diagnosis and appropriate treatment, cyanotic toes can progress to necrosis, gangrene, and even autoamputation (**Fig. 2**).

Neuro-ophthalmologic Complications of Myeloproliferative Neoplasms

The prevalence of ocular and neuro-ophthalmologic complications in the MPNs has been estimated to be between 7.5% and 25% in both treated and untreated patients.[65] Microvascular disturbances that are caused by impaired retinal or cerebral perfusion include monocular and transient blindness, amaurosis fugax, scintillating scotomas, hemianopsia, and migrainelike transient ischemic attacks. With prompt diagnosis of neuro-ophthalmologic complications of MPNs, the symptoms and signs can usually be reversed. Vaso-occlusion caused by central retinal artery or vein thrombosis can cause retinal ischemia and vision loss. It can be caused in the MPNs by increased whole-blood viscosity in PV and abnormal adhesion of JAK2-mutated blood cells to the vascular endothelium.

Some MPN therapeutic agents potentially have adverse effects on the eyes. Interferon-α has been associated with anterior ischemic optic neuropathy, although a causal relationship is not well established. The immunosuppressive actions of ruxolitinib can lead to retinitis secondary to opportunistic infections (eg, cytomegalovirus, toxoplasmosis).

Maternal and Fetal Vascular Events

Most pregnant women with MPNs deliver at term without complications. However, many, especially those with ET, have significant maternal morbidity and poor fetal outcomes. Complications include maternal thrombosis (especially during the third trimester and puerperium) and hemorrhage. Fetal complications include early spontaneous miscarriage, preeclampsia, intrauterine growth restriction, stillbirth, and prematurity. Placental histopathology can show microvascular thrombotic occlusions with infarction of the placental circulation, leading to uteroplacental dysfunction that is similar to what is seen in acquired and inherited thrombophilias with an associated miscarriage.[66] Published series have reported live birth rates of 50% to 70% and spontaneous abortion rates of 22% to 50% in mothers with MPNs, predominantly ET.[67,68] A systematic review and meta-analysis of 22 studies reporting on 1210 pregnancies found that the use of aspirin and interferon-α, but not heparin, was associated with higher odds of live births.[69]

BLEEDING COMPLICATIONS IN THE MYELOPROLIFERATIVE NEOPLASMS

Most bleeding problems in patients with MPN are superficial surface bleeds such as easy or spontaneous bruising, oral mucosal bleeding, epistaxis, hemoptysis, and mucosal bleeding from the gastrointestinal and genitourinary tracts. This pattern of bleeding is characteristic of abnormalities in primary hemostasis, associated with platelet–vessel wall interactions, in contrast with the typically deep tissue and organ bleeds seen in coagulation factor abnormalities (secondary hemostasis). In most studies, the estimated prevalence of bleeding problems as an initial symptom of MPN has been between 3% and 18% in ET, 3% and 8% in PV, and 12% in PMF.[70] In a more recent systematic review and meta-analysis, bleeding as the initial manifestation of MPN was noted to be 6.9% in PV, 7.3% in ET, and 8.9% in PMF. Major sites of bleeding at presentation were mucocutaneous (2.8%), gastrointestinal (2.1%), epistaxis (1.0%), and postoperative bleeding (1.1%).[5] There have been conflicting data about whether or not the use of aspirin in the MPNs increases bleeding risk.[2,70–72] Postsurgical bleeding episodes are increased in patients with MPN, affecting 7.3% of all patients, with antithrombotic prophylaxis increasing the risk.[73] In a retrospective study of bleeding and thrombosis of patients with MPN postoperatively, with about half of the 311 patient having major surgery, most on cytoreductive therapy, there were 12 arterial and 12 venous thrombotic events after 3 months of follow-up, and 23 major and 7 minor hemorrhages.[74]

The cause of bleeding in patients with MPN is not completely understood. Patients with MPNs have been reported to have a variety of functional platelet abnormalities (with or without thrombocytosis) in vitro, including some that seem to be practically diagnostic of an MPN (eg, platelet α-adrenergic receptor or 12-lipoxygenase deficiency). However, none of these platelet defects has been clearly associated with a clinical bleeding tendency. More recently, the finding of acquired von Willebrand disease (aVWD), especially in a substantial number of patients with ET, has been thought to be a major factor causing bleeding. The aVWD is related to loss of the highest-molecular-weight multimers of von Willebrand factor, which are the most hemostatically effective portion of the protein, because of their selective adsorption onto the surfaces of high numbers of functionally abnormal platelets. Loss of these multimers may also be caused by proteolysis associated with MPN platelets and leukocytes. To test for this, clinicians should order not only a von Willebrand panel but also analysis of multimer distribution. The latter can reveal the abnormality when other measures of von Willebrand disease do not. Until recently, the aVWD was thought to develop only when there was extreme thrombocytosis (ie, platelets >1 million). However, it is now known that patients with even near-normal platelet counts can have aVWD.[75,76]

PATHOBIOLOGY OF THROMBOSIS IN THE MYELOPROLIFERATIVE NEOPLASMS

In PV, the degree of erythrocytosis is clearly related to thrombotic risk as a function of increasing whole-blood viscosity.[77,78] However, that cannot be the sole basis for the vascular complications of PV because individuals with even higher levels of secondary erythrocytosis (eg, persons living at high altitude) have little or no increased risk of thrombosis. Functional alterations in red cells must coexist. For example, *JAK2(V617F)* mutation–bearing red cells show abnormally avid adhesion to vascular endothelial laminin because *JAK2(V617F)* triggers phosphorylation of the unique erythroid laminin receptor, Lu/BCAM.[79]

Leukocytosis has been reported to be a risk factor for thrombosis in MPNs in several studies that have used single time points for blood counts. More recently, using subgroup trajectory modeling, which analyzes multiple leukocyte counts measured longitudinally at regular intervals over up to 48 months of follow-up, reflecting trajectories and cumulative exposure to leukocytosis, persistent leukocytosis was not found to be associated with thrombosis.[80] Leukocytes in MPNs also circulate in blood in an activated state.[81,82] Neutrophil extracellular traps (NETs) consist of nuclear material released into the circulation by activated leukocytes to produce an extracellular mesh that promotes thrombosis in general and in the MPNs specifically.[83,84] NETs also provide a surface for activation of the IL-1 family cytokines,[85] and they stimulate endothelial cell activation as well as TF generation.[86] Moreover, activated neutrophils in patients with MPNs release proteolytic enzymes and reactive oxygen species that injure endothelial cells and trigger the coagulation cascade.[87]

The tenuous relationship between the level of thrombocytosis and thrombotic, vascular, and bleeding complications in the MPNs was discussed earlier. Direct platelet–red cell interactions have been noted to be mediated by FasL/FasR[88] in experimental thrombogenesis. Basal platelet hyperactivity has been found both in vitro and ex vivo, possibly contributing to the prothrombotic phenotype of MPNs.[89] However, increased platelet reactivity is also seen other non-MPN inflammatory disorders.

In the MPNs, the major cellular elements of blood (red cells, platelets, leukocytes) and the vascular endothelial cells that they encounter throughout the circulatory tree[41,42,90] become further activated by their mutual interactions. They then work in concert with inflammatory mediators and activated clotting factors to create a self-perpetuating prothrombotic and proadhesive milieu.[89] As indicated earlier, endothelial cells themselves, which originate from the same mesodermal pluripotent stem cells that give rise to hematopoietic lineages,[91] may bear the *JAK2* mutation in certain regions of the vasculature, thereby becoming active participants in this complex interplay.

PREVENTION AND TREATMENT OF THROMBOTIC, VASCULAR, AND BLEEDING COMPLICATIONS IN THE MYELOPROLIFERATIVE NEOPLASMS

In general, the armamentarium of antithrombotic drugs available for prevention or treatment of patients with MPN is no different than it is for general populations. The difference is that the use of these agents in patients without MPN with thrombosis is firmly based on high level of quality evidence from large, well-designed, randomized, double-blind, placebo-controlled clinical trials. However, this is not the case for managing comparable thrombotic complications in the MPNs specifically. Therefore, guidelines for the MPNs are often extrapolated from data generated from studies in non-MPN populations. Importantly, the concurrent treatment of these patients for the underlying MPN must be considered along with decisions concerning antithrombotic management.

First, the role of low-dose daily aspirin in preventing an initial thrombotic or vascular event must be seriously reassessed in light of new information about its hemorrhagic risks. Three large randomized clinical trials in the general population on risks and benefits of aspirin were published in 2018. The ASPREE trial for reducing vascular events in 19,114 elderly individuals found a 29% increase in major bleeds in patients taking aspirin compared with the placebo group (with a median follow-up of 4.7 years).[92] The ARRIVE trial of 12,546 individuals at moderate risk of cardiovascular disease found that aspirin compared with placebo nonsignificantly reduced the risk of nonfatal myocardial infarction, but doubled the risk of gastrointestinal bleeding (0.97% vs 0.46%; $P = .0007$; median follow-up 60 months).[93] The ASCEND trial of 15,480 patients with diabetes mellitus to determine the effects of aspirin versus placebo on cardiovascular complications found a 12% decrease in serious cardiovascular events in the aspirin group, accompanied by a 29% increase in major bleeding problems (approximately 41% gastrointestinal, 21% intraocular, and 17% intracranial bleeds), with a median follow-up of 7.4 years.[94] Subsequently published systematic reviews and meta-analyses concluded that, in contemporary practice, the routine use of aspirin for the primary prevention of cardiovascular events may have a net harmful effect.[95–97] It is important to point out that all of these studies were designed for primary prevention (ie, persons with no past history of a thrombotic or vascular event), not for secondary prevention in patients with previous clinical events. Therefore, clinicians now have to be more judicious in recommending aspirin to patients with MPN, taking into account each person's relative risks for thrombotic and vascular versus bleeding complications.

Second, hematologists may often overlook the critical need to control modifiable risk factors to prevent cardiovascular and thrombotic complications in patients with MPN (including smoking, obesity, hypertension, dyslipidemia, and physical activity). Whenever hematologists taking care of patients with MPN feel uncomfortable managing these chronic conditions, there should be assurance that they are being followed by a primary care physician or a preventive, general cardiologist, in concert with the hematologist.

With few exceptions,[77,98] studies to examine the efficacy and safety of cytoreduction to prevent thrombosis and bleeding in the MPNs have generally provided less than robust evidence. Based on the few high-quality studies available, the published opinions or consensus of experts, and the author's practice, **Figs. 3** and **4** provide algorithms for decision making to prevent thrombotic, vascular, and bleeding complications in patients with MPNs, with **Fig. 4** focusing specifically on antiplatelet therapy. As with any other algorithms, patient care must be personalized. The hematologist's experience and judgment should override any of these recommendations based on the individual patient's circumstances.

FUTURE DIRECTIONS

Understanding of the pathobiology of thrombotic, vascular, and bleeding problems in the MPNs has grown substantially over the past 2 decades, alongside spectacular progress in elucidating the molecular underpinnings of the MPNs in general.

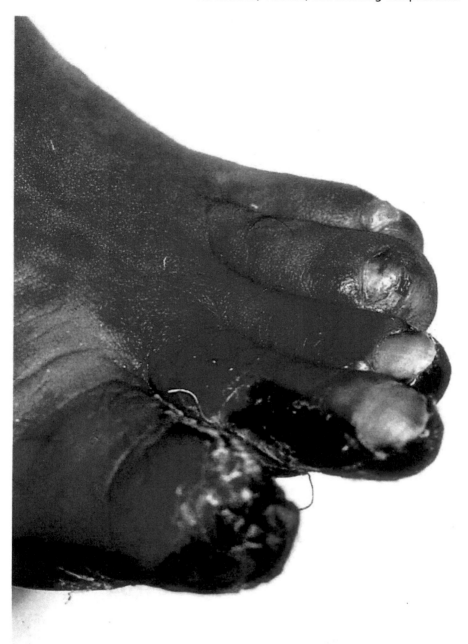

Fig. 2. Digital ischemia in MPN. This approximately 65-year-old homeless man was seen in consultation by the author in the emergency department. He had presented months prior at another hospital with symptoms and signs of digital ischemia, with toes of both feet showing cyanosis. On angiography, his major lower extremity arteries were essentially normal. Nonetheless, he underwent femoral-popliteal bypass, which did not improve blood flow to the feet. Only in retrospect, a platelet count of 850,000 was noted at that time. On this emergency department presentation, showing advanced gangrene and autoamputation of digits, his posterior tibial and dorsalis pedis pulses were still brisk, and his platelet count was greater than 1 million.

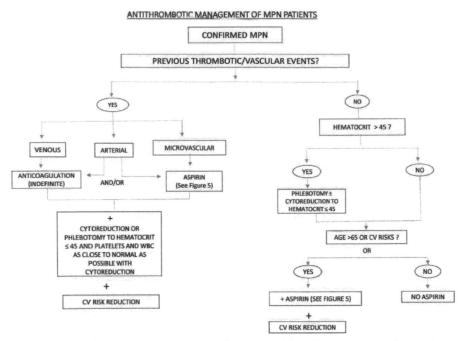

Fig. 3. An algorithm for the management of patients with MPN to prevent and treat thrombosis. CV, cardiovascular.

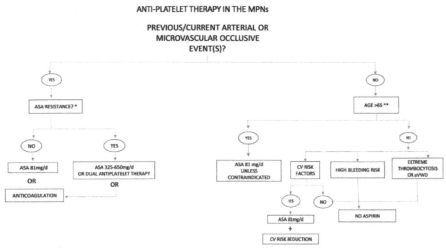

Fig. 4. An algorithm for antiplatelet therapy in the MPNs. This scheme was developed in light of recent clinical trials that indicate bleeding risk in patients without MPN that is higher than previously thought (see text). ASA (aspirin) resistance refers to either (1) failure of ASA to prevent clinical cardiovascular or cerebrovascular events (clinical resistance), or (2) failure of taking ASA to cause the ex vivo platelet defect expected (laboratory resistance). The latter can be readily performed by a point-of-care platelet function analyzer (PFA-100), a point-of-care turbidimetric optical detection of platelet aggregation in whole blood (VerifyNow Aspirin), or enzyme immunoassay of urinary 11-dehydro-thromboxane B_2.

Prevention and treatment have lagged behind but, with the establishment of expert cooperative study groups, strong evidence-based guidelines are anticipated. Moreover, the use of targeted therapy to prevent and treat these complications is rapidly approaching, based on studies that are summarized in this article. Antiinflammatory agents, such as ruxolitinib, seem to be crucial adjuncts to therapies targeting the MPN stem cell (see **Fig. 1**). For example, the CANTOS trials of the IL-1β inhibitor canakinumab[99] and of BET inhibitors[100] show much promise. The development of antithrombotic agents that prevent or treat MPN-associated thrombosis and vascular occlusive complications, based on what are now known to be key molecular and cellular events that occur specifically in the MPNs, will be another new direction. One example is P-selectin inhibition, which interferes with abnormal blood cell adhesion to endothelial cells.[101]

REFERENCES

1. Schafer AI. Bleeding and thrombosis in the myeloproliferative disorders. Blood 1984;64:1–12.
2. Marchioli R, Finazzi G, Landolfi R, et al. Vascular and neoplastic risk in a large cohort of patients with polycythemia vera. J Clin Oncol 2005;23:2224–32.
3. Cabot RC. A case of chronic cyanosis without discoverable cause, ending in cerebral hemorrhage. Boston Med Surg J 1899;141:574.
4. Hultcrantz M, Björkholm M, Dickman PW, et al. Risk of arterial and venous thrombosis in patients with myeloproliferative neoplasms. A population-based cohort study. Ann Intern Med 2018;168:317–25.
5. Rungjirajittranon T, Owattanapanich W, Ungprasert P, et al. A systematic review and meta-analysis of the prevalence of thrombosis and bleeding at diagnosis of Philadelphia-negative myeloproliferative neoplasms. BMC Cancer 2019; 19(1):184.
6. Kaifie A, Kirschner M, Wolf D, et al. Bleeding, thrombosis, and anticoagulation in myeloproliferative neoplasms (MPN): analysis from the german SAL-MPN-registry. J Hematol Oncol 2016;9:18.
7. Vristina SF, Polo B, Lacerda JF. Somatic mutations in Philadelphia chromosome-negative myeloproliferative neoplasms. Semin Hematol 2018;55:215–22.
8. Sankar K, Stein BL, Rampal RK. Thrombosis in the Philadelphia chromosome-negative myeloproliferative neoplasms. Cancer Treat Res 2019;179:159–1178.
9. Tefferi A, Barbui T. Polycythemia vera and essential thrombocythemia: 2019 update on diagnosis, risk-stratification and management. Am J Hematol 2019;94: 133–43.
10. Zin R, Guglielmelli P, Pietra D, et al. *CALR* mutational status identifies different disease subtypes of essential thrombocythemia showing distinct expression profiles. Blood Cancer J 2017;7:638.
11. Arber DA, Orazi A, Hasserjian R, et al. The 2016 revision of the World Health Organization classification of myeloid neoplasms and acute leukemia. Blood 2016; 127:2391–405.
12. Savage DG, Szydlo RM, Goldman JM. Clinical features at diagnosis in 430 patients with chronic myeloid leukaemia seen at a referral centre over a 16-year period. Br J Haematol 1997;96:111–6.
13. Wu Y-Y, Tang L, Wang M-H. Leukemia and risk of venous thromboembolism: a meta-analysis and systematic review of 144 studies comprising 162,126 patients. Sci Rep 2017;7(1):1167.

14. Manouchehri A, Kanu E, Mauro MJ, et al. Tyrosine kinase inhibitors in leukemia and cardiovascular events. From mechanism to patient care. Arterioscler Thromb Vasc Biol 2020;40:301–8.

15. Jain P, Kantarjian H, Boddu P, et al. Analysis of cardiovascular and arteriothrombotic adverse events in chronic-phase CML patients after frontline TKIs. Blood Adv 2019;3:851–61.

16. Liu Y, Meng X, Feng J, et al. Hypereosinophilia with concurrent venous thromboembolism: clinical features, potential risk factors, and short-term outcomes in a Chinese cohort. Sci Rep 2020;10(1):8359.

17. Moosbauer C, Morgenstern E, Civelier SL, et al. Eosinophils are a major intravascular location for tissue factor storage and exposure. Blood 2007;109:995–1002.

18. Uderhardt S, Ackermann JA, Fillep T, et al. Enzymatic lipid oxidation by eosinophils propagates coagulation, hemostasis, and thrombotic disease. J Exp Med 2017;214:2121–38 (Correction in J Exp Med 2018;215:1003.).

19. Lefèvre G, Leurs A, Gibier J-P, et al. "Idiopathic eosinophilic vasculitis": another side of hypereosinophilic syndrome? A comprehensive analysis of 117 cases in asthma-free patients. J Allergy Clin Immunol Pract 2020;8:1329–40.

20. Carvalhosa AB, Aouba A, Damaj G, et al. A French national survey on clotting disorders in mastocytosis. Medicine 2015;94:1–9.

21. Ponomaryov T, Payne H, Fabritz L, et al. Mast cell granular contents are crucial for deep vein thrombosis in mice. Circ Res 2017;121:941–50.

22. Jaiswal S, Fontanillas P, Flannick J, et al. Age-related clonal hematopoiesis associated with adverse outcomes. N Engl J Med 2014;371:2488–98.

23. Jaiswal S, Ebert BL. Clonal hematopoiesis in human aging and disease. Science 2019;366(6465):eaan4673.

24. Jaiswal S, Natarajan A, Silver J, et al. Clonal hematopoiesis and risk of atherosclerotic cardiovascular disease. N Engl J Med 2017;377:111–21.

25. Perner F, Perner C, Ernst T, et al. Roles of JAK2 in aging, inflammation, hematopoiesis and malignant transformation. Cells 2019;8(8):854.

26. Koschmieder S, Mughal TI, Hasselbalch HC, et al. Myeloproliferative neoplasms and inflammation: whether to target the malignant clone or the inflammatory process or both. Leukemia 2016;30:1018–24.

27. Lussana F, Rambaldi A. Inflammation and myeloproliferative neoplasms. J Autoimmun 2017;85:58–63.

28. Ridker PM, MacFayden JG, Everett BM, et al. Relationship of C-reactive protein reduction to cardiovascular event reduction following treatment with canakinumab: a secondary analysis from the CANTOS trial. Lancet 2018;391:319–28.

29. Bick AG, Pirruccello JM, Griffin GK, et al. Genetic IL6 signaling deficiency attenuates cardiovascular risk in clonal hematopoiesis. Circulation 2020;141:124–31.

30. Jackson SP, Darbousset R, Schoenwaelder SM. Thromboinflammation: challenges of therapeutically targeting coagulation and other host defense mechanisms. Blood 2019;133:906–18.

31. d'Alessandro E, Becker C, Bergmeier W, et al. Thrombo-inflammation in cardiovascular disease: an expert consensus document from the third Maastricht consensus conference on thrombosis. Thromb Haemost 2020;120:538–64.

32. Deitelzweig SB, Johnson BH, Lim J, et al. Prevalence of venous thromboembolism in the USA: current trends and future projections. Am J Hematol 2011;86:217–20.

33. Asada Y, Yamashita A, Sato Y, et al. Pathophysiology of atherothrombosis: mechanisms of thrombus formation on disrupted atherosclerotic plaques. Pathol Int 2020. https://doi.org/10.1111/pin.12921.
34. Bonafé M, Prattichizzo F, Giuliani A, et al. Inflamm-aging: why older men are the most susceptible to SARS-CoV-2 complicated outcomes. Cytokine Growth Factor Rev 2020;53:33–7.
35. Soysal P, Arik F, Smith L, et al. Inflammation, frailty and cardiovascular disease. Adv Exp Med Biol 2020;1216:55–64.
36. Prandoni P. Venous and arterial thrombosis: is there a link? Adv Exp Med Biol 2017;906:273–83.
37. Valeriani E, Riva N, Nisio M, et al. Splanchnic vein thrombosis: current perspectives. Vasc Health Risk Manag 2019;15:449–61.
38. Aird W. Phenotypic heterogeneity of the endothelium: II. Representative vascular beds. Circ Res 2007;100:174–90.
39. How J, Zhou A, Oh ST. Splanchnic vein thrombosis in myeloproliferative neoplasms: pathophysiology and molecular mechanisms of disease. Ther Adv Hematol 2017;8:107–18.
40. Sozer S, Fiel MI, Schiano T, et al. The presence of JAK2V617F mutation in the liver endothelial cells of patients with Budd-Chiari syndrome. Blood 2009;113:5246–9.
41. Guadall A, Lesteven E, Letort G, et al. Endothelial cells harbouring the JAK2^{V617F} mutation display pro-adherent and pro-thrombotic features. Thromb Haemost 2018;118:1586–99.
42. Guy A, Gourdou-Latyszenok V, Le Lay N, et al. Vascular endothelial cell expression of JAK2^{V617F} is sufficient to promote a pro-thrombotic state due to increased P-selectin expression. Haematologica 2019;104:70–81.
43. Van Bijnen S, van Heerde WL, Muus P. Mechanisms and clinical implications of thrombosis in paroxysmal nocturnal hemoglobinuria. J Thromb Haemost 2012;10:1–10.
44. Naymagon L, Tremblay T, Zubuzarreta N, et al. Portal vein thrombosis patients harboring *JAK2V617F* have poor long-term outcomes despite anticoagulation. J Thromb Thrombolysis 2020. https://doi.org/10.1007/s11239-020-02052-4.
45. Naymagon L, Tremblay D, Zubizarreta N, et al. The efficacy and safety of direct oral anticoagulants in noncirrhotic portal vein thrombosis. Blood Adv 2020;4:655–66.
46. Passamonti SM, Biguzzi E, Cazzola M, et al. The JAK2 V617F mutation in patients with cerebral venous thrombosis. J Thromb Haemost 2012;10:998–1003.
47. Martinelli I, De Stefano V, Carobbio A, et al. Cerebral vein thrombosis in patients with Philadelphia-negative myeloproliferative neoplasms. An European Leukemia Net study. Am J Hematol 2014;89:200–5.
48. Artoni A, Bucciarelli P, Martinelli I. Cerebral thrombosis and myeloproliferative neoplasms. Curr Neurol Neurosci Rep 2014;14(11):496.
49. Schafer AI, Kroll MH. Nonatheromatous arterial thrombosis. Annu Rev Med 1993;44:155–70.
50. Frederiksen H, Szépligeti S, Bak M, et al. Vascular diseases in patients with myeloproliferative neoplasms – impact on comorbidity. Clin Epidemiol 2019;11:955–67.
51. De Stefano V, Ghirardi A, Masciulli A, et al. Arterial thrombosis in Philadelphia-negative myeloproliferative neoplasms predicts second cancer: a case-control study. Blood 2020;135:381–6.

52. Lata K, Madiraju N, Levitt L. *JAK2* mutations and coronary ischemia. N Engl J Med 2010;363:396–7.

53. Cengiz B, Aytekin V, Bildirici U, et al. A rare cause of acute coronary syndrome in young adults – myeloproliferative neoplasms: a case series. Rev Port Cardiol 2019;38:613–7.

54. De Stefano V, Carobbio A, Di Lazzaro V, et al. Benefit-risk profile of cytoreductive drugs along with antiplatelet and antithrombotic therapy after transient ischemic attack of ischemic stroke in myeloproliferative neoplasms. Blood Cancer J 2018; 8(3):25.

55. Mann N, King T, Murphy R. Review of primary and secondary erythromelalgia. Clin Exp Dermatol 2019;44:477–82.

56. Kurzrock R, Cohen PR. Erythromelalgia and myeloproliferative disorders. Arch Intern Med 1989;149:105–9.

57. Davis MD, Weenig RH, Genebriera J, et al. Histopathologic findings in primary erythromelalgia are nonspecific: special studies show a decrease in small nerve fiber density. J Am Acad Dermatol 2006;55:519–22.

58. Leroux MB. Erythromelalgia: a cutaneous manifestation of neuropathy? An Bras Dermatol 2018;93:86–94.

59. Tham SW, Giles M. Current pain management strategies for patients with erythromelalgia: a critical review. J Pain Res 2018;11:1689–98.

60. Kraemer M, Linden D, Berlit P. The spectrum of differential diagnosis in neurological patients with livedo reticularis and livedo racemosa. A literature review. J Neurol 2005;252:1155–66.

61. Inoue S, Okiyama N, Okune M, et al. Clinical and histological characteristics of livedo racemose in essential thrombocythemia: a report of two cases and review of the published works. J Dermatol 2017;44:84–7.

62. Itin PH, Winkelmann RK. Cutaneous manifestations in patients with essential thrombocythemia. J Am Acad Dermatol 1991;24:59–63.

63. Samanta D, Cobb S, Arya K. Sneddon syndrome: a comprehensive overview. J Stroke Cerebrovasc Dis 2019;8:2098–108.

64. Hon JK, Chow A, Abdalla S, et al. Myeloproliferative disorder as the cause of peripheral ischemia in a young patient. Ann Vasc Surg 2008;22:456–8.

65. Liisborg C, Hasselbalch HC, Sørensen TL. Ocular manifestations in patients with Philadelphia-negative myeloproliferative neoplasms. Cancers 2020;12:573.

66. Robinson SE, Harrison CN. How we manage Philadelphia-negative myeloproliferative neoplasms in pregnancy. Br J Haematol 2020;189:625–34.

67. Lapoirie J, Contis A, Guy A, et al. Management and outcomes of 27 pregnancies in women with myeloproliferative neoplasms. J Matern Fetal Neonatal Med 2020; 33:49–56.

68. Yu Y, Zhang X, Shi Q, et al. Essential thrombocytosis with recurrent spontaneous abortion in the mid trimester. Medicine (Baltimore) 2019;98(26):e16203.

69. Maze D, Kazi S, Gupta V, et al. Association of treatments for myeloproliferative neoplasms during pregnancy with birth rates and maternal outcomes. JAMA Netw Open 2019;2(10):e1912666.

70. Martin K. Risk factors for and management of MPN-associated bleeding and thrombosis. Curr Hematol Malig Rep 2017;12:389–96.

71. Kander EM, Raza S, Zhou Z, et al. Bleeding complications in BCR-ABL negative myeloproliferative neoplasms: prevalence, type, and risk factors in a single-center cohort. Int J Hematol 2015;102:587–93.

72. Finazzi G, Carobbio A, Thiele J, et al. Incidence and risk factors for bleeding in 1104 patients with essential thrombocythemia or prefibrotic myelofibrosis diagnosed according to the 2008 WHO criteria. Leukemia 2012;26:716–9.
73. Appelmann I, Kreher S, Parmentier S, et al. Diagnosis, prevention, and management of bleeding episodes in Philadelphia-negative myeloproliferative neoplasms: recommendations of the hemostasis working party of the German society of hematology and medical oncology (DGHO) and the Society of thrombosis and hemostasis research (GTH). Ann Hematol 2016;95:707–18.
74. Ruggeri M, Rodeghiero F, Tosetto A, et al. Postsurgery outcomes in patients with polycythemia vera and essential thrombocythemia: a retrospective survey. Blood 2008;111:666–71.
75. Lancellotti S, Dragani A, Ranalli P, et al. Qualitative and quantitative modifications of von Willebrand factor in patients with essential thrombocythemia and controlled platelet count. J Thromb Haemost 2015;13:1226–37.
76. Rottenstreich A, Kleinstern G, Krichevsky S, et al. Factors related to the development of acquired von Willebrand syndrome in patients with essential thrombocythemia and polycythemia vera. Eur J Intern Med 2017;41:49–54.
77. Marchioli R, Finazzi G, Specchia G, et al. Cardiovascular events and intensity of treatment in polycythemia vera. N Engl J Med 2013;368:22–33.
78. Pearson TC, Wetherley-Mein G. Vascular occlusive episodes and venous haematocrit in primary proliferative polycythaemia. Lancet 1978;2:1219–22.
79. El Nemer W, De Grandis M, Brusson M. Abnormal adhesion of red blood cells in polycythemia vera: a prothrombotic effect? Thromb Res 2014;133:S107–11.
80. Ronner L, Podoltsev N, Gotlib J, et al. Persistent leukocytosis in polycythemia vera is associated with disease evolution but not thrombosis. Blood 2020;135:1696–703.
81. Nouboussie DF, Reeves DF, Strahl BN, et al. Neutrophils: back in the thrombosis spotlight. Blood 2019;133:2186–97.
82. Carobbio A, Ferrari A, Masciulli A, et al. Leukocytosis and thrombosis in essential thrombocythemia and polycythemia vera: a systematic review and meta-analysis. Blood Adv 2019;3:1729–37.
83. Papayannopoulos V. Neutrophil extracellular traps in immunity and disease. Nat Rev Immunol 2018;18:134–47.
84. Cedervall J, Hamidi A, Olsson AK. Platelets, NETs and cancer. Thromb Res 2018;164(Suppl 1):S148–52.
85. Clancy DM, Henry CM, Sullivan GP, et al. Neutrophil extracellular traps can serve as platforms for processing and activation of IL-1 family cytokines. FEBS J 2017;284:1712–25.
86. Folco EJ, Mawson TL, Vromman A, et al. Neutrophil extracellular traps induce endothelial cell activation and tissue factor production through interleukin-1α and cathepsin G. Arterioscler Thromb Vasc Biol 2018;38:1901–12.
87. Falanga A, Marchetti M, Evangelista V, et al. Polymorphonuclear leukocyte activation and hemostasis in patients with essential thrombocythemia and polycythemia vera. Blood 2000;96:4261–6.
88. Klatt C, Kruger I, Zay S, et al. Platelet-RBC interaction mediated by FasL/FasR induces procoagulant activity important for thrombosis. J Clin Invest 2018;128:3906–25.
89. Marin Oyarzún CP. Platelets as mediators of thromboinflammation in chronic myeloproliferative neoplasms. Front Immunol 2019;10:1373.
90. Ribatti D, Tamma R, Ruggieri S, et al. Surface markers: an identity card of endothelial cells. Microcirculation 2020;27(1):e12587.

91. Kobayashi I, Kobayashi-Sun J, Hirakawa Y, et al. Dual role of Jam3b in early hematopoietic and vascular development. Development 2020;147(1):dev181040.

92. McNeil JJ, Nelson MR, Woods RL, et al. ASPREE Investigator Group. Effect of aspirin on all-cause mortality in the healthy elderly. N Engl J Med 2018;379: 1519–28.

93. Gaziano JM, Brotons C, Coppolechia R, et al. ARRIVE executive committee. Use of aspirin to reduce risk of initial vascular events in patients at moderate risk of cardiovascular disease (ARRIVE): a randomised, double-blind, placebo-controlled trial. Lancet 2018;392:1036–46.

94. Bowman L, Mafham M, Wallendszus K, et al. ASCEND Study Collaborative Group. Effects of aspirin for primary prevention in persons with diabetes mellitus. N Engl J Med 2018;379:1529–39.

95. Shah R, Khan B, Latham SB, et al. A meta-analysis of aspirin for the primary prevention of cardiovascular diseases in the context of contemporary preventive strategies. Am J Med 2019;132:1295–304.

96. Veronese N, Demurtas J, Thompson T, et al. Effect of low-dose aspirin on health outcomes: an umbrella review of systematic reviews and meta-analyses. Br J Clin Pharmacol 2020. https://doi.org/10.1111/bcp.14310.

97. Ujjawal A, Gupta M, Ghosh RK, et al. Aspirin for primary prevention of coronary artery disease. Curr Probl Cardiol 2020;100553. https://doi.org/10.1016/j.cpcardiol.2020.100553.

98. Cortelazzo S, Finazzi G, Ruggeri M, et al. Hydroxyurea for patients with essential thrombocythemia and a high risk of thrombosis. N Engl J Med 1995;332:1132–6.

99. Ridker PM, Everett BM, Thuren T, et al. Antiinflammatory therapy with canakinumab for atherosclerotic disease. N Engl J Med 2017;377:1119–31.

100. Kleppe M, Koche R, Zou L, et al. Dual targeting of oncogenic activation and inflammatory signaling increases therapeutic efficacy in myeloproliferative neoplasms. Cancer Cell 2018;33:29–43.

101. Ataga KI, Kutlar A, Kanter J, et al. Crizanlizumab for the prevention of pain crises in sickle cell disease. N Engl J Med 2017;376:429–39.

Accelerated and Blast Phase Myeloproliferative Neoplasms

Tania Jain, MBBS[a],*, Raajit K. Rampal, MD, PhD[b]

KEYWORDS

- Myeloproliferative neoplasm • Accelerated phase • Blast phase
- Acute myeloid leukemia

KEY POINTS

- Blast phase myeloproliferative neoplasms (MPN) have inferior outcomes in comparison with *de novo* acute myeloid leukemia (AML) or postmyelodysplastic syndrome AML.
- High-risk cytogenetic and somatic mutations are enriched in patients with accelerated and blast phase MPN.
- Although enrollment on clinical trials should be encouraged, available treatment options include induction chemotherapy as used for *de novo* AML, hypomethylating agent–based therapy (with venetoclax or ruxolitinib) or targeted therapy based on mutational biomarkers.

INTRODUCTION
What Are Accelerated and Blast Phase Myeloproliferative Neoplasms?

Philadelphia negative myeloproliferative neoplasms (MPNs) are a heterogeneous group of myeloid disorders arising from dysregulated clonal hematopoiesis, driven by activating mutations in the Janus kinase-signal transducer and activator of transcription (JAK-STAT) pathway. These driver somatic mutations primarily include those in Janus kinase 2 gene (*JAK2*), thrombopoietin receptor gene (*MPL*), or calreticulin (*CALR*) gene. The resulting clinical phenotype in chronic phase is characterized by splenomegaly, constitutional symptoms, thrombovascular complications, aberrant counts, and risk for progression to advanced disease.

Advanced disease includes the following phases:

- *Accelerated phase*, defined as 10% to 19% myeloid blasts in the peripheral blood or bone marrow compartment

[a] Division of Hematological Malignancies and Stem Cell Transplantation, Department of Oncology, The Sidney Kimmel Comprehensive Cancer Center at Johns Hopkins University, 1650 Orleans Street, Baltimore, MD 21287, USA; [b] Leukemia Service, Department of Medicine, Memorial Sloan Kettering, 530 East 74th Street, New York, NY 10021, USA
* Corresponding author.
E-mail address: tjain2@jhmi.edu
Twitter: @TaniaJain11 (T.J.); @RaajitRampal (R.K.R.)

Hematol Oncol Clin N Am 35 (2021) 325–335
https://doi.org/10.1016/j.hoc.2020.12.008
hemonc.theclinics.com

- *Blast phase*, which refers to 20% or greater myeloid blasts in the peripheral blood or bone marrow

Evolution to advanced phase MPN in patients with polycythemia vera or essential thrombocythemia is usually preceded by myelofibrosis. The rate of blast phase transformation from polycythemia vera or essential thrombocythemia is significantly lower than primary myelofibrosis, with a cumulative incidence reported at 6.8%, 3.8%, and 14.2% in the Mayo Clinic cohort, respectively.[1] In addition, most of the patients who transform from chronic phase MPN to blast phase make this transition via the accelerated phase.[2] In addition to the percentage of blasts greater than or equal to 10%, platelet count less than 50×10^9/L, chromosome 17 abnormality, and lower performance status were independently significantly associated with increased risk to blast transformation.[2] Blast transformation of MPN is usually myeloid in nature, whereas cases of lymphoid transformation have been reported.[3]

Although the recent ongoing increment in the potential therapeutic options in chronic phase MPNs offers optimism, survival in patients with accelerated and blast phase MPNs has been grim historically.[4–11] Over the past decade, there has been minimal improvement in clinical outcomes of patients with blast phase MPN where median overall survival remains less than 6 months and despite allogeneic hematopoietic transplantation (HCT), survival at 5 years remains low at around 10%.[12,13] In smaller series of patients with accelerated phase disease, the reported median survival has been less than 2 years.[2,14,15]

In summary, both accelerated and blast phase diseases represent the advanced phase of the overall spectrum of myeloproliferative neoplasm and warrant immediate evaluation and management strategies.

DISCUSSION
Who Is at Risk?

Various risk factors have been identified over the years that can identify patients in chronic phase who have a higher likelihood of progressing into the advanced phase. Some of these are listed as follows:

Clinical/laboratory features: worsening splenomegaly (?), Dynamic International Prognostic Scoring System intermediate-2/high risk, transfusion dependence, platelets less than 50×10^9/L, increasing circulating blasts.

Karyotype: high-risk karyotype including 18, 27/7q, i(17q), 25/5q2, 12p2, inv(3), and 11q23 or chromosome 5, 7, or 17p abnormalities.

Somatic mutations: ASXL1, IDH1/2, EZH2, SRSF2, TET2, TP53, U2AF1; absence of CALR (in primary myelofibrosis), greater than or equal to 2 somatic mutations, germline duplication of ATG2B/GSKIP*.[13,16,17]

Although the natural history of chronic MPN, a stem cell origin clonal disorder, involves evolution to a more advanced disease including acute myeloid leukemia (AML), the process can be expedited with the use of some other agents of leukemogenic potential. Exposure to cytoreductive agents including ^{32}P, chlorambucil, pipobroman, and busulfan, previously used in management of chronic phase MPNs, has also been implicated in portending a higher risk for transformation.[18–22] The leukemogenic potential of hydroxyurea is disputable owing to some reports showing a potential implication, whereas others showing no difference with the use of hydroxyurea.[19,21,23]

It is of clinical relevance to identify patients at high risk, as they are usually considered candidates for an earlier intervention with an HCT, considering the poor prognosis once the progression actually occurs. At the same time, most studies done to evaluate these risk factors are retrospective studies, and some variables of this heterogeneous disease clinic-pathological phenotype have shown variable impact in different studies.

Biological Insights into Advanced Myeloproliferative Neoplasms

Biological features and mutational spectrum of blast phase MPN are remarkably distinct from de novo AML, suggesting a distinct molecular pathogenesis pathway. Poor-risk cytogenetics are more common in patients with blast phase MPN (38%) compared with de novo AML (23%).[14] Beyond the canonical mutations in JAK-STAT pathway, specific somatic mutations have been shown to be distinctly enriched in patients with accelerated or blast phase MPN including ASXL1, TET2, RUNX1, TP53, EZH2, and IDH1.[24–26] Contrarily, mutations in NPM1, cohesin complex, FLT3, and CEBPA, which are commonly represented in de novo AML, are infrequent in post-MPN AML.[27] Of these, more prominently studied and described are mutations in TP53 that are more frequently associated with blast phase MPN (~27%) than chronic phase (~3%).[27–29] Including gains of chromosome 1q that harbors MDM4, a potent TP53 inhibitor, as high as 45.5% patients with blast phase MPN have p53-related defect.[28] Similarly, mutational frequency of IDH1/2 is significantly higher in blast phase MPN (~21%) than in chronic phase (~4%).[30,31]

Genomic profiling of post-MPN AML samples, compared with chronic phase, has also demonstrated co-occurrence of TP53 mutation in patients with JAK2 V617F mutation but not in patients with CALR mutations.[27] It has also been demonstrated that low variant allele frequency TP53 mutation may be seen in chronic phase, and with loss of heterozygosity, the mutant clone can expand with clinical transformation to blast phase.[29] In another study, genomic evaluation of 17 matched chronic phase and blast phase MPN samples showed an average gain of one mutation, a worse comparative genomic hybridization profile, although no significant (>20%) variation in variant allele frequency was noted in samples in blast phase.[32] In addition, genes involved in RNA splicing (SRSF2), chromatin modification (ASXL1, EZH2), and signaling pathways (CBL, FLT3, RAS) were more commonly affected in transformed MPNs than in chronic MPNs.[32] Similarly, next generation sequencing in 17 paired chronic and blast phase samples from Mayo Clinic showed more frequent mutations in ASXL1, EZH2, LNK, TET2, TP53, and PTPN11 in the blast phase samples, whereas acquisition of JAK2, MPL, CALR, SRSF2, or U2AF1 mutations were not noted at the time of blast transformation.[25] These differences in the mutational profile at the time of transformation suggest a possible contribution of these acquired mutations in the pathogenesis of leukemia transformation (**Fig. 1**). If mutation analysis is performed clinically over the course of follow-up, it can potentially predict clinical evolution of the disease.

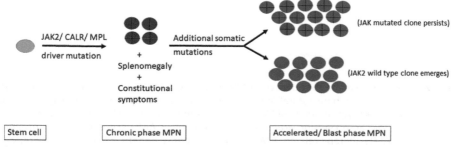

Fig. 1. Acquisition of mutations contributes to leukemic transformation in MPNs.

The sequence of mutation events in evolution of MPNs can vary and potentially have variable impact on stem cell biology and MPN progression. In serial MPN samples using DNA from single colonies, *TET2* and *DNMT3A* mutations preceded *JAK2 V617F* or co-existed as a different clone, whereas *IDH1* mutation occurred after JAK2V617F mutation.[29] Mutations in *ASXL1* and *EZH2* could occur before, after, or as a separate clone than JAK2V617F[29]. One study has shown that clinically, patients who develop *JAK2 V617F* mutations preceding *TET2* tend to be younger, present with polycythemia vera, increased risk of thrombosis, and increased sensitivity to ruxolitinib in vitro.[33] It is plausible that sequence of additional mutations with the driver mutation may influence the clinical phenotype in patients with MPN.

Treatment Paradigm in Advanced Myeloproliferative Neoplasms

Because the prognosis for both accelerated and blast phase remains relatively poor and because accelerated phase is an interim transition step to blast phase, similar treatment considerations are usually recommended (**Fig. 2**). The response rates to standard AML therapy in these patients have been discouraging, possibly the result of a more complex and higher risk genetic profile that renders the leukemia cells resistant to standard therapy. In theory, HCT remains the only potentially curative option but has limited applicability in patients with advanced age, comorbidities, or inadequate leukemia clearance before a planned HCT.[34,35]

Nontransplantation/chemotherapeutic options

Given the grim outlook in this space and the dire need to improve therapies, every effort must be made to treat these patients on clinical trials depending on availability (NCT04113616, NCT03289910). Outside of clinical trials, this decision primarily depends on anticipated ability to undergo high-dose chemotherapy such as high-dose induction chemotherapy with 7 + 3 regimen, used in *de novo* AML. Most patients with advanced phase MPN, by virtue of their age or comorbidities, are not candidates for induction-like chemotherapy. In 2 studies from Princess Margaret Cancer Center, the benefit of intensive therapy has been most prominent in patients who achieve a

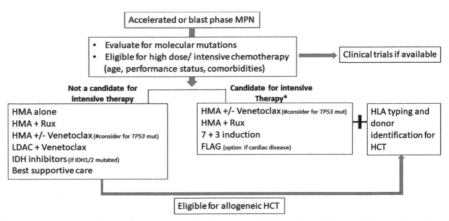

Fig. 2. Treatment schema for advanced MPN. AML-MRC, AML with myelodysplasia-related changes; FLAG, fludarabine, cytarabine, plus G-CSF; HCT, hematopoietic cell transplantation; HLA, human leukocyte antigen; HMA, hyomethylating agents; IDH, isocitrate dehydrogenase; LDAC, low-dose cytosine arabinoside (cytarabine); s-AML, secondary acute myeloid leukemia; t-AML, therapy-related AML. [a]Studies suggest benefit of intensive therapy is limited to patients who can undergo HCT.

remission and undergo an HCT compared with those who did not undergo an HCT (2-year overall survival 47% vs 15%).[26,36]

An emerging therapeutic option for patients with AML, and by extension, blast phase MPN has been a combination of hypomethylating agent with BCL-2 inhibitor, venetoclax. This option is being increasingly considered in patients with *TP53* mutation, which have historically demonstrated resistance or lower responses to chemotherapy.[37] Based on a phase 3 trial comparing the combination to hypomethylating agent alone, the combination of hypomethylating agent and venetoclax has received approval from Food and Drug Administration (FDA) for use in older patients ($\geq$75 years) or those in whom comorbidities preclude the use of high-intensity induction chemotherapy.[38] Of note though, data specifically for patients with post-MPN AML remains limited.[39] Azanucleosides are pyrimidine analogues that are potent inhibitors of DNA methylation and are commonly referred to as hypomethylating agents and have been a well-established alternative to induction chemotherapy with comparable outcomes in retrospective studies,[40,41] based on evidence implicating hypermethylation of P15^{INK4b} and P16^{INK4a} in leukemia transformation.[42] With 5-azacitidine, statistically similar response rates (54.6% vs 58.8% with induction chemotherapy) and medial overall survival (7.9 months vs 8.3 months with induction chemotherapy) were demonstrated.[41] Similarly, with decitabine, comparable median overall survival of 6.9 months was reported compared with 7.6 months with induction chemotherapy.[40]

Ruxolitinib-based therapies have also been studied although response rates remain rather low despite high doses of ruxolitinib. In a phase 2 study of patients with relapsed/refractory AML, 3/18 (17%) patients with post-MPN AML achieved a complete response and spleen size reduction with ruxolitinib at a dose of 25 or 50 mg twice a day.[43] *JAK2* allele burden reduction was not noted in these patients. In another trial, using higher doses of ruxolitinib (50, 100, or 200 mg twice a day), 0/5 patients with post-MPN AML was noted to have a meaningful response.[44] Hence, ruxolitinib alone is not recommended for use in patients with accelerated or blast phase disease.

Finally, combination of hypomethylating agents (decitabine and 5-azacitidine) with JAK inhibitors has been studied in a few recent studies. In vitro, post-MPN AML cells demonstrated sensitivity to both decitabine and ruxolitinib.[27] A phase 1 trial, based on this observation, studied decitabine with escalating doses of ruxolitinib (10, 15, 25, or 50 mg twice a day), showed a complete or partial response (by modified Cheson criteria) in 9/21 (43%) patients who had accelerated or blast phase disease.[45] A subsequent phase 2 study used the recommended phase 2 dose of 25 mg twice daily for induction followed by combination of decitabine and ruxolitinib, 10 mg twice daily, on days 8 to 12 and continuing ruxolitinib for the 28-day cycle,[46] which resulted in a complete or partial response in 11 out of 25 patients (44%) with a median overall survival of 9.5 months although response was not associated with improvement in survival.[46] Another phase 2 trial evaluated outcomes with decitabine and ruxolitinib (50 mg BID) in patients with post-MPN AML, and an overall response rate of 61% (including 11% complete response, 50% complete response with incomplete count recovery) was seen in the patients treated with the phase 2 dose.[47] Hematological and nonhematological toxicity was manageable. Azacitidine was also studied in combination with ruxolitinib where azacitidine was started at 25 mg/m^2 day 1 to 5 but could be introduced earlier or dose increased to 75 mg/m^2 in patients with accelerated phase disease.[48] Among 3 patients with accelerated phase MPN, one (33%) patient achieved clinical improvement in spleen and improved total symptoms score with reduction of blasts to 2%, which was maintained for 28 weeks.

Transplantation considerations

A recent study using registry data from Center for International Blood and Marrow Transplant Research (CIBMTR) demonstrated a worse overall survival following HCT in patients with blast phase MPN when compared with patients with de novo AML in remission at HCT (hazard ratio [HR] 1.40, 95% confidence interval [CI] 1.12–1.76) or postmyelodysplastic syndrome AML (HR 1.19, 95% CI 1.00–1.43).[14] This was mainly attributed to higher relapse in patients with blast phase MPN, yet again reflecting on the more aggressive biology of advanced phase MPN. The importance of disease control (reduction of blasts) before HCT has been highlighted in prior studies that repeatedly show superior outcomes in patients who are in remission or chronic phase at the HCT.[34,35,49] In a Japanese registry study where majority (82%) of patients were not in remission at the time of HCT, overall survival at 2 years was 29%,[50] similar to the overall survival reported in the earlier studies among patients who had active disease at HCT. In addition, patients with a chronic malignancy such as MPN can accumulate comorbidities over the course of the disease (attributed to MPN or not) rendering them a less favorable candidate for HCT. Hence, the optimal timing or window for HCT is before transformation. A variety of conditioning regimens and donor choices have been described without a clear or consistent indication of improved outcomes in general although specific clinical scenarios may warrant specific considerations in chronic or advanced phase MPN.[34,35,49–54] Peripheral blood graft source was associated with a lower risk of relapse in the CIBMTR registry study.[14]

Future Directions

Emerging knowledge of the mutational landscape in advanced phase MPN would help identify patients at higher risk of progression and hence, be considered for an earlier intervention. In addition, the role of targeted agents such as IDH inhibitors is being explored further not only in blast phase or accelerated phase MPN but also in chronic phase MPN with IDH1/2 mutations (4% in chronic phase MPN vs ~20% blast phase).[11,31] In a single-center experience, 8 patients with accelerated or blast phase MPN were treated with IDH2 inhibitor as upfront therapy (n = 6) or in relapsed/refractory setting (n = 2).[55] Of 6 patients with complete/partial response, 3 remained on therapy at last follow-up, 2 were subsequently stopped following progression after more than 400 days, whereas another one experienced an early toxicity. Notable toxicity was with grade 5 differentiation syndrome in 2 patients. MD Anderson Cancer Center has also reported their experience with various IDH1/2 inhibitors (FDA approved and under investigation) in 12 patients with newly diagnosed or relapsed/refractory post-MPN AML.[56] Among, the 7 newly diagnosed, 3 (43%) had a CR (in combination with induction/venetoclax/azacitidine) that lasted a median 17.5 months, and median overall survival for these patients was 19 months. Of the relapsed/refractory, none had CR although 3 patients had a stable disease with greater than 50% blast reduction that lasted for more than 8 months. Based on preclinical efficacy of combination of isocitrate dehydrogenase (IDH) inhibitor and JAK inhibitor,[57] a clinical trial to systematically study safety and efficacy of combination therapy with IDH inhibitor and JAK inhibitors is planned (NCT04281498).

Similarly, mutations in TP53 are also enriched in patients with MPN at the time of leukemic transformation, and hence, role of investigational drugs such as APR-246, with the potential ability to restore function of point mutant TP53 in tumor cells, is currently being explored in TP53-mutated myeloid malignancies in combination with azacitidine (NCT03072043). Early data also suggest promising response of anti-47 antibody, magrolimab, in patients with TP53-mutated AML.[58]

SUMMARY

Philadelphia chromosome-negative MPNs are the result of a driver mutation in JAK-STAT pathway and manifests as a constellation of splenomegaly, aberrant counts, constitutional symptoms, and other resulting complications. These can progress into blast phase (myeloid blasts ≥20% in peripheral blood or bone marrow), and this progression usually occurs via an accelerated phase (myeloid blasts 10%–19%). Poor-risk cytogenetics as well as specific somatic mutations are specifically seen at higher frequency in patients with accelerated or blast phase MPN. These include chromatin modifiers (*ASXL1*, *EZH2*), DNA methylation genes (*TET2*, *IDH1* and *IDH2*), transcription factors (*RUNX1*), and tumor suppressor genes (*TP53*). The enrichment of these mutations in patients with advanced phase disease suggests possible involvement in pathogenesis of this leukemia transformation. In addition, sequence of mutations in context of driver mutations can vary and potentially affect clinical phenotype and prognosis of these patients. For all these patients, consideration for earlier intervention, including the potentially curative HCT, is warranted. Therapeutic approach in both accelerated and blast phase is similar, given the predicted transformation to leukemic phase from accelerated phase disease. Options include induction chemotherapy and hypomethylating based therapies (in combination with venetoclax or ruxolitinib), whereas the role of mutational biomarkers in predicting responses to treatment options is emerging.

CLINICS CARE POINTS

- Accelerated phase MPN is defined as 10% to 19% myeloid blasts and blast phase MPN as 20% or greater myeloid blasts in peripheral blood or bone marrow.

- Poor-risk cytogenetics and specific somatic mutations are enriched in patients who progress to accelerated or blast phase MPN such as ASXL1, TET2, RUNX1, TP53, EZH2, IDH1, or IDH2.

- Therapeutic options depend on age, performance status, and comorbidities, which can determine if patient can tolerate high-dose induction chemotherapy.

- Hypomethylating agents have shown similar responses compared with intensive chemotherapy and can be used in combination with venetoclax or ruxolitinib.

- Emerging data will further elucidate the role of targeted agents (such as IDH inhibitors) or use of biomarkers to predict responses to therapy.

DISCLOSURE

T. Jain, consultancy for Targeted Oncology, Advisory board for CareDx and Bristol Myers Squibb; R.K. Rampal, consulting fees from: Constellation, Incyte, Celgene, Promedior, CTI, Jazz Pharmaceuticals, Blueprint, Stemline, Abbvie, Disc Medicines, and research funding from Incyte, Constellation, Stemline.

REFERENCES

1. Tefferi A, Guglielmelli P, Larson DR, et al. Long-term survival and blast transformation in molecularly annotated essential thrombocythemia, polycythemia vera, and myelofibrosis. Blood 2014;124(16):2507–13 [quiz 2615].
2. Tam CS, Kantarjian H, Cortes J, et al. Dynamic model for predicting death within 12 months in patients with primary or post-polycythemia vera/essential thrombocythemia myelofibrosis. J Clin Oncol 2009;27(33):5587–93.

3. Alhuraiji A, Naqvi K, Huh YO, et al. Acute lymphoblastic leukemia secondary to myeloproliferative neoplasms or after lenalidomide exposure. Clin Case Rep 2018;6(1):155–61.

4. Al-Ali HK, Delgado RG, Lange A, et al. KRT-232, a first-in-class, murine double minute 2 inhibitor (MDM2i), for myelofibrosis (MF) relapsed or refractory (R/R) to janus-associated kinase inhibitor (JAKi) treatment (TX). EHA Library 2020;S215.

5. Harrison C, Kiladjian JJ, Al-Ali HK, et al. JAK inhibition with ruxolitinib versus best available therapy for myelofibrosis. N Engl J Med 2012;366(9):787–98.

6. Harrison CN, Garcia JS, Mesa RA, et al. Results from a Phase 2 study of navito-clax in combination with ruxolitinib in patients with primary or secondary myelo-fibrosis. Blood 2019;134(Supplement_1):671.

7. Harrison CN, Patriarca A, Mascarenhas J, et al. Preliminary report of MANIFEST, a Phase 2 study of CPI-0610, a bromodomain and extraterminal domain inhibitor (BETi), in combination with ruxolitinib, in JAK inhibitor (JAKi) treatment naïve myelofibrosis patients. Blood 2019;134(Supplement_1):4164.

8. Harrison CN, Schaap N, Vannucchi AM, et al. Janus kinase-2 inhibitor fedratinib in patients with myelofibrosis previously treated with ruxolitinib (JAKARTA-2): a single-arm, open-label, non-randomised, phase 2, multicentre study. Lancet Hae-matol 2017;4(7):e317–24.

9. Mascarenhas J, Hoffman R, Talpaz M, et al. Pacritinib vs best available therapy, including ruxolitinib, in patients with myelofibrosis: a randomized clinical trial. JAMA Oncol 2018;4(5):652–9.

10. Mesa RA, Vannucchi AM, Mead A, et al. Pacritinib versus best available therapy for the treatment of myelofibrosis irrespective of baseline cytopenias (PERSIST-1): an international, randomised, phase 3 trial. Lancet Haematol 2017;4(5): e225–36.

11. Pardanani A, Harrison C, Cortes JE, et al. Safety and efficacy of fedratinib in pa-tients with primary or secondary myelofibrosis: a randomized clinical trial. JAMA Oncol 2015;1(5):643–51.

12. Mesa RA, Li CY, Ketterling RP, et al. Leukemic transformation in myelofibrosis with myeloid metaplasia: a single-institution experience with 91 cases. Blood 2005; 105(3):973–7.

13. Tefferi A, Mudireddy M, Mannelli F, et al. Blast phase myeloproliferative neoplasm: Mayo-AGIMM study of 410 patients from two separate cohorts. Leuke-mia 2018;32(5):1200–10.

14. Gupta V, Kim S, Hu ZH, et al. Comparison of outcomes of HCT in blast phase of BCR-ABL1- MPN with de novo AML and with AML following MDS. Blood Adv 2020;4(19):4748–57.

15. Mudireddy M, Gangat N, Hanson CA, et al. Validation of the WHO-defined 20% circulating blasts threshold for diagnosis of leukemic transformation in primary myelofibrosis. Blood Cancer J 2018;8(6):57.

16. Guglielmelli P, Lasho TL, Rotunno G, et al. The number of prognostically detri-mental mutations and prognosis in primary myelofibrosis: an international study of 797 patients. Leukemia 2014;28(9):1804–10.

17. Vannucchi AM, Lasho TL, Guglielmelli P, et al. Mutations and prognosis in primary myelofibrosis. Leukemia 2013;27(9):1861–9.

18. Berk PD, Goldberg JD, Silverstein MN, et al. Increased incidence of acute leuke-mia in polycythemia vera associated with chlorambucil therapy. N Engl J Med 1981;304(8):441–7.

19. Bjorkholm M, Derolf AR, Hultcrantz M, et al. Treatment-related risk factors for transformation to acute myeloid leukemia and myelodysplastic syndromes in myeloproliferative neoplasms. J Clin Oncol 2011;29(17):2410–5.

20. Finazzi G, Caruso V, Marchioli R, et al. Acute leukemia in polycythemia vera: an analysis of 1638 patients enrolled in a prospective observational study. Blood 2005;105(7):2664–70.

21. Kiladjian JJ, Chevret S, Dosquet C, et al. Treatment of polycythemia vera with hydroxyurea and pipobroman: final results of a randomized trial initiated in 1980. J Clin Oncol 2011;29(29):3907–13.

22. Najean Y, Rain JD. Treatment of polycythemia vera: use of 32P alone or in combination with maintenance therapy using hydroxyurea in 461 patients greater than 65 years of age. The French polycythemia study group. Blood 1997;89(7): 2319–27.

23. Noor SJ, Tan W, Wilding GE, et al. Myeloid blastic transformation of myeloproliferative neoplasms–a review of 112 cases. Leuk Res 2011;35(5):608–13.

24. Abdel-Wahab O, Manshouri T, Patel J, et al. Genetic analysis of transforming events that convert chronic myeloproliferative neoplasms to leukemias. Cancer Res 2010;70(2):447–52.

25. Lasho TL, Mudireddy M, Finke CM, et al. Targeted next-generation sequencing in blast phase myeloproliferative neoplasms. Blood Adv 2018;2(4):370–80.

26. McNamara CJ, Panzarella T, Kennedy JA, et al. The mutational landscape of accelerated- and blast-phase myeloproliferative neoplasms impacts patient outcomes. Blood Adv 2018;2(20):2658–71.

27. Rampal R, Ahn J, Abdel-Wahab O, et al. Genomic and functional analysis of leukemic transformation of myeloproliferative neoplasms. Proc Natl Acad Sci U S A 2014;111(50):E5401–10.

28. Harutyunyan A, Klampfl T, Cazzola M, et al. p53 lesions in leukemic transformation. N Engl J Med 2011;364(5):488–90.

29. Lundberg P, Karow A, Nienhold R, et al. Clonal evolution and clinical correlates of somatic mutations in myeloproliferative neoplasms. Blood 2014;123(14):2220–8.

30. Pardanani A, Lasho TL, Finke CM, et al. IDH1 and IDH2 mutation analysis in chronic- and blast-phase myeloproliferative neoplasms. Leukemia 2010;24(6): 1146–51.

31. Tefferi A, Lasho TL, Abdel-Wahab O, et al. IDH1 and IDH2 mutation studies in 1473 patients with chronic-, fibrotic- or blast-phase essential thrombocythemia, polycythemia vera or myelofibrosis. Leukemia 2010;24(7):1302–9.

32. Courtier F, Carbuccia N, Garnier S, et al. Genomic analysis of myeloproliferative neoplasms in chronic and acute phases. Haematologica 2017;102(1):e11–4.

33. Ortmann CA, Kent DG, Nangalia J, et al. Effect of mutation order on myeloproliferative neoplasms. N Engl J Med 2015;372(7):601–12.

34. Alchalby H, Zabelina T, Stubig T, et al. Allogeneic stem cell transplantation for myelofibrosis with leukemic transformation: a study from the myeloproliferative neoplasm subcommittee of the CMWP of the European group for blood and marrow transplantation. Biol Blood Marrow Transplant 2014;20(2):279–81.

35. Cherington C, Slack JL, Leis J, et al. Allogeneic stem cell transplantation for myeloproliferative neoplasm in blast phase. Leuk Res 2012;36(9):1147–51.

36. Kennedy JA, Atenafu EG, Messner HA, et al. Treatment outcomes following leukemic transformation in Philadelphia-negative myeloproliferative neoplasms. Blood 2013;121(14):2725–33.

37. Rucker FG, Schlenk RF, Bullinger L, et al. TP53 alterations in acute myeloid leukemia with complex karyotype correlate with specific copy number alterations, monosomal karyotype, and dismal outcome. Blood 2012;119(9):2114–21.

38. DiNardo CD, Jonas BA, Pullarkat V, et al. Azacitidine and venetoclax in previously untreated acute myeloid leukemia. N Engl J Med 2020;383(7):617–29.

39. Winters AC, Gutman JA, Purev E, et al. Real-world experience of venetoclax with azacitidine for untreated patients with acute myeloid leukemia. Blood Adv 2019; 3(20):2911–9.

40. Badar T, Kantarjian HM, Ravandi F, et al. Therapeutic benefit of decitabine, a hypomethylating agent, in patients with high-risk primary myelofibrosis and myeloproliferative neoplasm in accelerated or blastic/acute myeloid leukemia phase. Leuk Res 2015;39(9):950–6.

41. Venton G, Courtier F, Charbonnier A, et al. Impact of gene mutations on treatment response and prognosis of acute myeloid leukemia secondary to myeloproliferative neoplasms. Am J Hematol 2018;93(3):330–8.

42. Wang JC, Chen W, Nallusamy S, et al. Hypermethylation of the P15INK4b and P16INK4a in agnogenic myeloid metaplasia (AMM) and AMM in leukaemic transformation. Br J Haematol 2002;116(3):582–6.

43. Eghtedar A, Verstovsek S, Estrov Z, et al. Phase 2 study of the JAK kinase inhibitor ruxolitinib in patients with refractory leukemias, including postmyeloproliferative neoplasm acute myeloid leukemia. Blood 2012;119(20):4614–8.

44. Pemmaraju N, Kantarjian H, Kadia T, et al. A phase I/II study of the Janus kinase (JAK)1 and 2 inhibitor ruxolitinib in patients with relapsed or refractory acute myeloid leukemia. Clin Lymphoma Myeloma Leuk 2015;15(3):171–6.

45. Rampal RK, Mascarenhas JO, Kosiorek HE, et al. Safety and efficacy of combined ruxolitinib and decitabine in accelerated and blast-phase myeloproliferative neoplasms. Blood Adv 2018;2(24):3572–80.

46. Mascarenhas JO, Rampal RK, Kosiorek HE, et al. Phase 2 study of ruxolitinib and decitabine in patients with myeloproliferative neoplasm in accelerated and blast phase. Blood Adv 2020;4(20):5246–56.

47. Bose P, Verstovsek S, Cortes JE, et al. A phase 1/2 study of ruxolitinib and decitabine in patients with post-myeloproliferative neoplasm acute myeloid leukemia. Leukemia 2020;34(9):2489–92.

48. Masarova L, Verstovsek S, Hidalgo-Lopez JE, et al. A phase 2 study of ruxolitinib in combination with azacitidine in patients with myelofibrosis. Blood 2018; 132(16):1664–74.

49. Cahu X, Chevallier P, Clavert A, et al. Allo-SCT for Philadelphia-negative myeloproliferative neoplasms in blast phase: a study from the Societe Francaise de Greffe de Moelle et de Therapie Cellulaire (SFGM-TC). Bone Marrow Transplant 2014;49(6):756–60.

50. Takagi S, Masuoka K, Uchida N, et al. Allogeneic hematopoietic cell transplantation for leukemic transformation preceded by Philadelphia chromosome-negative myeloproliferative neoplasms: a nationwide survey by the adult acute myeloid leukemia working group of the japan society for hematopoietic cell transplantation. Biol Blood Marrow Transplant 2016;22(12):2208–13.

51. Gupta V, Malone AK, Hari PN, et al. Reduced-intensity hematopoietic cell transplantation for patients with primary myelofibrosis: a cohort analysis from the center for international blood and marrow transplant research. Biol Blood Marrow Transplant 2014;20(1):89–97.

52. Jain T, Kunze KL, Temkit M, et al. Comparison of reduced intensity conditioning regimens used in patients undergoing hematopoietic stem cell transplantation for myelofibrosis. Bone Marrow Transplant 2019;54(2):204–11.

53. McLornan D, Szydlo R, Koster L, et al. Myeloablative and reduced-intensity conditioned allogeneic hematopoietic stem cell transplantation in myelofibrosis: a retrospective study by the chronic malignancies working party of the european society for blood and marrow transplantation. Biol Blood Marrow Transplant 2019; 25(11):2167–71.

54. Robin M, Porcher R, Wolschke C, et al. Outcome after transplantation according to reduced-intensity conditioning regimen in patients undergoing transplantation for myelofibrosis. Biol Blood Marrow Transplant 2016;22(7):1206–11.

55. Patel AA, Cahill K, Charnot-Katsikas A, et al. Clinical outcomes of IDH2-mutated advanced-phase Ph-negative myeloproliferative neoplasms treated with enaside-nib. Br J Haematol 2020;190(1):e48–51.

56. Chifotides HT, Masarova L, Alfayez M, et al. Outcome of patients with IDH1/2-mutated post-myeloproliferative neoplasm AML in the era of IDH inhibitors. Blood Adv 2020;4(21):5336–42.

57. McKenney AS, Lau AN, Somasundara AVH, et al. JAK2/IDH-mutant-driven myeloproliferative neoplasm is sensitive to combined targeted inhibition. J Clin Invest 2018;128(2):789–804.

58. Sallman DA, Asch AS, Al Malki MM, et al. The first-in-class anti-CD47 antibody magrolimab (5F9) in combination with azacitidine is effective in MDS and AML patients: ongoing phase 1b results. Blood 2019;134(Supplement_1):569.

Traipsing Through Muddy Waters

A Critical Review of the Myelodysplastic Syndrome/Myeloproliferative Neoplasm (MDS/MPN) Overlap Syndromes

Andrew T. Kuykendall, MD[a],*, Franco Castillo Tokumori, MD[b],
Rami S. Komrokji, MD[a]

KEYWORDS

- Myelodysplastic • Myeloproliferative • Overlap • Myelomonocytic • Atypical
- Ring sideroblasts

KEY POINTS

- MDS/MPNs are a group of diseases with overlapping clinical and genomic features.
- Clinical trials focusing specifically on MDS/MPNs are lacking, and the rationale for treatment is largely extrapolated from other diseases.
- The emergence of readily accessible genomic data has led to a better understanding of MDS/MPNs and laid the foundation for molecularly targeted therapies.

INTRODUCTION

Myelodysplastic/myeloproliferative neoplasms (MDS/MPNs) are hematologic malignancies that demonstrate increased and dysfunctional production of myeloid cells.[1,2] The category of MDS/MPN includes chronic myelomonocytic leukemia (CMML), juvenile myelomonocytic leukemia (JMML), atypical chronic myeloid leukemia (aCML), myelodysplastic syndrome/myeloproliferative neoplasm with ring sideroblasts and thrombocytosis (MDS/MPN-RS-T), and MDS/MPN-unclassifiable (MDS/MPN-U). Historically categorized as either MDSs or MPNs, the emergence of MDS/MPNs as an independent diagnostic category acknowledges the spectrum on which myeloid malignancies exist. Acceptance of MDS/MPNs as a distinct entity has been strengthened by an increased reliance on molecular information for diagnostic purposes.[3] Although increased availability of molecular information provides clarity in some

[a] Moffitt Cancer Center, 12902 USF Magnolia Drive, CSB 7th Floor, Tampa, FL 33612, USA;
[b] University of South Florida, 17 Davis Boulevard, Suite 308, Tampa, FL 33606, USA
* Corresponding author.
E-mail address: Andrew.Kuykendall@moffitt.org
Twitter: @KuykendallMD (A.T.K.); @CTFrancoMD (F.C.T.); @Ramikomrokji (R.S.K.)

Hematol Oncol Clin N Am 35 (2021) 337–352
https://doi.org/10.1016/j.hoc.2020.12.005
0889-8588/21/© 2020 Elsevier Inc. All rights reserved.

cases, overlapping genomic features between diagnostic entities highlights the artificial nature of our strict criteria.[4–6] MDS/MPNs pose a therapeutic challenge due to their hybrid phenotypes, molecular complexity, and a lack of focused clinical research from which to draw conclusions. Consequently, treatment approaches are varied and are largely extrapolated from experience in MDS and MPNs.[7]

Herein, we review the group of diseases enveloped within the MDS/MPN category, save for JMML, which is primarily a pediatric disease, focusing on the molecular abnormalities that drive these diseases as well as emerging therapeutic strategies.

HISTORICAL PERSPECTIVE

In 1997, the Society for Hematopathology and the European Association of Hematopathologists worked together to develop a classification of hematological neoplasms for the World Health Organization (WHO). Hematological malignancies were stratified primarily according to lineage: myeloid neoplasms, lymphoid neoplasms, mast cell disorders, and histiocytic neoplasms.[8,9] Myeloid neoplasms included 3 broad categories: acute leukemia, MPNs, and MDS.[9]

The 2002 revision of the WHO classification for myeloid neoplasms introduced the MDS/Myeloproliferative Disease (MPD) category, acknowledging that myeloid diseases often present with proliferative and dysplastic features.[10,11] Originally, the category included CMML, aCML, JMML, and MDS/MPD-U. Clinicians were encouraged to treat these diseases according to whether the dysplastic or proliferative component predominated. Concurrently, MDS/MPNs were also incorporated into the third edition of the International Classification of Diseases for Oncology (ICD-O-3). Before the publishing of ICD-O-3 in 2000, several MPNs were not considered malignant and thus were not reportable to cancer registries in the United States, thereby hindering the understanding of these diseases and the development of specific therapies.[12]

The 2008 WHO classification further refined the MDS/MPN category. In terms of nomenclature, MPD was replaced by MPN and aCML was renamed atypical CML, BCR-ABL1-negative. Refractory anemia with ring sideroblasts and thrombocytosis (RARS-T) was included as a provisional entity within the MDS/MPN-U subgroup. As a harbinger to the next decade of manuscripts, considerable attention within the commentary was given to molecular basis of MDS/MPNs.[13] In successive revisions of the WHO classification systems, the category has remained largely intact, although RARS-T is now termed MDS/MPN-RS-T and is included as a full entity.[3,14]

DIAGNOSTIC CONSIDERATIONS
Chronic Myelomonocytic Leukemia

The diagnosis of CMML requires a persistent absolute ($\geq 1 \times 10^9$/L) and relative ($\geq 10\%$) monocytosis in the peripheral blood. Alternative diagnoses that could account for a monocytosis must be ruled out and a prior MPN excludes a CMML diagnosis. Myeloid dysplasia and clonal abnormalities are preferred, but not required if the monocytosis is persistent and otherwise unexplained.[3] Recently, the requirement for an absolute and relative monocytosis has been challenged with a proposal for inclusion of special CMML variants and early phases of CMML. Special variants of CMML would account for instances in which a relative, but not absolute, monocytosis is present (termed "oligomonocytic CMML") and situations in which CMML occurs with molecular findings suggestive of an alternative MPN. Cases in which CMML coexists with another hematologic malignancy such as mastocytosis or an MPN would also be included as a special variant. Pre-CMML phases would aim to capture premalignant states with increased risk of CMML development. These would include the aforementioned oligomonocytic CMML as well as idiopathic monocytosis of unknown significance and clonal monocytosis of unknown significance.[15] Within this proposal, the authors further advocate for amending the current diagnostic criteria for so-called "classic" CMML to require either significant dysplasia or clonal markers to accompany a persistent relative and absolute monocytosis in the peripheral blood.[15]

The diagnosis of CMML is further refined by leukocyte count and blast percentage in the peripheral blood or bone marrow. White blood cell count $\geq 13 \times 10^9$/L indicates proliferative CMML, with the remaining patients being classified as dysplastic CMML.[3] Patients with proliferative CMML typically exhibit organomegaly and constitutional symptoms, are enriched with *RAS*-pathway mutations, and have worse outcomes than their dysplastic counterparts.[16] Dysplastic CMML, on the other hand, tends to present with cytopenias and transfusion dependence and frequently harbors *TET2* mutations.[17] Subclassification based on blast percentage yields CMML-0 (<2% peripheral blood blasts and <5% bone marrow blasts), CMML-1 (2%–4% peripheral blood blasts or 5%–9% bone marrow blasts), and CMML-2 (>5% peripheral blood blasts or 10%–19% bone marrow blasts). For the purposes of this classification, promonocytes are considered blasts and the presence of Auer rods indicates CMML-2.[3]

Atypical Chronic Myeloid Leukemia

A diagnosis of aCML relies on the presence of a peripheral blood leukocytosis with prevalent immature myeloid cells and evidence of dysfunctional granulocyte production.[3] Incorporation of molecular abnormalities has helped to distinguish aCML from frequent mimickers such as myelofibrosis, CMML, and chronic neutrophilic leukemia (CNL), although it is unclear if this distinction exists more for diagnostic convenience rather than reflecting true biologic differences.[6] The presence of an MPN driver mutation involving *JAK2*, *MPL*, or *CALR* suggests an MPN, whereas the presence of a *CSF3R* mutation is more commonly seen in cases of CNL. *SETBP1* and/or *ETKN1* mutations are enriched in aCML and, within the appropriate clinical context, support this diagnosis. Within these confines exists considerable gray area evidenced by cases in which MPN driver mutations are present at low allele frequencies in conjunction with *SETBP1* mutations and cases of so-called triple-negative myelofibrosis (lacking a mutation in *JAK2*, *MPL*, and *CALR*) that otherwise meet criteria for a diagnosis of aCML.

Myelodysplastic Syndrome/Myeloproliferative Neoplasm with Ring Sideroblasts and Thrombocytosis

A disease whose name reflects its diagnostic criteria, MDS/MPN-RS-T is characterized by the presence of anemia, $\geq 15\%$ ring sideroblasts, and platelets $\geq 450 \times 10^9$/L. The dual presence of an *SF3B1* mutation and an MPN driver mutation is highly suggestive of MDS/MPN-RS-T but must occur within the appropriate clinical context. Acquired causes of ring sideroblasts can mimic MDS/MPN-RS-T and include alcoholism, lead toxicity, zinc and copper deficiency, and medications such as isoniazid, chloramphenicol, and linezolid.[18] Additional nonmalignant mimickers include iron deficiency anemia and anemia of chronic inflammation, which often feature anemia and thrombocytosis but lack clonal markers or morphologic dysplasia. Iron deficiency has also been shown to mask the appearance of ring sideroblasts.[19] MDS with isolated del(5q) can mimic MDS/MPN-RS-T, as it frequently presents with anemia, dyserythropoiesis and thrombocytosis. In addition, patients with MDS with isolated del(5q) have been shown to harbor *SF3B1* and MPN driver mutations in 19% and 6% to 10% of cases, respectively.[20,21]

Myelodysplastic/Myeloproliferative Neoplasm–Unclassifiable

Myeloid malignancies exhibiting proliferative and dysplastic features that fail to meet diagnostic criteria for CMML, JMML, aCML, or MDS/MPN-RS-T are thereby deemed MDS/MPN-U. Although dysplasia is characterized morphologically, proliferative features can include leukocytosis, thrombocytosis, or splenomegaly. Previously, MDS/MPN-RS-T was included as provisional entity within the MDS/MPN-U diagnosis; however, improved molecular characterization and demonstration of comparably better outcomes led to its categorization as a distinct entity. This experience suggests that within this wastebasket disease category, further investigation may reveal additional distinct disease entities.[22,23]

MOLECULAR CHARACTERIZATION AND MANAGEMENT IMPLICATIONS

Increasingly, MDS/MPNs have become defined and distinguished based on molecular details. The 2008 revision of the WHO classification of myeloid neoplasms alluded to the prevalence of RAS-pathway mutations in CMML, aCML, and JMML while commenting on the frequent presence of *JAK2* V617F mutations in MDS/MPN-RS-T. The 2016 WHO classification built on this, linking CMML to *TET2*, *SRSF2*, *ASXL1*, and *SETBP1* mutations; aCML to *SETBP1* and *ETNK1* mutations; and MDS/MPN-RS-T to *SF3B1* and MPN driver mutations. Genomic investigations have proliferated over the past decade as investigators have attempted to link genetic abnormalities to diagnosis, clinical phenotype, prognosis, and treatment response. Ultimately, these investigations have revealed a molecular overlap that mirrors what is seen clinically. Still, unique genotype-phenotype associations have been shown to hold prognostic and therapeutic significance.

Cell Signaling Mutations (CSF3R, RAS-Pathway, JAK2)

CSF3R mutations were initially reported to be prevalent in cohort of patients with aCML and CNL; however, they appear to be relatively specific to CNL and have been incorporated into the diagnostic criteria accordingly.[3,24,25] The presence of a *CSF3R* mutation is associated with relative neutrophilia, monocytopenia and the presence of splenomegaly. *CSF3R* mutations commonly co-occur with *ASXL1* and *SETBP1* mutations and can vary in order of acquisition.[6] Ruxolitinib, a JAK1/2 inhibitor has demonstrated efficacy in patients harboring membrane proximal *CSF3R* mutations, which lead to upregulated signaling through the JAK-STAT pathway. Co-occurring *SETBP1* or *RAS*-pathway mutations may negatively impact response to treatment.[24,26–29] Truncation mutations in *CSF3R* preferentially activate SRC family kinases and may be sensitive to dasatinib, though this needs formal clinical evaluation.[24,30]

RAS-pathway genes include *KRAS*, *NRAS*, *CBL*, *PTPN11*, and *NF1*, with mutations occurring frequently in MDS/MPNs, with the notable exception of MDS/MPN-RS-T. *RAS*-pathway mutations are estimated to occur in 30% to 53% of CMML cases, 30% to 40% of aCML cases, and 10% to 15% of MDS/MPN-U and are associated with monocytosis, anemia, thrombocytopenia, and relative neutropenia.[5,6,31–33] Although *RAS*-pathway mutations play the predominant role in initiating JMML, they are usually secondary events in adult MDS/MPNs, occurring after mutations associated with age-related clonal hematopoiesis and often driving disease progression.[34] Recently, *RAS*-pathway mutations have been implicated in resistance to therapies targeting IDH and FLT3 mutations as well as the JAK/STAT pathway.[35–37]

RAS mutations are the most common dominant lesions in human cancer. Nevertheless, rational targeting of mutant *RAS* has proved exceedingly difficult. Drug discovery efforts have largely focused on inhibiting downstream kinase components, though recent efforts to specifically target mutant RAS in solid tumors have demonstrated promising results.[38,39] Efforts to target downstream Raf/MEK/ERK and PI3K/Akt/mTOR in MDS/MPN are actively being pursued.[40] A phase 1/2 study assessing the use of the MEK inhibitor, trametinib, in relapsed/refractory myeloid diseases showed preferential activity in patients with RAS mutations, with response rates ranging from 20% to 27% in RAS-mutant patients compared with 3% in patients with wild-type or unknown mutations status. Despite low response rates, this study demonstrated proof of concept for targeting the RAS-pathway MDS/MPNs.[41] More recently, KRAS G12D mutations have been shown to induce proliferative effects through activation of the NLRP3 inflammasome, which may confer sensitivity to interleukin-1/NLRP3 inhibition.[42] Direct targeting of Ras via inhibition of processing and activation or induction of synthetic lethality is being investigated.[43]

JAK2 mutations are seen in most patients with polycythemia vera, essential thrombocythemia, and primary myelofibrosis and lead to hyperactive JAK-STAT signaling. The prevalence of JAK2 mutations in MDS/MPNs varies, estimated at 5% to 10% in CMML, less than 5% in aCML cases, greater than 50% of MDS/MPN-RS-T, and 25% in MDS/MPN-U.[5,32,44] Expectedly, JAK2 mutations are associated with proliferative features such as erythrocytosis, thrombocytosis, and splenomegaly; however, their presence does not appear to impact clinical outcomes.[45] Although MPL and CALR mutations commonly occur in patients with MPN lacking JAK2 mutations, they occur less frequently in MDS/MPN-RS-T.[18,46] Hyperactive JAK/STAT signaling can be targeted with approved JAK inhibitors such as ruxolitinib or fedratinib. In a phase 1/2 study, ruxolitinib treatment resulted in spleen size reduction and symptom improvements in patients with CMML.[47,48] A subsequent phase 2 expansion focusing on patients with proliferative CMML is ongoing (NCT03722407). Additional JAK inhibitors such as momelotinib and pacritinib are in late-stage development in MPNs and may have clinical activity in MDS/MPNs.

Epigenetic Modification (ASXL1, EZH2, TET2, DNMT3A, IDH1, IDH2)

Mutations in genes regulating epigenetic modifications are common across MDS/MPNs and correlate with older age. TET2 mutations are seen in 26% to 60% of patients with MDS/MPN, regardless of subtype, although they occur with increased frequency in CMML and aCML.[5,17,49] TET2 mutations are associated with higher hemoglobin levels, lower platelet counts, lower percentage of circulating blasts, and lower likelihood of being transfusion dependent.[49] Although the prognostic significance of TET2 mutations is not clear, they may be prognostically beneficial in patients with CMML who lack ASXL1 mutations.[17,50] In MDS and CMML, the presence of a TET2 mutation in the absence of an ASXL1 mutation has been associated with response to hypomethylating agents.[51,52]

Along with TET2, mutations involving ASXL1 are among the most frequent in MDS/MPNs, occurring in 20% to 60% of patients. They occur more commonly in aCML and CMML than MDS/MPN-RS-T.[5] ASXL1 mutations lead to dysregulated transcription and oncogenesis and are associated with leukocytosis and a need for platelet transfusions.[6,53] ASXL1 mutations frequently co-occur with mutations in CSF3R, SETBP1, TET2.[6,50,54] Frameshift and nonsense ASXL1 mutations independently and adversely impact prognosis in CMML, and co-occurring mutations can further modify their prognostic influence.[50,55]

DNMT3A mutations occur less frequently than TET2 and ASXL1 mutations, ranging from 2% to 18% with a bias toward MDS/MPN-RS-T. Accordingly, DNMT3A mutations frequently occur with SF3B1 mutations and in the absence of SRSF2 mutations. In CMML, DNMT3A mutations have been associated with shortened leukemia-free and overall survival, although they occur in only ~6% of cases.[56] The role of *DNMT3A* mutations in predicting response to hypomethylating agent (HMA) therapy is not clear at this point.[57,58]

Mutations involving *IDH1*, *IDH2*, and *EZH2* occur infrequently in MDS/MPNs, suggesting a limited role for currently approved *IDH* inhibitors and *EZH2* inhibitors in development. *EZH2* mutations typically occur later in the disease process and within a molecularly complex context.[6] In CMML, *EZH2* mutations occur almost exclusively in the presence of *ASXL1* mutations and appear to adversely impact prognosis in these patients.[55]

Splicing Mutations (SRSF2, SF3B1, U2AF1, ZRSR2)

Mutations involving pre–messenger RNA splicing are seen in excess of 50% of MDS/MPNs, with an incidence exceeding 80% in MDS/MPN-RS-T due to the ubiquitous nature of *SF3B1* mutations in this disease.[5,6] In aCML, CMML, and MDS/MPN-U, *SRSF2* mutations predominate, with *U2AF1* and *ZRSR2* mutations occurring less frequently. Most *U2AF1* mutations occur at the Q157 codon, which is favored in MPNs, as compared with the S34 codon, which is more frequently mutated in MDS and acute meylid leukemia (AML). *U2AF1* mutations are often acquired by an early founder clone, while *SRSF2* mutations can occur in the founder clone or be acquired later.[6] Although *SRSF2* and *U2AF1* mutations have been shown to have prognostic implications in myelofibrosis, splicing mutations have not been shown to be independently prognostic in MDS/MPNs.[31,59]

Currently, there are no approved therapies that selectively target splicing mutations; however, this is an area of considerable interest. Mutations involving splicing machinery are mutually exclusive and consistently heterozygous, suggesting the wild-type allele of the mutated splicing factor is required. Efforts to leverage this requirement by inducing synthetic lethality are actively being pursued.[60] Recently presented results of a phase 1 clinical trial investigating the splicing modulator, H3B-8800, in patients with MDS, AML, or CMML harboring splicing mutations demonstrated safety in the absence of significant efficacy.[61] Alternative methods to target splicing are actively being explored.

Transcription and Nucleosome Assembly Mutations (RUNX1, SETBP1)

Mutations in *RUNX1* have been reported in 2% to 21% of MDS/MPNs, preferentially occurring in patients with aCML and CMML.[5] Although the impact of *RUNX1* mutations on survival is conflicting, *RUNX1* is associated with an inferior leukemia-free survival.[62,63] *RUNX1* mutations frequently co-occur with *RAS*-pathway mutations and correlate with thrombocytopenia and monocytosis. *SETBP1* mutations occur in 23% to 32% of aCML cases and lend support to this diagnosis based on the most recent revision of the WHO classification.[3,54,64] *SETBP1* mutations occur with less frequency in CMML (5%–15%) and MDS/MPN-U (9%) and are virtually absent in MDS/MPN-RS-T.[5,54,65] In CMML, *SETBP1* mutations confer an increased risk of leukemic transformation and have been incorporated in the molecularly updated CMML-specific prognostic scoring system (CPSS-Mol) along with *RUNX1*, *NRAS* and *ASXL1*.[66] Therapeutic strategies targeting *RUNX1* or *SETBP1* mutations have not been well-defined, although BET inhibitors may hold therapeutic potential for the former.[67]

PROGNOSIS AND RISK STRATIFICATION

MDS/MPNs are aggressive myeloid malignancies with median overall survival estimated to be between 1 and 3 years.[45,68,69] The lone exception is MDS/MPN-RS-T, which is associated with more favorable outcomes.[70] Disease progression and blast transformation are the main drivers of poor prognosis. In one study of 274 patients with CMML, 13% progressed to acute leukemia with a median follow-up of 17.1 months. Median survival after blast transformation was 4.7 months.[71] Numerous prognostic scoring systems have been established for CMML with comparable performance.[72] Among these systems, variables with adverse prognostic implications include older age, anemia, circulating immature myeloid cells, marked monocytosis, increase peripheral blood or bone marrow blasts, thrombocytopenia, transfusion dependence, adverse cytogenetics, and mutations involving *ASXL1, NRAS, SETBP1,* and *RUNX1*.[53]

The median overall survival in aCML has been estimated between 12 and 25 months, with transformation to acute leukemia seen in approximately 40% of patients within 11 to 18 months.[22,73–76] Predictors of inferior outcomes in aCML include female sex, older age, anemia, marked leukocytosis, increased immature precursors, and *SETBP1* mutations.[22,64,73,77]

MDS/MPN-U appears to have a favorable prognosis compared with aCML, though this is still estimated at 19 to 26 months with 16% of patients transforming to acute leukemia with a median follow-up of approximately 5 years.[22,33] In this heterogeneous group of patients, age, adverse cytogenetics (complex or involving chromosome 7), increased blood or bone marrow blasts, and mutations in *CBL* or *TP53* have been independently linked to adverse outcomes.[22]

Among MDS/MPNs, MDS/MPN-RS-T has the most favorable prognosis with median survival estimated at 76 months, which is better than MDS-RS but worse than essential thrombocythemia (ET). Leukemic transformation rate has been estimated at 1.8 per 100 years.[78] Adverse prognostic features include abnormal karyotype, anemia, and the presence of *SETBP1* and *ASXL1* mutations. Incorporating these prognostic features into a hazard ratio-weighted prognostic model stratifies patients into 3 risk categories with median survivals ranging from 11 to 80 months, underscoring the significant prognostic heterogeneity within this disease.[70] Given the favorable clinical outcomes expected for most patients, attention must be paid to thrombotic risk which is similar to that of ET.[78] Multivariate analysis has shown the presence of *SF3B1* mutations to be associated with an increased risk of thrombotic events.[79]

TREATMENT APPROACH

The current approach to the treatment of MDS/MPNs is largely extrapolated from the experience in MDS and MPNs.[7] In patients with high-risk disease by clinical or molecular models, allogeneic hematopoietic cell transplantation (AHCT) should be considered in fit patients as this represents the only treatment with curative potential. Retrospective analyses of transplant outcomes in MDS/MPNs estimate 2-year and 5-year posttransplant survival from 42% to 51% and 41% to 47%, respectively with disease relapses being common.[80–83] Unfortunately, most MDS/MPN patients with high-risk disease will not undergo AHCT due to age, comorbidities, or interval disease progression.

In patients not receiving AHCT, treatment for MDS/MPNs is largely symptom-directed. Molecular abnormalities should be assessed at diagnosis as they may present therapeutic opportunities, as reviewed earlier. Azacitidine and decitabine are often used based on positive results in trials that primarily enrolled patients with MDS.[84–86] Although less robust and often retrospective, the experience of HMA use in MDS/MPNs is associated with an overall response rate of 30% to 48%, with complete responses in 10% to 20% and a median survival less than 2 years.[87–89] A phase 2 study comparing low-dose azacitidine to low-dose decitabine in low-risk MDS and MDS/MPN suggested superiority of decitabine for MDS/MPN patients, although the sample of MDS/MPN patients was low.[90] In high-risk cases with excess peripheral blood or bone marrow blasts, HMAs represent a reasonable option. A retrospective analysis suggested improved transplant outcomes following HMA treatment compared with intensive chemotherapy, although the retrospective nature of this analysis makes it susceptible to selection bias.[91] Future studies will also need to address the impact of venetoclax when added to HMA in MDS/MPNs given the benefit of this combination in AML and emerging data in high-risk MDS.[92]

In cases marked by clinically significant cytopenias, a variety of agents have been used. Lenalidomide is profoundly effective in MDS with del(5q) with more moderate activity when del(5q) is absent.[93–95] Favorable responses to lenalidomide have been reported in case series of MDS/MPN-RS-T and the combination of lenalidomide and azacitidine was associated with impressive overall response rates in a small cohort of patients with CMML.[96,97] Recently, luspatercept, an activin receptor ligand trap, demonstrated superior rates of transfusion independence compared with placebo in patients with MDS-RS and was approved with an indication extending to MDS/MPN-RS-T.[98] Thrombopoietin-receptor agonists such as eltrombopag may provide benefit in the case of marked thrombocytopenia; however, due to concerns of increased peripheral blasts and proliferative disease, further use of these agents should be limited to clinical trials.[99] Cytoreductive therapy with hydroxyurea can be considered in cases of proliferative disease, and may be required in cases of MDS/MPN-RS-T that are high risk for thrombosis.[100]

DISCUSSION AND FUTURE DIRECTIONS

A growing understanding of the molecular basis of MDS/MPNs has paved the way for rationally designed clinical trials focused on patients with MDS/MPNs. The establishment of uniform response criteria is critical for drug development as it identifies meaningful endpoints that can be used across trials.[101] Collaborative groups are necessary to align efforts and combine patient populations in disease states that are extremely rare. Although the inclusion of MDS/MPN patients in larger trials that primarily enroll MDS or MPN patients provides therapeutic options for patients with unmet clinical needs, efforts should be made to develop clinical trials that focus specifically on these patient populations.

Increasingly, CMML, aCML, MDS/MPN-U, and CNL appear to exist on a spectrum, as rigorous attempts to distinguish between them using mutational patterns and gene expression analysis have failed.[6] These diseases are hallmarked by molecular complexity and co-occurring mutations leading to deregulating signaling, epigenetics, and splicing. Diagnostic differentiation rests on morphologic assessments and laboratory thresholds that are of dubious significance.[3]

Beyond genetic similarities, these diseases are prognostically similar with abbreviated survival and frequent leukemic transformation that is influenced by older age, cytopenias, increased blasts, and genetic abnormalities. Going forward, it will be important to shift the focus away from determining how these diseases differ; instead, focusing on therapeutic strategies that target shared features. Accordingly, it will be vital for clinical trials to incorporate biologically significant translational correlatives into their study design. Response rates of 20% to 40% are demonstrated all too often; leading to persistent debate regarding the clinical relevance of these results. Identifying predictive variables will be critical in designing later stage clinical trials that may lead to drug registration.

Overall, MDS/MPNs pose a daunting therapeutic challenge. For one, they are aggressive, molecularly complex diseases that are difficult to target. Second, they are clinically heterogeneous diseases that have defied standard classification, thus making them difficult to study. Last, they are exceedingly rare, requiring collaborative efforts to accrue the patient populations necessary for clinical investigation. Yet, despite these challenges, MDS/MPNs present numerous therapeutic opportunities, which, through rational study design and collaborative efforts, can be exploited to better serve patients afflicted with the diseases.

SUMMARY

MDS/MPNs represent a group of molecularly complex, clinically heterogeneous diseases that have poor clinical outcomes and limited treatment options. Most treatment options have been coopted from other disease states without rigorous investigation in MDS/MPNs. With the recent incorporation of routine molecular sequencing into the clinical evaluation of patients with aggressive myeloid diseases, therapeutic opportunities have been identified. The mutational landscape of MDS/MPNs has increasingly come into focus; however, instead of distinct disease entities, a spectrum of disease has emerged. Preclinical efforts have proposed novel mechanisms to target defects in signaling, splicing and epigenetics and these concepts are beginning to translate to the clinic. Hopefully, this will lead to disease-modifying therapies that will replace our current treatment, which is largely symptom-directed. Development of uniform response criteria and disease-based cooperative groups has laid the groundwork on which clinical investigation can commence.

CLINICS CARE POINTS

- MDS/MPNs are a group of diseases with overlapping clinical and genomic features.
- MDS/MPNs includes CMML, aCML, JMML, MDS/MPN-RS-T, and MDS/MPN-U.
- The presence of specific gene mutations or combinatorial mutation patters can aid in the diagnosis of specific MDS/MPNs.
- CMML, aCML, and MDS/MPN-U are associated with median survival less than 3 years, whereas MDS/MPN-RS-T is typically associated with a more indolent course.
- The prognosis for MDS/MPNs is influenced by the presence of increased peripheral blood or bone marrow blasts, cytopenias, adverse cytogenetics and specific gene mutations.
- Targeted therapies have considerable therapeutic potential. Ruxolitinib has been shown to be effective in patients with specific *CSF3R* mutations and in diseases that activate the JAK/STAT pathway.
- Luspatercept, an activating receptor ligand trap, is approved for MDS/MPN-RS-T.

DISCLOSURE

A.T. Kuykendall has performed consulting work, served on advisory boards/speakers bureau, or received research funding from Incyte, Novartis, Celgene/Bristol-Myers Squibb, and Blueprint Medicines. R.S. Komrokji has performed consulting work, served on advisory boards/speakers bureau, or received research funding from Agios

Pharmaceuticals, Daiichi Sankyo, Janssen Biotech, Jazz Pharmaceuticals, Novartis, Pfizer, Alexion Pharmaceuticals, and Celgene/Bristol-Myers Squibb.

REFERENCES

1. Cazzola M, Malcovati L, Invernizzi R. Myelodysplastic/myeloproliferative neoplasms. Hematology Am Soc Hematol Educ Program 2011;2011:264–72.
2. Hyjek E, Vardiman JW. Myelodysplastic/myeloproliferative neoplasms. Semin Diagn Pathol 2011;28(4):283–97. WB Saunders.
3. Arber DA, Orazi A, Hasserjian R, et al. The 2016 revision to the World Health Organization classification of myeloid neoplasms and acute leukemia. Blood 2016; 127(20):2391–405.
4. Meggendorfer M, Haferlach T, Alpermann T, et al. Specific molecular mutation patterns delineate chronic neutrophilic leukemia, atypical chronic myeloid leukemia, and chronic myelomonocytic leukemia. Haematologica 2014;99(12): e244–6.
5. Meggendorfer M, Jeromin S, Haferlach C, et al. The mutational landscape of 18 investigated genes clearly separates four subtypes of myelodysplastic/myeloproliferative neoplasms. Haematologica 2018;103(5):e192–5.
6. Zhang H, Wilmot B, Bottomly D, et al. Genomic landscape of neutrophilic leukemias of ambiguous diagnosis. Blood 2019;134(11):867–79.
7. Talati C, Padron E. An exercise in extrapolation: clinical management of atypical CML, MDS/MPN-unclassifiable, and MDS/MPN-RS-T. Curr Hematol Malig Rep 2016;11(6):425–33.
8. Harris NL, Jaffe ES, Stein H, et al. A revised European–American classification of lymphoid neoplasms: a proposal from the International Lymphoma Study Group. Blood 1994;84:1361–92.
9. Harris NL, Jaffe ES, Diebold J, et al. The World Health Organization classification of neoplastic diseases of the hematopoietic and lymphoid tissues: report of the Clinical Advisory Committee meeting, Airlie House, Virginia, November, 1997. Ann Oncol 1999;10(12):1419–32.
10. Vardiman JW, Harris NL, Brunning RD. The World Health Organization (WHO) classification of the myeloid neoplasms. Blood 2002;100(7):2292–302.
11. Vardiman JW, Thiele J, Arber DA, et al. The 2008 revision of theWorld Health Organization (WHO) classification of myeloid neoplasms and acute leukemia: rationale and important changes. Blood 2009;114(5):937–51.
12. Fritz AG, Percy C, Jack A, et al. International classification of diseases for oncology: ICD-O - 3rd edition, 1st revision. Geneva (Switzerland): World Health Organization; 2013.
13. Swerdlow S. WHO classification of tumours of haematopoietic and lymphoid tissues. In: Swerdlow S, Campo E, Harris N, et al, editors. Lyon (France): IARC; 2008.
14. Kuykendall AT, Padron E. Treatment of MDS/MPN and the MDS/MPN IWG international trial: ABNL MARRO. Curr Hematol Malig Rep 2019;14(6):543–9.
15. Valent P, Orazi A, Savona MR, et al. Proposed diagnostic criteria for classical CMML, CMML variants and pre-CMML conditions. Haematologica 2019; 104(10):1935–49.
16. Ricci C, Fermo E, Corti S, et al. RAS mutations contribute to evolution of chronic myelomonocytic leukemia to the proliferative variant. Clin Cancer Res 2010; 16(8):2246–56.

17. Coltro G, Mangaonkar AA, Lasho TL, et al. Clinical, molecular, and prognostic correlates of number, type, and functional localization of TET2 mutations in chronic myelomonocytic leukemia (CMML)-a study of 1084 patients. Leukemia 2020;34(5):1407–21.

18. Patnaik MM, Tefferi A. Refractory anemia with ring sideroblasts (RARS) and RARS with thrombocytosis (RARS-T): 2017 update on diagnosis, risk-stratification, and management. Am J Hematol 2017;92(3):297–310.

19. Minuk LA, Hsia CC. Refractory anemia with ring sideroblasts masked by iron deficiency anemia. Blood 2011;117(22):5793.

20. Meggendorfer M, Haferlach C, Kern W, et al. Molecular analysis of myelodysplastic syndrome with isolated deletion of the long arm of chromosome 5 reveals a specific spectrum of molecular mutations with prognostic impact: a study on 123 patients and 27 genes. Haematologica 2017;102(9):1502–10.

21. Patnaik MM, Lasho TL, Finke CM, et al. WHO-defined 'myelodysplastic syndrome with isolated del(5q)' in 88 consecutive patients: survival data, leukemic transformation rates and prevalence of JAK2, MPL and IDH mutations. Leukemia 2010;24(7):1283–9.

22. Wang SA, Hasserjian RP, Fox PS, et al. Atypical chronic myeloid leukemia is clinically distinct from unclassifiable myelodysplastic/myeloproliferative neoplasms. Blood 2014;123(17):2645–51.

23. Shallis RM, Zeidan AM. Myelodysplastic/myeloproliferative neoplasm, unclassifiable (MDS/MPN-U): more than just a "catch-all" term? Best Pract Res Clin Haematol 2020;33(2):101132.

24. Maxson JE, Gotlib J, Pollyea DA, et al. Oncogenic CSF3R mutations in chronic neutrophilic leukemia and atypical CML. N Engl J Med 2013;368(19):1781–90.

25. Maxson JE, Tyner JW. Genomics of chronic neutrophilic leukemia. Blood 2017; 129(6):715–22.

26. Dao KT, Gotlib J, Deininger MMN, et al. Efficacy of ruxolitinib in patients with chronic neutrophilic leukemia and atypical chronic myeloid leukemia. J Clin Oncol 2020;38(10):1006–18.

27. Gunawan AS, McLornan DP, Wilkins B, et al. Ruxolitinib, a potent JAK1/JAK2 inhibitor, induces temporary reductions in the allelic burden of concurrent CSF3R mutations in chronic neutrophilic leukemia. Haematologica 2017;102(6): e238–40.

28. Lasho TL, Mims A, Elliott MA, et al. Chronic neutrophilic leukemia with concurrent CSF3R and SETBP1 mutations: single colony clonality studies, in vitro sensitivity to JAK inhibitors and lack of treatment response to ruxolitinib. Leukemia 2014;28(6):1363–5.

29. Stahl M, Xu ML, Steensma DP, et al. Clinical response to ruxolitinib in CSF3R T618-mutated chronic neutrophilic leukemia. Ann Hematol 2016;95(7): 1197–200.

30. Schwartz MS, Wieduwilt MJ. CSF3R truncation mutations in a patient with B-cell acute lymphoblastic leukemia and a favorable response to chemotherapy plus dasatinib. Leuk Res Rep 2020;14:100208.

31. Itzykson R, Kosmider O, Renneville A, et al. Prognostic score including gene mutations in chronic myelomonocytic leukemia. J Clin Oncol 2013;31(19): 2428–36.

32. Bose P, Nazha A, Komrokji RS, et al. Mutational landscape of myelodysplastic/myeloproliferative neoplasm-unclassifiable. Blood 2018;132(19):2100–3.

33. Mangaonkar AA, Swoboda DM, Coltro G, et al. Clinicopathologic characteristics, prognostication and treatment outcomes for myelodysplastic/

myeloproliferative neoplasm, unclassifiable (MDS/MPN-U): Mayo Clinic-Moffitt Cancer Center study of 135 consecutive patients. Leukemia 2020;34(2):656–61.

34. Itzykson R, Kosmider O, Renneville A, et al. Clonal architecture of chronic myelomonocytic leukemias. Blood 2013;121(12):2186–98.

35. Coltro G, Rotunno G, Mannelli L, et al. RAS/MAPK pathway mutations are associated with adverse survival outcomes and may predict resistance to JAK inhibitors in myelofibrosis. Presented at the 25th EHA Annual Congress (Abstract S211). (Virtual), June 11-21, 2020.

36. Stein EM, DiNardo CD, Fathi AT, et al. Molecular remission and response patterns in patients with mutant-IDH2 acute myeloid leukemia treated with enasidenib. Blood 2019;133(7):676–87.

37. McMahon CM, Ferng T, Canaani J, et al. Clonal selection with RAS pathway activation mediates secondary clinical resistance to selective FLT3 inhibition in acute myeloid leukemia. Cancer Discov 2019;9(8):1050–63.

38. Schubbert S, Shannon K, Bollag G. Hyperactive Ras in developmental disorders and cancer. Nat Rev Cancer 2007;7(4):295–308.

39. Canon J, Rex K, Saiki AY, et al. The clinical KRAS(G12C) inhibitor AMG 510 drives anti-tumour immunity. Nature 2019;575(7781):217–23.

40. Akutagawa J, Huang TQ, Epstein I, et al. Targeting the PI3K/Akt pathway in murine MDS/MPN driven by hyperactive Ras. Leukemia 2016;30(6):1335–43.

41. Borthakur G, Popplewell L, Boyiadzis M, et al. Activity of the oral mitogen-activated protein kinase kinase inhibitor trametinib in RAS-mutant relapsed or refractory myeloid malignancies. Cancer 2016;122(12):1871–9.

42. Hamarsheh S, Osswald L, Saller BS, et al. Oncogenic Kras(G12D) causes myeloproliferation via NLRP3 inflammasome activation. Nat Commun 2020;11(1): 1659.

43. Ward AF, Braun BS, Shannon KM. Targeting oncogenic Ras signaling in hematologic malignancies. Blood 2012;120(17):3397–406.

44. Patnaik MM, Tefferi A. Cytogenetic and molecular abnormalities in chronic myelomonocytic leukemia. Blood Cancer J 2016;6:e393.

45. Patnaik MM, Pophali PA, Lasho TL, et al. Clinical correlates, prognostic impact and survival outcomes in chronic myelomonocytic leukemia patients with the JAK2V617F mutation. Haematologica 2019;104(6):e236–9.

46. Broseus J, Lippert E, Harutyunyan AS, et al. Low rate of calreticulin mutations in refractory anaemia with ring sideroblasts and marked thrombocytosis. Leukemia 2014;28(6):1374–6.

47. Padron E, DeZern A, Niyongere S, et al. Promising results of a phase 1/2 clinical trial of ruxolitinib in patients with chronic myelomonocytic leukemia. Blood 2017; 130(Suppl 1):162.

48. Padron E, Dezern A, Andrade-Campos M, et al. A multi-institution phase I trial of ruxolitinib in patients with chronic myelomonocytic leukemia (CMML). Clin Cancer Res 2016;22(15):3746–54.

49. Coltro G, Antelo G, Lasho TL, et al. Phenotypic correlates and prognostic outcomes of TET2 mutations in myelodysplastic syndrome/myeloproliferative neoplasm overlap syndromes: a comprehensive study of 504 adult patients. Am J Hematol 2020. [epub ahead of print].

50. Patnaik MM, Lasho TL, Vijayvargiya P, et al. Prognostic interaction between ASXL1 and TET2 mutations in chronic myelomonocytic leukemia. Blood Cancer J 2016;6:e385.

51. Patnaik MM, Wassie EA, Padron E, et al. Chronic myelomonocytic leukemia in younger patients: molecular and cytogenetic predictors of survival and treatment outcome. Blood Cancer J 2015;5:e280.

52. Bejar R, Lord A, Stevenson K, et al. TET2 mutations predict response to hypomethylating agents in myelodysplastic syndrome patients. Blood 2014;124(17): 2705–12.

53. Patnaik MM, Tefferi A. Chronic Myelomonocytic leukemia: 2020 update on diagnosis, risk stratification and management. Am J Hematol 2020;95(1):97–115.

54. Meggendorfer M, Bacher U, Alpermann T, et al. SETBP1 mutations occur in 9% of MDS/MPN and in 4% of MPN cases and are strongly associated with atypical CML, monosomy 7, isochromosome i(17)(q10), ASXL1 and CBL mutations. Leukemia 2013;27(9):1852–60.

55. Patnaik MM, Vallapureddy R, Lasho TL, et al. EZH2 mutations in chronic myelomonocytic leukemia cluster with ASXL1 mutations and their co-occurrence is prognostically detrimental. Blood Cancer J 2018;8(1):12.

56. Patnaik MM, Barraco D, Lasho TL, et al. DNMT3A mutations are associated with inferior overall and leukemia-free survival in chronic myelomonocytic leukemia. Am J Hematol 2017;92(1):56–61.

57. Metzeler KH, Walker A, Geyer S, et al. DNMT3A mutations and response to the hypomethylating agent decitabine in acute myeloid leukemia. Leukemia 2012; 26(5):1106–7.

58. DiNardo CD, Patel KP, Garcia-Manero G, et al. Lack of association of IDH1, IDH2 and DNMT3A mutations with outcome in older patients with acute myeloid leukemia treated with hypomethylating agents. Leuk Lymphoma 2014;55(8): 1925–9.

59. Patnaik MM, Lasho TL, Finke CM, et al. Spliceosome mutations involving SRSF2, SF3B1, and U2AF35 in chronic myelomonocytic leukemia: prevalence, clinical correlates, and prognostic relevance. Am J Hematol 2013;88(3):201–6.

60. Lee SC, Abdel-Wahab O. Therapeutic targeting of splicing in cancer. Nat Med 2016;22(9):976–86.

61. Seiler M, Yoshimi A, Darman R, et al. H3B-8800, an orally available small-molecule splicing modulator, induces lethality in spliceosome-mutant cancers. Nat Med 2018;24(4):497–504.

62. Tsai SC, Shih LY, Liang ST, et al. Biological activities of RUNX1 mutants predict secondary acute leukemia transformation from chronic myelomonocytic leukemia and myelodysplastic syndromes. Clin Cancer Res 2015;21(15):3541–51.

63. Kuo MC, Liang DC, Huang CF, et al. RUNX1 mutations are frequent in chronic myelomonocytic leukemia and mutations at the C-terminal region might predict acute myeloid leukemia transformation. Leukemia 2009;23(8):1426–31.

64. Piazza R, Valletta S, Winkelmann N, et al. Recurrent SETBP1 mutations in atypical chronic myeloid leukemia. Nat Genet 2013;45(1):18.

65. Patnaik MM, Itzykson R, Lasho TL, et al. ASXL1 and SETBP1 mutations and their prognostic contribution in chronic myelomonocytic leukemia: a two-center study of 466 patients. Leukemia 2014;28(11):2206–12.

66. Elena C, Galli A, Such E, et al. Integrating clinical features and genetic lesions in the risk assessment of patients with chronic myelomonocytic leukemia. Blood 2016;128(10):1408–17.

67. Mill CP, Fiskus W, DiNardo CD, et al. RUNX1-targeted therapy for AML expressing somatic or germline mutation in RUNX1. Blood 2019;134(1):59–73.

68. DiNardo C, Daver N, Jain N, et al. Myelodysplastic/myeloproliferative neoplasms, unclassifiable (MDS/MPN, U): natural history and clinical outcome by treatment strategy. Leukemia 2014;28(4):958–61.
69. Giri S, Pathak R, Martin MG, et al. Characteristics and survival of BCR/ABL negative chronic myeloid leukemia: a retrospective analysis of the Surveillance, Epidemiology and End Results database. Ther Adv Hematol 2015;6(6):308–12.
70. Patnaik MM, Lasho TL, Finke CM, et al. Predictors of survival in refractory anemia with ring sideroblasts and thrombocytosis (RARS-T) and the role of next-generation sequencing. Am J Hematol 2016;91(5):492–8.
71. Patnaik MM, Wassie EA, Lasho TL, et al. Blast transformation in chronic myelomonocytic leukemia: risk factors, genetic features, survival, and treatment outcome. Am J Hematol 2015;90(5):411–6.
72. Padron E, Garcia-Manero G, Patnaik MM, et al. An international data set for CMML validates prognostic scoring systems and demonstrates a need for novel prognostication strategies. Blood Cancer J 2015;5:e333.
73. Breccia M, Biondo F, Latagliata R, et al. Identification of risk factors in atypical chronic myeloid leukemia. Haematologica 2006;91(11):1566–8.
74. Kurzrock R, Bueso-Ramos CE, Kantarjian H, et al. BCR rearrangement-negative chronic myelogenous leukemia revisited. J Clin Oncol 2001;19(11):2915–26.
75. Martiat P, Michaux JL, Rodhain J. Philadelphia-negative (Ph-) chronic myeloid leukemia (CML): comparison with Ph+ CML and chronic myelomonocytic leukemia. The Groupe Francais de Cytogenetique Hematologique. Blood 1991;78(1): 205–11.
76. Hernandez JM, del Canizo MC, Cuneo A, et al. Clinical, hematological and cytogenetic characteristics of atypical chronic myeloid leukemia. Ann Oncol 2000; 11(4):441–4.
77. Onida F, Ball G, Kantarjian HM, et al. Characteristics and outcome of patients with Philadelphia chromosome negative, bcr/abl negative chronic myelogenous leukemia. Cancer 2002;95(8):1673–84.
78. Broseus J, Florensa L, Zipperer E, et al. Clinical features and course of refractory anemia with ring sideroblasts associated with marked thrombocytosis. Haematologica 2012;97(7):1036–41.
79. Patnaik MM, Lasho TL, Finke CM, et al. Vascular events and risk factors for thrombosis in refractory anemia with ring sideroblasts and thrombocytosis. Leukemia 2016;30(11):2273–5.
80. Mittal P, Saliba RM, Giralt SA, et al. Allogeneic transplantation: a therapeutic option for myelofibrosis, chronic myelomonocytic leukemia and Philadelphia-negative/BCR-ABL-negative chronic myelogenous leukemia. Bone Marrow Transplant 2004;33(10):1005–9.
81. Lim SN, Lee JH, Lee JH, et al. Allogeneic hematopoietic cell transplantation in adult patients with myelodysplastic/myeloproliferative neoplasms. Blood Res 2013;48(3):178–84.
82. Onida F, de Wreede LC, van Biezen A, et al. Allogeneic stem cell transplantation in patients with atypical chronic myeloid leukaemia: a retrospective study from the Chronic Malignancies Working Party of the European Society for Blood and Marrow Transplantation. Br J Haematol 2017;177(5):759–65.
83. Sharma P, Shinde SS, Damlaj M, et al. Allogeneic hematopoietic stem cell transplant in adult patients with myelodysplastic syndrome/myeloproliferative neoplasm (MDS/MPN) overlap syndromes. Leuk Lymphoma 2017;58(4):872–81.

84. Kantarjian H, Oki Y, Garcia-Manero G, et al. Results of a randomized study of 3 schedules of low-dose decitabine in higher-risk myelodysplastic syndrome and chronic myelomonocytic leukemia. Blood 2007;109(1):52–7.

85. Silverman LR, Demakos EP, Peterson BL, et al. Randomized controlled trial of azacitidine in patients with the myelodysplastic syndrome: a study of the cancer and leukemia group B. J Clin Oncol 2002;20(10):2429–40.

86. Kantarjian H, Issa JP, Rosenfeld CS, et al. Decitabine improves patient outcomes in myelodysplastic syndromes: results of a phase III randomized study. Cancer 2006;106(8):1794–803.

87. Braun T, Itzykson R, Renneville A, et al. Molecular predictors of response to decitabine in advanced chronic myelomonocytic leukemia: a phase 2 trial. Blood 2011;118(14):3824–31.

88. Santini V, Allione B, Zini G, et al. A phase II, multicentre trial of decitabine in higher-risk chronic myelomonocytic leukemia. Leukemia 2018;32(2):413–8.

89. Al-Kali A, Abou Hussein AK, Patnaik M, et al. Hypomethylating agents (HMAs) effect on myelodysplastic/myeloproliferative neoplasm unclassifiable (MDS/MPN-U): single institution experience. Leuk Lymphoma 2018;59(11):2737–9.

90. Jabbour E, Short NJ, Montalban-Bravo G, et al. Randomized phase 2 study of low-dose decitabine vs low-dose azacitidine in lower-risk MDS and MDS/MPN. Blood 2017;130(13):1514–22.

91. Kongtim P, Popat U, Jimenez A, et al. Treatment with hypomethylating agents before allogeneic stem cell transplant improves progression-free survival for patients with chronic myelomonocytic leukemia. Biol Blood Marrow Transplant 2016;22(1):47–53.

92. DiNardo CD, Pratz K, Pullarkat V, et al. Venetoclax combined with decitabine or azacitidine in treatment-naive, elderly patients with acute myeloid leukemia. Blood 2019;133(1):7–17.

93. List A, Dewald G, Bennett J, et al. Lenalidomide in the myelodysplastic syndrome with chromosome 5q deletion. N Engl J Med 2006;355(14):1456–65.

94. Shallis RM, Zeidan AM. Lenalidomide in non-deletion 5q lower-risk myelodysplastic syndromes: a glass quarter full or three quarters empty? Leuk Lymphoma 2018;59(9):2015–7.

95. Santini V, Almeida A, Giagounidis A, et al. Randomized phase III study of lenalidomide versus placebo in RBC transfusion-dependent patients with lower-risk Non-del(5q) Myelodysplastic syndromes and ineligible for or refractory to erythropoiesis-stimulating agents. J Clin Oncol 2016;34(25):2988–96.

96. Nicolosi M, Mudireddy M, Vallapureddy R, et al. Lenalidomide therapy in patients with myelodysplastic syndrome/myeloproliferative neoplasm with ring sideroblasts and thrombocytosis (MDS/MPN-RS-T). Am J Hematol 2018;93(1):E27–30.

97. Sekeres MA, Othus M, List AF, et al. Randomized phase II study of azacitidine alone or in combination with lenalidomide or with vorinostat in higher-risk myelodysplastic syndromes and chronic myelomonocytic leukemia: North American Intergroup Study SWOG S1117. J Clin Oncol 2017;35(24):2745.

98. Fenaux P, Platzbecker U, Mufti GJ, et al. Luspatercept in patients with lower-risk myelodysplastic syndromes. N Engl J Med 2020;382(2):140–51.

99. Ramadan H, Duong VH, Al Ali N, et al. Eltrombopag use in patients with chronic myelomonocytic leukemia (CMML): a cautionary tale. Clin Lymphoma Myeloma Leuk 2016;16(Suppl):S64–6.

100. Hunter AM, Zhang L, Padron E. Current management and recent advances in the treatment of chronic myelomonocytic leukemia. Curr Treat Options Oncol 2018;19(12):67.

101. Savona MR, Malcovati L, Komrokji R, et al. An international consortium proposal of uniform response criteria for myelodysplastic/myeloproliferative neoplasms (MDS/MPN) in adults. Blood 2015;125(12):1857–65.

Current Clinical Investigations in Myelofibrosis

Sangeetha Venugopal, MD[a,b], John Mascarenhas, MD[c,d],*

KEYWORDS

- Myelofibrosis • JAK-STAT • Ruxolitinib • Fedratinib • Pacritinib • CPI-0610
- Imetelstat

KEY POINTS

- Ruxolitinib and fedratinib are the two Janus Associated Kinase 2 (JAK2) inhibitors currently approved for the treatment of intermediate-2 and high-risk myelofibrosis (MF).
- Pacritinib, a dual JAK2/IRAK1 (interleukin-1 receptor-associated kinase 1) inhibitor may prove effective in patients with myelodepletive MF phenotype.
- CPI-0610, a bromodomain inhibitor is under phase III clinical evaluation for JAK inhibitor-treatment naive MF.
- Imetelstat, the telomerase inhibitor has compelling phase II data for extension of survival and will now be tested in a phase III study in JAK inhibitor refractory MF with overall survival as the primary endpoint.

INTRODUCTION

Myelofibrosis (MF) is a clonal hematopoietic *BCR-ABL1*–negative myeloproliferative neoplasm (MPN) characterized by constitutional symptoms, extramedullary hematopoiesis including symptomatic splenomegaly, bone marrow fibrosis, and megakaryocytic hyperplasia.[1] MF may be primary or secondary to polycythemia vera (PV) or essential thrombocytopenia (ET)[2] with a heterogeneous clinical course ranging from

a Division of Hematology/Oncology, Tisch Cancer Institute, Icahn School of Medicine at Mount Sinai, New York, NY, USA; b Department of Leukemia, University of Texas MD Anderson Cancer Center, 1400 Holcombe Blvd, FC4.3039, Houston, TX, 77030, USA; c Adult Leukemia Program, Division of Hematology/Oncology, Tisch Cancer Institute, Icahn School of Medicine at Mount Sinai, One Gustave L Levy Place, Box 1079, New York, NY 10029, USA; d Myeloproliferative Disorders Clinical Research Program, Division of Hematology/Oncology, Tisch Cancer Institute, Icahn School of Medicine at Mount Sinai, One Gustave L Levy Place, Box 1079, New York, NY 10029, USA
* Corresponding author. Adult Leukemia Program, Division of Hematology/Oncology, Tisch Cancer Institute, Icahn School of Medicine at Mount Sinai, One Gustave L Levy Place, Box 1079, New York, NY 10029.
E-mail address: john.mascarenhas@mssm.edu

Hematol Oncol Clin N Am 35 (2021) 353–373
https://doi.org/10.1016/j.hoc.2020.12.003
0889-8588/21/© 2020 Elsevier Inc. All rights reserved.

a chronic asymptomatic state to acute leukemic transformation. The management of patients with MF is personalized and may be focused on alleviation of the spleen and/ or systemic symptom burden, improvement in cytopenias, prevention of leukemic transformation, and prolongation of overall survival (OS)[3] (**Fig. 1**). Janus Associated Kinase (JAK) inhibitors were developed on the premise that hyperactivation of the JAK–signal transducers and activators of transcription (STAT) pathway is central to the pathogenesis of MF. Abrogation of this hyperactive intracellular signaling pathway was anticipated to lead to pathologic, cytogenetic, and molecular responses.[4] The JAK1/2 inhibitors ruxolitinib[5] and fedratinib[6] currently are approved for the treatment of MF patients with intermediate or high-risk disease by modern prognostic scoring systems. Although ruxolitinib and fedratinib mitigate cytokine-driven symptom burden and reduce burdensome splenomegaly associated with MF, they neither clearly alter the natural disease trajectory nor convincingly halt leukemic transformation. Hematopoietic cell transplantation remains the only curative therapy for MF, which may not be a viable option in many patients, owing to advanced age and competing comorbidities. Therefore, there is a relentless need to improve upon existing management strategies in MF with novel therapeutics that leverage complementary disease-related pathways involved in the complex pathogenesis of MF (**Fig. 2**).

OVERVIEW OF THE PATHOBIOLOGY OF MYELOFIBROSIS

Approximately 90% of patients harbor 1 of the 3 driver mutations involving *JAK2*, *MPL*, or *CALR* that result in constitutive activation of JAK-STAT signaling as well as several downstream signaling pathways, including ERK/mitogen-activated protein kinase and phosphatidylinositol 3-kinase (PI3K)/AKT pathways.[7–9] The JAK-STAT pathway plays an obligatory role in normal hematopoiesis and facilitates the transcription of key regulators of cellular proliferation, differentiation, and apoptosis (eg, p21, *BCL-XL*, *BCL-2*, *cyclin D1*, and *PIM1*).[10] Other nondriver mutations frequently found in patients with MF include mutated *ASXL1*, *SRSF2*, *EZH2*, *IDH1/2*, and *U2AF1*. These high-molecular-risk genetic alterations encode proteins involved in epigenetic control of gene expression through histone modification (*ASXL1*), RNA splicing (*SRSF2* and *U2AF1*), and DNA methylation (*IDH1/2*).[11]

The pathogenesis of reactive bone marrow fibrosis in MF is incompletely understood and remains an area of ongoing translational investigation. Abnormal megakaryocytes (MKs) within the bone marrow of MF contribute to the pathologic deposition of collagen and reticulin fibers through altered expression of cell adhesion molecules. The abnormal localization of P-selectin is believed to lead to impaired emperipolesis and, ultimately, elaboration of inflammatory and fibrogenic cytokines, including

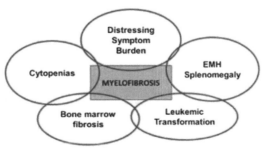

Fig. 1. Interrelated clinical features of myelofibrosis that constitute therapeutic targets. EMH, Extramedullary hematopoiesis.

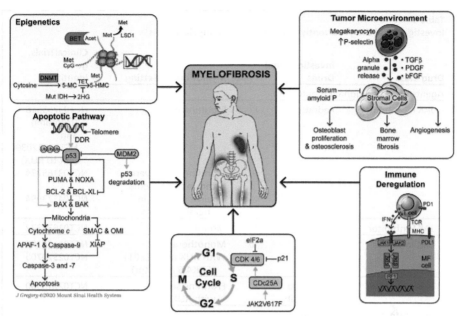

Fig. 2. Interconnected network of complementary pathways amenable for therapeutic exploitation in MF. Broad therapeutic domains include the epigenome, immune regulation, cell cycling, and apoptosis pathway. 2HG, 2-hydroxyglutarate; 5-HMC, 5-hydroxymethylcytosine; 5-MC, 5-methylcytosine; Acet, acetylated; APAF, *apoptotic* protease activating factor; Acet - acetylated; BAK, Bcl-2 homologous antagonist/killer; BAX, BCL2-associated X; BCL, B-cell lymphoma; bFGF, basal fibroblast growth factor; DDR, DNA damage response; DNMT, DNA methyl transferase; elF, eukaryotic translation initiation factor; elF2a- Eukaryotic translation initiation factor 2a; IDH, isocitrate dehydrogenase; Met, Methylated; Mut, mutated; MDM, murine double minute; MHC, major histocompatibility complex; Met - Methylated; Mut - mutated; PDGF, platelet-derived growth factor; TCR, T-cell receptor; Ub, ubiquitylation; XIAP, X-linked IAP.

transforming growth factor (TGF)-β from the MF MK[12,13] These activated cytokine pathways lead to deregulated fibrosis, neoangiogenesis, and osteosclerosis in MF and offer potential therapeutic targets to restore the bone marrow microenvironmental niche.[14]

In the past decade, several researchers have described an interconnection between chronic inflammation and the evolution of MF.[15–17] One intriguing hypothesis is that chronic inflammation may both actuate and drive clonal evolution.[18] These inflammatory cytokines also activate the JAK-STAT pathway, providing a survival advantage to various cells, including the neoplastic monocyte-macrophages and hematopoietic progenitors, which in turn perpetuate the inflammatory signaling of nuclear factor (NF)-κB, JAK1-STAT, and hypoxia-inducible factor 1α, thus propagating the cycle of a heightened inflammatory milieu in MF.[19] Inflammatory cytokines, namely tumor necrosis factor (TNF)-α, interleukin (IL)-6, IL-8, IL-2R, IL-12, and IL-15, are up-regulated in the plasma of patients with MF. Constitutional symptoms, such as fever, weight loss, night sweats, and bone pain, are believed to be mediated by these circulating inflammatory cytokines and have been shown to be independent predictors of poor survival in MF.[17]

Current clinical investigation in MF is focused on harnessing the various pathways governing the pathobiology of MF that may be complementary to JAK-STAT signaling and, in some cases, added to a JAK inhibitor (**Table 1**).

Table 1
Investigational drugs currently in clinical trials in myelofibrosis

Drug Class	Investigational Drugs	Phase	Myelofibrosis Setting	ClinicalTrials.gov Identifier
Agents targeting signaling pathways				
JAK1/2 inhibitor	Fedratinib	III	Frontline and R/R	NCT03755518 (frontline) and NCT03952039 (R/R to RUX)
	Pacritinib	III	Frontline and severe thrombocytopenia	NCT03165734
	Momelotinib	III	Against danazol in anemic patients	NCT04173494
JAK1 inhibitor	Itacitinib	II	Monotherapy	NCT01633372
PIM inhibitor	TP-3654	Ib	Monotherapy	NCT04176198
	PIM447	I	With RUX and LEE011 (CDK4/6 inhibitor)	NCT02370706
PI3Kδ inhibitor	Parsaclisib	II	Frontline setting	NCT02718300
	Umbralisib		with RUX	NCT02493530
Agents targeting epigenetic regulation				
HMA	Azacitidine	II	Frontline setting with RUX	NCT01787487
IDH inhibitor	Enasidenib	II	Frontline setting with RUX	NCT04281498
BET inhibitor	CPI-0610	II	± RUX in frontline setting	NCT02158858
LSD1 inhibitor	Bomedemstat	II	Monotherapy	NCT03136185
Agents targeting the apoptotic pathway				
BH3 mimetic	Navitoclax		± RUX in frontline setting	NCT03222609
	APG-1252 (parenteral)	I/II	± RUX in frontline setting	NCT04354727
MDM2 inhibitor	KRT-232	II	R/R to RUX	NCT03662126
	Siremadlin	I/II	Platform study design	NCT04097821
SMAC mimetic	LCL-161	II	R/R to RUX	NCT02098161
TRAIL inducer	ONC201	I	R/R to RUX	Not yet assigned
Agents targeting the tumor microenvironment				
TGF-β trap	AVID200	I	Frontline setting	NCT03895112
Recombinant human fibrocyte inhibitor	PRM-151 (pentraxin)	II	Frontline setting	NCT01981850
Hsp90 inhibitor	PU-H71	I	Frontline setting with RUX	NCT03373877
MAB against P-selectin	Crizanlizumab	I/II	Platform study design	NCT04097821

(continued on next page)

Table 1
(continued)

Drug Class	Investigational Drugs	Phase	Myelofibrosis Setting	ClinicalTrials.gov Identifier
AURKA inhibitor	Alisertib	I/II	R/R to RUX	NCT02530619
GSK-3β inhibitor	9-ING-41	II	± RUX in frontline setting	NCT04218071
NCT inhibitor	Selinexor	II	R/R to RUX	NCT03627403
NEDD8 inhibitor	Pevonedistat	I	Frontline setting with RUX	NCT03386214
Agents targeting cytokine/host immunity				
CD123 targeted	Tagraxofusp	II	Frontline setting with RUX	NCT02268253
Interferon	Pegylated IFN alfa-2a	II	Frontline setting with RUX	NCT02742324
Checkpoint inhibitor	MBG453	I/II	Platform study MBG453 + NIS793, MBG453 + NIS793 + decitabine, and MBG453+ NIS793 + spartalizumab	NCT04097821 NCT04283526
Telomerase inhibitor	Imetelstat	III	R/R to RUX	NA
Agents targeting cytopenias				
Immunomodulatory imide drug	Thalidomide	II	With RUX to mitigate thrombocytopenia	NCT03069326
	Pomolidamide		With RUX to mitigate anemia	NCT01644110
Agents targeting erythropoiesis	Sotatercept Luspatercept	II	To mitigate anemia	NCT01712308 NCT03194542

Abbreviations: HMA, hypomethylating agent; IDH, isocitrate dehydrogenase; R/R, relapse/refractory; RUX, ruxolitinib.

JANUS ASSOCIATED KINASE INHIBITORS

Momelotinib, pacritinib, and itacitinib (INCB039110) are JAK inhibitors actively being investigated in late-phase clinical trials in MF. Momelotinib is a JAK1/2 and type I activin A receptor (ACVR1) inhibitor shown to inhibit bone morphogenic protein receptor kinase ACVR1–mediated hepcidin expression in the liver. This is thought to increase the mobilization of sequestered iron from cellular stores and stimulate erythropoiesis.[20] Momelotinib did not meet its key secondary endpoint (>50% total symptom score [TSS] reduction) and primary endpoint (>35% spleen volume reduction [SVR]) in the phase III SIMPLIFY 1 and 2 trials that compared momelotinib to ruxolitinib and best available therapy (BAT), respectively.[21,22] More patients in the momelotinib arm, however, attained transfusion independence (TI) at week 24 than those in the BAT arm (43% vs 21%, respectively; nominal $P = .0012$), and 40% of momelotinib-treated patients required no red blood cell (RBC) transfusions over the treatment period compared with 27% of patients in the BAT group (nominal $P = .10$).[22] MO-MENTUM, a randomized, double-blind, active control phase III study, is currently enrolling patients with MF previously treated with an approved JAK inhibitor and randomizing them to either momelotinib or danazol, with TSS reduction as a primary endpoint (NCT04173494).

Pacritinib is a selective JAK2/*fms*-like tyrosine kinase 3 inhibitor in advanced-stage clinical development for patients with MF and severe thrombocytopenia (platelet count <50,000/μL). Pacritinib was placed on clinical hold in February 2016 due to concerns centered on increased hemorrhagic risk and excess mortality in the phase III PERSIST-1 and PERSIST-2 randomized controlled trials that compared pacritinib to BAT and to a dose-comparison study in thrombocytopenic patients (baseline platelet count ≤100 × 10⁹/L), respectively.[23,24] After an independent data review deemed that the rates of cardiac and hemorrhagic events were not significantly different between the study arms, the phase II PAC203 (NCT03165734) dose-finding (100 mg, daily; 100 mg, twice daily; and 200 mg, twice daily) study was conducted. This trial evaluated pacritinib with risk mitigation strategies for cardiac and hemorrhagic events, including the avoidance of anticoagulant/antiplatelet and QT-prolonging agents. Pacritinib was well tolerated and the most significant rate of SVR35% was observed in the 200-mg, twice daily, cohort with no excess cardiac or hemorrhagic events compared with the lower doses tested. Spleen responses in the 200 mg, twice daily, cohort was predominant in patients with severe thrombocytopenia (<50 × 10⁹/L) at 17%.[25] The ongoing phase III PACIFICA trial will evaluate the safety and efficacy of pacritinib (200 mg, twice daily) compared with physician's choice (low-dose ruxolitinib, corticosteroids, hydroxyurea, or danazol) in patients with MF and severe thrombocytopenia (<50 × 10⁹/L) and less than 12 weeks of prior JAK inhibitor therapy[26] (NCT03165734).

Itacitinib is a selective JAK1 inhibitor that curtails JAK1-mediated cytokine dysregulation while sparing the myelosuppressive effects of JAK2 inhibition. Itacitinib was evaluated in a phase II dose-expansion (100 mg, twice daily; 200 mg, twice daily; and 600 mg, once daily) trial in intermediate-risk or high-risk patients with MF, with the primary endpoint greater than or equal to 50% reduction in TSS at week 12. A total of 35.7% and 32.3% of patients achieved the primary endpoint in the 200-mg, twice-daily, and 600-mg, once-daily, cohorts, respectively. Most importantly, 53.8% of RBC transfusion-dependent (TD) patients achieved greater than or equal to 50% reduction in TD during the study period.[27] Itacitinib currently is being evaluated in combination with low-dose ruxolitinib or as monotherapy in patients with MF (NCT03144687).

SIGNAL CROSSTALK-BASED MONOTHERAPY AND COMBINATORIAL THERAPY

Murine and human MF hematopoietic stem and progenitor cells significantly overexpress PIM1, a serine/threonine kinase induced by JAK-STAT activation that is known to regulate hematopoietic stem cell growth and apoptosis.[28] TP-3654, a second-generation pan-PIM kinase inhibitor, abrogated the cellular proliferation and enhanced apoptosis of murine Ba/F3-EpoR cells expressing *Jak2* V617F or human *JAK2* V617F–positive HEL and UKE-1 cells. Although TP-3654 monotherapy in *Jak2* V617F homozygous mice restricted leukocytosis and splenomegaly, combined treatment of TP-3654 and ruxolitinib almost normalized the leukocyte count and spleen size in addition to reversing bone marrow fibrosis. Post-treatment RNA sequencing analysis on murine purified LSK (Lin⁻Sca-1⁺c-kit⁺) cells showed that TP-3654 alone or in combination with ruxolitinib down-regulated TNF-α and WNT signaling–related genes.[29] Accordingly, a phase Ib study is evaluating TP-3654 monotherapy in MF patients ineligible or refractory to JAK inhibitors (NCT04176198).

In addition to PIM1 kinase overexpression, JAK2-STAT5 activation promotes CDC25A transcription, down-regulates p27 expression, and activates cyclin-dependent kinases (CDKs) 4/6. Triple therapy with ruxolitinib, PIM447 (pan-PIM inhibitor), and LEE011 (CDK4/6 inhibitor) demonstrated synergistic antitumor activity in allografted Ba/F3 cells expressing EPOR-*JAK2* V617F and prolonged the survival of an *MPL*W515L-mediated murine retroviral transplant model. No additive toxicity was observed in triple-therapy treated mice.[30] This concept has been evaluated in a phase I trial; however, results have not yet been published (NCT02370706).

Given that *JAK2* V617F activates several signaling pathways, including the PI3K-AKT pathway, Bartalucci and colleagues[31] sought to evaluate the efficacy of BEZ235, a dual PI3K/MTOR inhibitor in combination with ruxolitinib. This combination strategy exhibited strong synergy by inhibiting more than 50% cell proliferation in Ba/F3-EPOR *JAK2* V617F and human SET2 cell lines. Furthermore, combined PI3K and JAK inhibition reduced splenomegaly and prolonged survival in a *JAK2* V617F–driven murine model.[31] Moreover, Choong and colleagues,[32] in a cell-screen (Ba/F3 cells expressing TpoR JAK2 V617F) assay, demonstrated that the synergistic effects of PI3K and JAK inhibition are enhanced only in the presence of JAK inhibition, thus attesting that hyperactive PI3K signaling likely is secondary to constitutive JAK2 activation and PI3K inhibitor monotherapy may not be beneficial in MF. Because PI3Kδ isoform is the predominant isoform expressed in MF CD34$^+$ progenitor cells,[33] a phase II study evaluated the safety and efficacy of umbralisib, a dual PI3Kδ/CK1 epsilon inhibitor, in combination with ruxolitinib in MF patients with suboptimal response to ruxolitinib monotherapy. Among the 23 evaluable patients, 9% (2/23) achieved complete response and 56% (13/23) clinical improvement by International Working Group for Myeloproliferative Neoplasms Research and Treatment (IWG-MRT) criteria. Although hepatotoxicity (class effect) was rare with umbralisib, 9% (2/23) patients had greater than grade 3 asymptomatic lipase elevation and 4% (1/23) had colitis in the setting of preexisting mesenteric ischemia. Pneumonitis was not observed.[34] Most recently, a phase II study evaluated parsaclisib (INCB050465), a highly selective PI3Kδ inhibitor, in combination with ruxolitinib in MF patients with suboptimal response to ruxolitinib monotherapy. Given the preliminary efficacy of parsaclisib (daily for 8 weeks followed by weekly) add-on strategy to ruxolitinib in MF,[35] a recently presented randomized dose-expansion study evaluated the add-on strategy with parsaclisib in 2 groups: daily/weekly (10 mg or 20 mg parsaclisib daily for 8 weeks/same dose weekly, thereafter; n = 33) or all daily (n = 18). The median percent change in SVR and MFSAF TSS at week 12 was better with daily cohort compared with the daily/weekly cohort (−2.3% [n = 30] in daily/weekly and −13.0% [n = 11] in daily; −14.0% [n = 21] in daily/weekly and −51.4% [n = 6] in daily cohorts, respectively). Parsaclisib was reasonably well tolerated and 1 patient each in the daily/weekly cohort had grade 3/4 nonhematologic treatment-emergent adverse event (TEAE): disseminated tuberculosis, varicella zoster virus infection, enteritis, fatigue, hypertension, and transaminase elevation. No colitis, dose-limiting diarrhea, or rash (inherent to PI3K inhibitors) was observed. Because daily dosing appears more efficacious than the daily/weekly combination, daily parsaclisib add on to ruxolitinib will be further evaluated in this ongoing trial in MF patients who had a suboptimal response to ruxolitinib monotherapy[36] (NCT02718300).

EPIGENETIC TARGETED THERAPIES

Given the perturbed methylation status identified in MF, azacitidine, a hypomethylating agent, was evaluated in a sequential combination approach with ruxolitinib (ruxolitinib monotherapy for the first 3 cycles followed by combination therapy with azacitidine from cycle 4 onwards with a gradual dose titration from 25 mg/m^2 to 75 mg/m^2 on days 1–5). Seventy percent (n = 54) of treated patients achieved an overall response rate (ORR) by the IWG-MRT criteria. Improvement in bone marrow fibrosis was observed in 60% of patients, with a median time to response of 12 (6–18) months, which suggests a disease-modifying effect of this combination regimen. As expected, additive myelosuppression is the most common TEAE (grade ≥3 anemia [35%], thrombocytopenia [26%], and neutropenia [24%]), which led to treatment discontinuation in 8% of treated patients[37] (NCT01787487).

Mutations in epigenetic regulators, such as *IDH*, are associated with poor outcomes in MF.[11] McKenney and colleagues[38] demonstrated that combined double-mutant JAK2-IDH expression in murine models altered progenitor cell function, impaired differentiation, and impelled MPN progression and was sensitive to IDH pharmacologic inhibition. Combined JAK2/IDH2 inhibition in a double-mutant *jak2/idh2* murine transplant model ameliorated myeloproliferation with complete resolution of splenomegaly, thus suggesting that this combination may offer a potential therapeutic advantage in this high-risk MPN subtype.[38] This concept is being evaluated with combination enasidenib and ruxolitinib in a clinic, in patients with MF and MPN–blast phase harboring an *IDH2* mutation (MPN-RC-119) (NCT04281498).

MPNs are characterized by a chronic state of inflammation. In this regard, Kleppe and colleagues, through integrated RNA-seq and ChIP-seq data, identified an NF-κB–dependent transcriptional network that fuels the MPN-associated inflammatory state. The bromodomain and extraterminal motif (BET) proteins are histone readers that may have a key epigenetic role in aberrant NF-κB activation as well as the downstream consequences of *TGF-β* and *C-MYC* target gene expression in MPNs and, therefore, an attractive therapeutic target. BET inhibitor monotherapy, or more importantly combined BET/JAK inhibitor treatment, reduced inflammatory signaling and disease burden and reversed bone marrow reticulin fibrosis in an *MPL*-driven murine model.[39] Based on this preclinical rationale, MANIFEST, an open-label phase II trial, is evaluating the oral pan-BET inhibitor CPI-0610 as monotherapy or as an add-on strategy to ruxolitinib in MF patients who are refractory/intolerant to ruxolitinib. The primary endpoint is SVR35% for non-TD patients or conversion to TI in TD patients. In a cohort of JAK inhibitor–naïve patients (arm 3), 67% (n = 15) achieved SVR35% with combination therapy[40] and 36.8% (7/19) of TD patients converted to TI (median TI duration: 14.1 weeks) accompanied by an improvement in bone marrow fibrosis by greater than or equal to 1 grade in 64% (9/14) of evaluable TD patients, suggesting potential disease-modifying activity with combination CPI-0610 and ruxolitinib.[41] CPI-0610 was well tolerated and included low-grade gastrointestinal-related TEAEs (diarrhea and nausea) and minimal myelosuppression in less than 10% (grade 3/4 anemia and thrombocytopenia).[42] Further expansion of the combination therapy cohort for TD patients and JAK inhibitor–naïve patients is ongoing (NCT02158858). A randomized, double-blind, phase III trial comparing combination CPI-0610 and ruxolitinib to placebo and ruxolitinib in JAK inhibitor–naïve MF patients is planned to activate in the fourth quarter of 2020.

Another epigenetic target of interest in MF is lysine-specific demethylase 1 (LSD1). LSD1 is an epigenetic enzyme critical for steady-state hematopoiesis and is overexpressed in patients with MF.[43] Jutzi and colleagues[44] showed that IMG-7289 (bomedemstat), an irreversible LSD1 inhibitor, selectively inhibited proliferation and induced apoptosis of *JAK2 V617F* cells by disrupting the balance between proapoptotic (increased p53 up-regulated modulator of apoptosis [PUMA] levels) and antiapoptotic proteins (BCL-XL) with concurrent increase in p53 expression. Although IMG-7289 decreased spleen volumes, improved blood counts, and prolonged survival in PV-like *Jak2* V617F murine model, it reduced bone marrow fibrosis in the ET/MF-like *MPL* W515L–driven murine model. Bomedemstat reduced Nuclear Factor, Erythroid 2 protein levels, a transcription factor critical for thrombopoiesis, leading to on-target dose-dependent thrombocytopenia. Moreover, low doses of combination bomedemstat and ruxolitinib exhibited synergistic efficacy in abrogating SET-2 cell proliferation, inhibiting stem and progenitor cell expansion, and markedly decreasing splenomegaly in a *Jak2* V617F mouse.[44] Accordingly, bomedemstat is being evaluated in a phase I/IIa dose-finding study of patients with intermediate-2 or high-risk MF resistant to or intolerant of ruxolitinib Given the expected for dose-dependent thrombocytopenia, bomedemstat was slowly dose-titrated from a subtherapeutic dose to achieve the target platelet count of $50 \times 10^9/L$ to $100 \times 10^9/L$. The platelet count was used as a biomarker for dose titration, and 85% patients (17/20) achieved the target platelet count in approximately 45 days. Despite underdosing and slow dose escalation, 50% (7/14) of patients treated with bomedemstat achieved modest SVR (median SVR: −14%; Range: −2% to −30%). Bomedemstat was reasonably well tolerated and is being evaluated as a second-line agent in patients with MF[45] (NCT03136185).

AGENTS TARGETING THE APOPTOTIC PATHWAY

The JAK2/STAT5/BCL-XL axis is a crucial survival pathway for *JAK2 V617F*–driven MPN cells, and combined targeting of JAK2 and BCL-2/BCL-XL exhibited synergism in a *JAK2* V617F MPN murine model and overcame acquired resistance to JAK2 inhibition.[46,47] Nonselective BCL2 inhibition (navitoclax) is limited by profound thrombocytopenia because platelets are dependent on BCL-XL for survival. In a phase II evaluation of combination navitoclax and ruxolitinib therapy in MF, 29% (7/24) of evaluable patients achieved SVR35%; 25% (6/24) of patients had greater than or equal to 1 grade bone marrow fibrosis reduction; and the median TSS at response was 7.4 (range 0–23), a 20% improvement from baseline. Although combination navitoclax and ruxolitinib showed preliminary efficacy, 77% of patients (26/34) developed grade 3 TEAEs or worse thrombocytopenia[48] (NCT03222609). APG-1252, a parenteral BH3 mimetic administered as weekly infusions, also will be evaluated as monotherapy and in combination with daily ruxolitinib in patients with MF (NCT04354727).

The tumor suppressor protein p53 is a master regulator of DNA repair, apoptosis, and cancer surveillance. Murine double minute 2 (MDM2) is an E3 ubiquitin ligase that negatively regulates p53 through multiple mechanisms, including ubiquitin-dependent degradation of p53. Therefore, MDM2 not only facilitates p53 degradation but also binds p53 and inhibits its transcriptional activity.[49] MDM2 is up-regulated in Primary Myelofibrosis (PMF) CD34$^+$ stem/progenitor cells, supporting a possible therapeutic role for MDM2 inhibitors in this patient population.[50] The MDM2 inhibitor idasanutlin demonstrated safety and on-target clinical activity in patients with refractory PV in a proof-of-concept study.[51] KRT-232, a potent, small-molecule, oral MDM2 inhibitor, currently is being evaluated in an open-label phase II study in patients with advanced MF who relapsed on or are refractory to JAK inhibitors.[52] Given the preliminary efficacy (SVR35% in 16% [4/25] of patients) in the higher-dose cohort, the recommended phase IIb dose of KRT-232 was deemed to be 240 mg daily, for 7 days, in a 28-day cycle. A total of 98% of treated patients experienced TEAEs, of which 51% were grade 3 and 24% were grade 4. Gastrointestinal adverse events (AEs) were most common (diarrhea [62%], nausea [38%], and vomiting [21%])[53] (NCT03662126). Siremadlin, another selective inhibitor of p53-MDM2 interaction, is being evaluated in the ADORE trial, a platform study exploring novel combinations with ruxolitinib in patients with MF (NCT04097821).

Overexpression of the inhibitor of apoptosis proteins (IAP) allows cancer cells to circumvent apoptosis by inhibition of proapoptotic caspases.[54] When a cell is primed to undergo apoptosis, second mitochondria-derived activator of caspases (SMACs) are released into the cytosol and bind directly to IAPs, promoting their degradation and facilitating caspase-mediated apoptosis.[55] Preclinical studies in solid tumors have shown that NF-κB activation is critical for SMAC mimetic–induced apoptosis,[56] which sensitizes cancer cells to TNF-α–induced cell death.[57] Given that MF is a chronic inflammatory disease characterized by elevated TNF-α levels and NF-κB hyperactivation, Fleishman and colleagues sought to evaluate the role of an SMAC mimetic in MPN.[58] They demonstrated that murine and human JAK2 V617F cell lines (HEL) and Jak2 V617F knock-in mice exhibited hypersensitivity to LCL-161–mediated apoptosis. Adding a JAK2 inhibitor (ruxolitinib or pacritinib) to JAK2 V617F+ cells in vitro rendered them insensitive to LCL-161, suggesting that the constitutive activation of JAK2 is critical for MPN cell sensitivity to SMAC mimetic–mediated apoptosis.[58] In a phase II study of LCL-161 in patients with MF resistant/intolerant to ruxolitinib, 32% (15/47) achieved an ORR by IWG-MRT 2013 criteria. Weekly oral dosing schedule was well tolerated, and fatigue was a common cause for dose reduction in 36% of treated patients.[59] Further clinical evaluation is ongoing (NCT02098161).

ONC201 is a novel small molecule that promotes apoptosis through a p53-independent mechanism. In solid tumors, ONC201 inhibits MEK-AKT signaling and resultant activation of the transcription factor FOXO3 promotes TNF-related apoptosis-inducing ligand (TRAIL) gene transcription and induces caspase-mediated apoptosis (extrinsic) through TRAIL death receptor 5.[60] In hematological malignancies (Acute myeloid leukemia [AML] and mantle cell lymphoma), however, ONC201 also was shown to facilitate apoptosis through an intrinsic mechanism utilizing the eukaryotic translation Initiation factor eIF2α–transcription factor ATF4 pathway, akin to an unfolded protein response and integrated stress response. Most importantly, ONC201 exerted an antileukemic effect on AML stem and progenitor cells while sparing normal cells independent of p53 status.[61] A recently presented abstract showed that idasanutlin, an MDM2 antagonist, and ONC201 acted synergistically to decrease MF CD34+ colonies while sparing normal CD34+ cells, suggesting a potential therapeutic role for ONC201 in MF.[62] The MPN-RC 122 trial will evaluate the safety and efficacy of ONC201 in patients with MF.

AGENTS TARGETING THE TUMOR MICROENVIRONMENT

MK-derived TGF-β is implicated in the pathogenesis of bone marrow fibrosis and collagen deposition as well as in altering the dynamic balance between malignant and normal hematopoiesis in MF.[63] TGF-β1 has been shown to be elevated in bone marrow of patients with MF,[64] and MPN hematopoietic stem cells appear to be resistant to the repressive signals of TGF-β.[65] Among the 3 isoforms of TGF-β (TGF-β1, TGF-β2, and TGF-β3), AVID200 is a selective TGF-β trap with specificity to TGF-β1/β3 sparing TGF-β2 and can release the repressive effects of TGF-β1 on normal hematopoiesis while decreasing bone marrow fibrosis and splenomegaly in a GATA1low murine model of MF. Varricchio and colleagues[66] demonstrated that AVID200 selectively suppressed TGF-β1 signaling associated with mesenchymal stem cell proliferation and type I collagen synthesis and depleted JAK2 V617F+ progenitors in MF mononuclear cell cultures. This concept is actively being explored as multicenter phase Ib trial (MPN-RC 118) (NCT03895112).

Monocyte-derived fibrocyte proliferation is observed in the bone marrow of patients with MF, and Verstovsek and colleagues[67] demonstrated that MF bone marrow harbors neoplastic derived functionally distinct fibrocytes. Immunodeficient mice transplanted with bone marrow cells from patients with MF developed a lethal MF-like phenotype. Xenograft mice treated with recombinant human fibrocyte inhibitor, serum amyloid protein P (SAP; pentraxin-2; PRM-151) prolonged survival and mitigated bone marrow fibrosis in these treated mice. Recently presented results of the first stage of phase II, open-label, extension study showed that PRM-151 was well tolerated as a monthly infusion either alone or in combination with ruxolitinib and no unexpected AEs were observed in patients with MF (NCT01981850).[68] In the stage 2, randomized, double-blind evaluation of PRM-151 monotherapy, greater than 1 grade bone marrow fibrosis reduction was observed across all tested dose levels (0.3 mg/kg: 30% [10/33]; 3 mg/kg: 28% [9/31]; and 10 mg/kg: 25% [8/32]); 26% of patients experienced greater than or equal to 25% reduction in TSS, and SVR35% was observed in only 1 patient. Up to 9 cycles of PRM-151 were reasonably well tolerated; fatigue, cough, and weight loss were the most common AEs observed.[69]

The epichaperome is an integrated cellular network that regulates cell homeostasis (protein folding and macromolecule assembly) during cellular stress. The 90-kDa heat shock protein (Hsp90) is essential for epichaperome function and cell viability in addition to stabilizing protein folding of client proteins. *Hsp90* is up-regulated in response to cellular stress and DNA damage (hallmarks of malignant transformation), and Hsp90 overexpression correlates with malignant cell proliferation. Among others, JAK2 is a client protein of Hsp90.[70] AUY922, an intravenous HSP90 inhibitor, demonstrated clinical activity in MPNs, but the trial was terminated due to significant drug specific toxicity (gastrointestinal bleeding, night blindness, and altered mental status).[71] PU-H71 is a first-in-class epichaperome-specific Hsp90 inhibitor that inhibits cancer cells through epichaperome disruption and degradation of JAK2 as well as other relevant client proteins.[72] This concept is being evaluated in the clinic in combination with ruxolitinib in patients with MF[73] (NCT03373877).

MF patient-derived MKs overexpress P-selectin, the adhesion receptor for neutrophils and other cell types. In a GATA1[low] murine model of MF, Spangrude and colleagues[13] demonstrated that perturbed *P-selectin* expression fosters pathologic emperipolesis between neutrophils and MKs, resulting in TGF-β accumulation in MK, favoring a supportive microenvironment for MF hematopoietic stem cells in the spleen, which may sustain extramedullary hematopoiesis in MF. Crizanlizumab, a monoclonal antibody selective for P-selectin, approved for the prevention of vaso-occlusive crisis in patients with sickle cell anemia,[74] is being evaluated in MF as part of the multiarm ADORE trial, discussed previously (NCT04097821).

MKs are among the rare cells that undergo polyploidization, an endomitotic process during their terminal differentiation process.[75] Wen and colleagues,[76] through an integrated proteomic and short hairpin (sh) RNA target screening approach, identified that Aurora kinase A (AURKA) is a negative regulator of polyploidization, and alisertib, a selective AURKA inhibitor, facilitated polyploidization and induced terminal differentiation of MKs. In PMF CD34[+] cells, AURKA expression was found to be up-regulated, which was mediated through increased C-Myc expression. In *Jak2* V617F knock-in and *Mpl* W515L murine models, alisertib ameliorated myeloproliferation, decreased TGF-β, and reduced bone marrow fibrosis. Furthermore, combination alisertib and ruxolitinib acted synergistically to decrease colony formation in vitro and eradicated bone marrow fibrosis in a *Mpl* W515L transplant model.[77] Accordingly, alisertib was evaluated in an investigator-initiated phase I pilot study in MF patients who were intolerant or refractory to JAK inhibitors, including ruxolitinib. Among 22 evaluable patients with MF, 29% (4/14) achieved a spleen response (greater than 50% SVR in 12 weeks), and 32% (7/22) experienced symptom response (greater than 50% reduction in TSS); more than grade 1 bone marrow fibrosis reduction was observed in 71% (5/7) after 5 cycles of alisertib. Alisertib was reasonably well tolerated. Diarrhea, nausea, vomiting, fatigue, and alopecia were the most common nonhematologic grade 1/2 TEAEs, occurring in greater than 10% of patients[78] (NCT02530619).

Glycogen synthase kinase-3β (GSK-3β) is a serine/threonine kinase associated with aggressive tumor growth and chemotherapy resistance in advanced malignancies.[79] Furthermore, GSK-3β inhibition blocked fibroblast activation, promoted myofibroblast differentiation, and reversed pulmonary and pleural fibrosis in bleomycin and TGF-β–induced pulmonary fibrosis murine models.[80] 9-ING-41 is a first-in-class, intravenously administered, maleimide-based, small-molecule, selective GSK-3β inhibitor with significant preclinical and clinical anticancer activity without significant myelosuppression.[81] This concept will be evaluated as monotherapy and in combination with ruxolitinib in patients with MF (NCT04218071).

Yan and colleagues,[82] through lentiviral shRNA screening, identified that HEL and SET-2 cell lines and primary MF cells are exquisitely dependent on nuclear-cytoplasmic transport (NCT) for survival and proliferation. Selinexor, an NCT inhibitor, selectively suppressed colony formation of MF CD34+ cells compared with healthy cells and enhanced ruxolitinib-mediated growth inhibition and apoptosis. In a *JAK2* V617F–driven MPN murine model, combination selinexor and ruxolitinib synergistically acted to reduce disease burden, spleen volume, and suppress resistance to JAK inhibitors in vivo.[82] Selinexor is being evaluated in patients with refractory MF (ESSENTIAL; NCT03627403).

Pevonedistat, a first-in-class inhibitor of NEDD8 activating enzyme, induced free radical–mediated DNA damage and inhibited NF-κB activity in *JAK2* mutant HEL cells.[83] A phase I trial of combination pevonedistat and ruxolitinib is under way in patients with MF (NCT03386214).

AGENTS TARGETING CYTOKINES/HOST IMMUNITY

CD123 (IL-3 receptor) is expressed in most myeloid malignancies, including MF. High-expressing CD123+ plasmacytoid dendritic cells [(pDC)cell of origin of blastic plasmacytoid dendritic cell neoplasm (BPDCN)], have been identified in MF, which may play a role in disease progression.[84] Tagraxofusp is a CD123-directed cytotoxin consisting of human IL-3 fused to truncated diphtheria toxin, approved for the treatment of blastic plasmacytoid dendritic cell neoplasm.[85] Given that plasmacytoid dendritic cells and monocytes derive from a common precursor and monocytosis is reported to be a poor prognostic factor in MF, tagraxofusp was hypothesized to be clinically active in relapsed/refractory MF with monocytosis. In an open-label phase I/II study of tagraxofusp monotherapy in patients with relapsed/refractory MF, objective IWG-MRT responses were observed in 40% (7/17) of patients and 80% (n = 5) with monocytosis (>1 × 10^9/L monocytes) experienced spleen reductions. The most common greater than or equal to grade 3 TEAEs include thrombocytopenia (8%) and anemia (15%). Capillary leak syndrome was reported in 1 patient (grade 3). Tagraxofusp was reasonably well tolerated and further evaluation is ongoing[86] (NCT02268253).

RUXOPEG, a multicenter bayesian phase I/II adaptive trial, is evaluating the safety and efficacy of combination ruxolitinib and pegylated interferon alfa-2a (IFN-a) in patients with PMF and post-PV or ET-related MF. The phase I part will enroll 9 cohorts of 3 patients each, with increasing doses of both drugs, to evaluate 3 dose levels of ruxolitinib (10 mg, 15 mg, and 20 mg, twice daily) and IF-Na (45 μg/wk, 90 μg/wk, and 135 μg/wk). The 2 effective dose combinations selected from phase I will be randomized in phase II. No dose-limiting toxicity has been observed thus far in the first 5 cohorts enrolled. Ruxolitinib and IFN-a combination demonstrated preliminary efficacy in 10 evaluable patients, of whom 7 experienced hematological improvement per IWG-MRT response assessment. Further evaluation is ongoing (NCT02742324).[87]

Prestipino and colleagues[88] showed that *JAK2* V617F up-regulated programmed death receptor 1 ligand (PD-L1) protein expression in primary MPN patient-derived monocytes, MKs, and platelets, and PD-L1–programmed cell death protein 1 (PD-L1-PD-1) inhibition prolonged survival of the human MPN xenograft and primary MPN murine models in a T-cell–dependent manner, thereby establishing a preclinical rationale for the clinical evaluation of PD-1 pathway inhibitors in MF, with a goal of reversing immune escape by tumor-directed T-cell reactivation.[88] Two phase II trials of pembrolizumab (NCT03065400) and nivolumab (NCT02421354) in advanced MF have been conducted with results expected to be reported in 2021. Several phase I studies targeting the immune milieu in MF also are under active clinical evaluation. T-cell immunoglobulin domain and mucin domain 3 (TIM-3) is an immune checkpoint protein with a complex regulatory role in both adaptive and innate immune responses.[89] MBG453, a high-affinity humanized anti–TIM-3 IgG4 antibody, currently is under evaluation in MF as part of the ADORE platform trial (NCT04097821). MBG453 also is being evaluated in a multiagent combination strategy approach with NIS793, an anti–TGF-β monoclonal antibody, with or without decitabine or spartalizumab, a humanized monoclonal antibody against PD-1 (NCT04283526). This concept is based on restoration of disease directed immunity through release of different immune checkpoints across the genetic diversity that underlies MF biology.

IMETELSTAT

Human telomeres are structures of tandem (5′-TTAGGG-3′) repeats that cap chromosome ends and prevent cells from replicative senescence, thereby maintaining chromosome integrity. Telomerase is the enzyme complex that retains telomere caps. Two major subunits contribute to the enzymatic activity of telomerase: a structural RNA template and a catalytic subunit with reverse transcriptase (hTERT) activity. Telomerase activity is up-regulated in proliferating myeloid stem cells, and shortened telomeres frequently are a feature of MPN stem cells, which is associated with poor prognosis.[90] Imetelstat is a 13-mer lipid-conjugated oligonucleotide, telomerase inhibitor that competitively targets the RNA template of hTERT. The initial single-institution proof-of-concept trial involved 33 advanced MF patients, with an ORR of 21% (7/33) a median response duration of 18 months in complete responders and 10 months in partial responders. Three of the 7 patients who attained a clinicopathologic response also achieved TI, and reversal of bone marrow fibrosis was observed in all 4 patients who had a complete response with imetelstat.[91] Despite these encouraging results, imetelstat was placed on full clinical hold in 2014 due to persistent low-grade liver test abnormalities and concern for chronic irreversible liver injury noted in an ET trial.[92] After an independent data review and full resolution of liver test abnormalities in these patients, imetelstat development in MF resumed in 2015.

IMbark (MYF2001; NCT02426086), a randomized phase II clinical study, evaluated 2 dose levels of imetelstat in patients with MF who were relapsed or refractory to JAK inhibitor therapy. Imetelstat, at 9.4 mg/kg intravenously, administered every 3 weeks, demonstrated modest clinical activity (SVR35% in 10% and TSS50% in 30%) in MF but was associated with a notable median OS that approached 30 months, twice as long as the reported survival of a similar population of ruxolitinib failure patients.[93] Greater than 50% reduction of telomerase activity or hTERT expression correlated with clinical responses and longer OS, and a greater proportion of patients treated with the active dose arm attained a 25% or greater reduction in driver mutation burden.[94] In light of these promising results, with evidence of target engagement and reduction of clonal burden,[95,96] a randomized phase III registration trial will accrue JAK inhibitor refractory MF patients, with a primary endpoint of OS.[97,98]

AGENTS TARGETED AT MITIGATION OF MYELOFIBROSIS-RELATED CYTOPENIAS

Anemia and thrombocytopenia in MF patients may be related to either disease or therapy. Disease-related cytopenias are associated with a poor prognosis,[3] and cytopenias, regardless of etiology, contribute to reduced quality of life and can restrict treatment in this patient subset, who already have limited available therapeutic options. Immunomodulatory imide agents, such as thalidomide (NCT03069326) and pomalidomide[99] (NCT01644110), are being evaluated in combination with ruxolitinib to mitigate cytopenias. A phase II study is evaluating combination ruxolitinib and thalidomide in patients with MF, and responses were assessed according to the IWG-MRT/European Leukemia Net 2013 criteria. The ORR was 60% (9/15), and 75% (6/8) of patients with baseline thrombocytopenia experienced a platelet response. Combination ruxolitinib and thalidomide appears to be well tolerated; events of interest included thromboembolic event and grade 3 neutropenia observed in 1 patient each.[100]

Bone marrow stroma–derived ligands of the TGF-β superfamily inhibit the terminal stages of erythropoiesis in myeloid malignancies. The activin receptor ligand traps, sotatercept and luspatercept, administered subcutaneously every 3 weeks, prevent the ligand binding to activin receptors IIA (sotatercept) and IIB (luspatercept), reduce aberrant SMAD signaling, and promote erythrocyte maturation.[101,102] The primary endpoints in the clinical trial evaluation of these erythroid maturation agents include a sustained hemoglobin increase greater than or equal to 1.5 g/dL for greater than or equal to 12 consecutive weeks in TI patients or achieving RBC-TI in TD patients. In a phase II study of sotatercept (NCT01712308) in MF patients with anemia, 35% (7/20) of patients responded to sotatercept monotherapy, of whom 3 patients achieved RBC-TI; 23% (3/13) responded to combination therapy with ruxolitinib; and all were TI at baseline.[103] The recently presented study of luspatercept monotherapy and combination therapy with ruxolitinib evaluated TI and TD patients with MF. Among the TI patients, 10% (2/20) in the luspatercept monotherapy arm and 21% (3/14) in the combination therapy arm achieved a sustained hemoglobin increase greater than or equal to 1.5 g/dL at greater than or equal to 12 weeks. Among the TD patients, 10% (2/21) in the monotherapy arm and 32% (6/19) in the combination arm achieved RBC-TI for greater than or equal to 12 consecutive weeks (NCT03194542).[104] Sotatercept and luspatercept were reasonably well tolerated and TEAEs (hypertension and bone pain) were common to both drugs (class effect). Further evaluation is ongoing, both as monotherapy and in combination with ruxolitinib.

SUMMARY

In the past decade, ruxolitinib and fedratinib are the only 2 agents to have gained approval for MF. Approximately 15% of patients with MF are unable to receive the currently approved JAK inhibitors due to disease-related severe cytopenias or therapy-related myelosuppression.[3] Significantly, a majority of MF patients treated with ruxolitinib fail after 3 years of therapy,[105] and these patients are typified by dismal outcomes, with a median survival of approximately 1 year.[106] Therefore, an unmet need for new agents targeting interdependent pathways that can alleviate cytopenias, reduce extramedullary disease burden, reverse bone marrow fibrosis, and extend survival are urgently needed. Advances in next-generation sequencing and expanded understanding of the molecular underpinnings of MF have propelled the development of mechanism-based targeted therapeutics in MF. Preclinical modeling supports the current cutting-edge clinical investigations, with an emphasis on non-JAK pathway–based targeted approaches, rational combination therapy regimens, and modulation of the tumor microenvironment in order to achieve more meaningful clinical responses with an ultimate goal of cure.

DISCLOSURE

S. Venugopal has nothing to disclose. J. Mascarenhas receives research support paid to the institution from Inycte, Roche, Forbius, CTI Bio, Promedior, Geron, Janssen, Merck, PharmaEssentia, Roche and consulting for Incyte, Constellation, PharmaEssentia, Roche, Geron, Celgene, and BMS.

REFERENCES

1. Vainchenker W, Kralovics R. Genetic basis and molecular pathophysiology of classical myeloproliferative neoplasms. Blood 2017;129(6):667–79.
2. Barosi G, Mesa RA, Thiele J, et al. Proposed criteria for the diagnosis of post-polycythemia vera and post-essential thrombocythemia myelofibrosis: a consensus statement from the International Working Group for Myelofibrosis Research and Treatment. Leukemia 2008;22(2):437–8.
3. Tefferi A, Lasho TL, Jimma T, et al. One thousand patients with primary myelofibrosis: the mayo clinic experience. Mayo Clin Proc 2012;87(1):25.
4. Cazzola M, Kralovics R. From Janus kinase 2 to calreticulin: the clinically relevant genomic landscape of myeloproliferative neoplasms. Blood 2014; 123(24):3714–9.
5. Verstovsek S, Mesa RA, Gotlib J, et al. A double-blind, placebo-controlled trial of ruxolitinib for myelofibrosis. N Engl J Med 2012;366(9):799–807.
6. Harrison CN, Schaap N, Vannucchi AM, et al. Janus kinase-2 inhibitor fedratinib in patients with myelofibrosis previously treated with ruxolitinib (JAKARTA-2): a single-arm, open-label, non-randomised, phase 2, multicentre study. Lancet Haematol 2017;4(7):e317–24.
7. Levine RL, Wadleigh M, Cools J, et al. Activating mutation in the tyrosine kinase JAK2 in polycythemia vera, essential thrombocythemia, and myeloid metaplasia with myelofibrosis. Cancer Cell 2005;7(4):387–97.
8. Lu X, Levine R, Tong W, et al. Expression of a homodimeric type I cytokine receptor is required for JAK2V617F-mediated transformation. Proc Natl Acad Sci U S A 2005;102(52):18962–7.
9. Akada H, Yan D, Zou H, et al. Conditional expression of heterozygous or homozygous Jak2V617F from its endogenous promoter induces a polycythemia vera-like disease. Blood 2010;115(17):3589–97.
10. Kiu H, Nicholson SE. Biology and significance of the JAK/STAT signalling pathways. Growth Factors 2012;30(2):88–106.
11. Tefferi A, Guglielmelli P, Lasho TL, et al. MIPSS70+ version 2.0: mutation and karyotype-enhanced international prognostic scoring system for primary myelofibrosis. J Clin Oncol 2018;36(17):1769–70.
12. Le Bousse-Kerdiles MC, Martyre MC. Involvement of the fibrogenic cytokines, TGF-β and bFGF, in the pathogenesis of idiopathic myelofibrosis. Pathologie Biologie 2001;49(2):153–7.

13. Spangrude GJ, Lewandowski D, Martelli F, et al. P-Selectin sustains extramedullary hematopoiesis in the gata1 low model of myelofibrosis. Stem Cells 2016; 34(1):67–82.

14. Zahr AA, Salama ME, Carreau N, et al. Bone marrow fibrosis in myelofibrosis: pathogenesis, prognosis and targeted strategies. Haematologica 2016;101(6): 660–71.

15. Hasselbalch HC. Perspectives on chronic inflammation in essential thrombocythemia, polycythemia vera, and myelofibrosis: is chronic inflammation a trigger and driver of clonal evolution and development of accelerated atherosclerosis and second cancer? Blood 2012;119(14):3219–25.

16. Skov V, Larsen TS, Thomassen M, et al. Whole-blood transcriptional profiling of interferon-inducible genes identifies highly upregulated IFI27 in primary myelofibrosis. Eur J Haematol 2011;87(1):54–60.

17. Tefferi A, Vaidya R, Caramazza D, et al. Circulating interleukin (IL)-8, IL-2R, IL-12, and IL-15 levels are independently prognostic in primary myelofibrosis: a comprehensive cytokine profiling study. J Clin Oncol 2011;29(10):1356–63.

18. Hasselbalch HC. Chronic inflammation as a promotor of mutagenesis in essential thrombocythemia, polycythemia vera and myelofibrosis. A human inflammation model for cancer development? Leuk Res 2013;37(2):214–20.

19. Mantovani A, Allavena P, Sica A, et al. Cancer-related inflammation. Nature 2008;454(7203):436–44.

20. Asshoff M, Petzer V, Warr MR, et al. Momelotinib inhibits ACVR1/ALK2, decreases hepcidin production, and ameliorates anemia of chronic disease in rodents. Blood 2017;129(13):1823–30.

21. Mesa RA, Kiladjian JJ, Catalano JV, et al. SIMPLIFY-1: A Phase III randomized trial of momelotinib versus ruxolitinib in janus kinase inhibitor-naïve patients with myelofibrosis. J Clin Oncol 2017;35(34):3844–50.

22. Harrison CN, Vannucchi AM, Platzbecker U, et al. Momelotinib versus best available therapy in patients with myelofibrosis previously treated with ruxolitinib (SIMPLIFY 2): a randomised, open-label, phase 3 trial. Lancet Haematol 2018;5(2):e73–81.

23. Mesa RA, Vannucchi AM, Mead A, et al. Pacritinib versus best available therapy for the treatment of myelofibrosis irrespective of baseline cytopenias (PERSIST-1): an international, randomised, phase 3 trial. Lancet Haematol 2017;4(5): e225–36.

24. Mascarenhas J, Hoffman R, Talpaz M, et al. Pacritinib vs best available therapy, including ruxolitinib, in patients with myelofibrosis: A randomized clinical trial. JAMA Oncol 2018;4(5):652–9.

25. Gerds AT, Savona MR, Scott BL, et al. Results of PAC203: a randomized phase 2 dose-finding study and determination of the recommended dose of pacritinib. Blood 2019;134(Supplement_1):667.

26. Harrison CN, Gerds AT, Kiladjian J-J, et al. Pacifica: a randomized, controlled phase 3 study of pacritinib vs. physician's choice in patients with primary myelofibrosis, post polycythemia vera myelofibrosis, or post essential thrombocytopenia myelofibrosis with severe thrombocytopenia (platelet count <50,000/ mL). Blood 2019;134(Supplement_1):4175.

27. Mascarenhas JO, Talpaz M, Gupta V, et al. Primary analysis of a phase II open-label trial of INCB039110, a selective JAK1 inhibitor, in patients with myelofibrosis. Haematologica 2017;102(2):327–35.

28. Narlik-Grassow M, Blanco-Aparicio C, Carnero A. The PIM family of serine/threonine kinases in cancer. Med Res Rev 2014;34(1):136–59.

29. Dutta A, et al. Abstract 1874: The PIM kinase inhibitor TP-3654 demonstrates efficacy in a murine model of myelofibrosis. Cancer Res 2018;78(13 Supplement): 1874.

30. Rampal RK, Maria P-O, Amritha Varshini HS, et al. Synergistic therapeutic efficacy of combined JAK1/2, Pan-PIM, and CDK4/6 inhibition in myeloproliferative neoplasms. Blood 2016;128(22):634.

31. Bartalucci N, Tozzi L, Bogani C, et al. Co-targeting the PI3K/mTOR and JAK2 signalling pathways produces synergistic activity against myeloproliferative neoplasms. J Cell Mol Med 2013;17(11):1385–96.

32. Choong ML, Pecquet C, Pendharkar V, et al. Combination treatment for myeloproliferative neoplasms using JAK and pan-class I PI3K inhibitors. J Cell Mol Med 2013;17(11):1397–409.

33. Meadows SA, Nguyen H, Queva C, et al. PI3Kδ inhibitor idelalisib inhibits AKT signaling in myelofibrosis patients on chronic JAK inhibitor therapy. Blood 2013;122(21):4065.

34. Moyo T, et al. Resurrecting response to ruxolitinib: a phase i study testing the combination of ruxolitinib and the pi3k delta inhibitor umbralisib in ruxolitinib-experienced myelofibrosis, in EHA. 2018.

35. Daver NG, Kremyanskaya M, O'Connell C, et al. A Phase 2 Study of the Safety and Efficacy of INCB050465, a Selective PI3Kδ inhibitor, in combination with ruxolitinib in patients with myelofibrosis. Blood 2018;132(Supplement 1):353.

36. Yacoub A, et al. ADDITION OF PARSACLISIB, A PI3KDELTA INHIBITOR, IN PATIENTS (PTS) WITH SUBOPTIMAL RESPONSE TO RUXOLITINIB (RUX): A PHASE 2 STUDY IN PTS WITH MYELOFIBROSIS (MF), in EHA 2020.

37. Masarova L, Verstovsek S, Hidalgo-Lopez JE, et al. A phase 2 study of ruxolitinib in combination with azacitidine in patients with myelofibrosis. Blood 2018; 132(16):1664–74.

38. McKenney AS, Lau AN, Somasundara AVH, et al. JAK2/IDH-mutant-driven myeloproliferative neoplasm is sensitive to combined targeted inhibition. J Clin Invest 2018;128(2):789–804.

39. Kleppe M, Koche R, Zou L, et al. Dual targeting of oncogenic activation and inflammatory signaling increases therapeutic efficacy in myeloproliferative neoplasms. Cancer cell 2018;33(1):29–43.e7.

40. Mascarenhas J, et al. CPI-0610, A BROMODOMAIN AND EXTRATERMINAL DOMAIN PROTEIN (BET) INHIBITOR, IN COMBINATION WITH RUXOLITINIB, IN JAK INHIBITOR TREATMENT NAÏVE MYELOFIBROSIS PATIENTS: UPDATE FROM MANIFEST PHASE 2 STUDY, in EHA25. 2020: Virtual.

41. Verstovsek S, et al. CPI-0610, BROMODOMAIN AND EXTRATERMINAL DOMAIN PROTEIN (BET) INHIBITOR, AS 'ADD-ON' TO RUXOLITINIB (RUX), IN ADVANCED MYELOFIBROSIS PATIENTS WITH SUBOPTIMAL RESPONSE: UPDATE OF MANIFEST PHASE 2 STUDY, in EHA25. 2020: Virtual.

42. Mascarenhas J, Kremyanskaya M, Hoffman R, et al. MANIFEST, a Phase 2 Study of CPI-0610, a Bromodomain and Extraterminal Domain Inhibitor (BETi), As Monotherapy or "Add-on" to Ruxolitinib, in Patients with Refractory or Intolerant Advanced Myelofibrosis. Blood 2019;134(Supplement_1):670.

43. Niebel D, Kirfel J, Janzen V, et al. Lysine-specific demethylase 1 (LSD1) in hematopoietic and lymphoid neoplasms. Blood 2014;124(1):151–2.

44. Jutzi JS, Kleppe M, Dias J, et al. LSD1 inhibition prolongs survival in mouse models of MPN by selectively targeting the disease clone. HemaSphere 2018; 2(3):e54.

45. Pettit K, Gerds AT, Yacoub A, et al. A Phase 2a Study of the LSD1 Inhibitor Img-7289 (bomedemstat) for the treatment of myelofibrosis. Blood 2019; 134(Supplement_1):556.

46. Will B, Siddiqi T, Jordà MA, et al. Apoptosis induced by JAK2 inhibition is mediated by Bim and enhanced by the BH3 mimetic ABT-737 in JAK2 mutant human erythroid cells. Blood 2010;115(14):2901–9.

47. Koppikar P, Bhagwat N, Kilpivaara O, et al. Heterodimeric JAK-STAT activation as a mechanism of persistence to JAK2 inhibitor therapy. Nature 2012; 489(7414):155–9.

48. Harrison CN, Garcia JS, Mesa RA, et al. Results from a phase 2 study of navitoclax in combination with ruxolitinib in patients with primary or secondary myelofibrosis. Blood 2019;134(Supplement_1):671.

49. Lu M, Hoffman R. p53 as a target in myeloproliferative neoplasms. Oncotarget 2012;3(10):1052–3.

50. Lu M, Xia L, Li Y, et al. The orally bioavailable MDM2 antagonist RG7112 and pegylated interferon α 2a target JAK2V617F-positive progenitor and stem cells. Blood 2014;124(5):771–9.

51. Mascarenhas J, Lu M, Kosiorek H, et al. Oral idasanutlin in patients with polycythemia vera. Blood 2019;134(6):525–33.

52. Garcia-Delgado R, McLornan DP, Rejtő L, et al. An open-label, phase 2 study of KRT-232, a first-in-class, oral small molecule inhibitor of MDM2, for the treatment of patients with myelofibrosis (MF) who have previously received treatment with a JAK inhibitor. Blood 2019;134(Supplement_1):2945.

53. Al-Ali HK, et al. KRT-232, A FIRST-IN-CLASS, MURINE DOUBLE MINUTE 2 INHIBITOR (MDM2I), FOR MYELOFIBROSIS (MF) RELAPSED OR REFRACTORY (R/R) TO JANUS-ASSOCIATED KINASE INHIBITOR (JAKI) TREATMENT (TX). 2020.

54. Silke J, Meier P. Inhibitor of apoptosis (IAP) proteins-modulators of cell death and inflammation. Cold Spring Harb Perspect Biol 2013;5(2):a008730.

55. Chen DJ, Huerta S. Smac mimetics as new cancer therapeutics. Anticancer Drugs 2009;20(8):646–58.

56. Berger R, Jennewein C, Marschall V, et al. NF-κB is required for smac mimetic-mediated sensitization of glioblastoma cells for γ-irradiation–induced apoptosis. Mol Cancer Ther 2011;10(10):1867–75.

57. Welsh K, Milutinovic S, Ardecky RJ, et al. Characterization of potent SMAC mimetics that sensitize cancer cells to TNF family-induced apoptosis. PLoS One 2016;11(9):e0161952.

58. Craver BM, Nguyen T, Nguyen J, et al. The SMAC mimetic LCL-161 selectively targets JAK2V617F mutant cells. Exp Hematol Oncol 2020;9(1):1.

59. Pemmaraju N, Carter BZ, Kantarjian HM, et al. Final Results of Phase 2 Clinical Trial of LCL161, a Novel Oral SMAC Mimetic/IAP Antagonist, for Patients with Intermediate to High Risk Myelofibrosis. Blood 2019;134(Supplement_1):555.

60. Allen JE, Krigsfeld G, Mayes PA, et al. Dual inactivation of Akt and ERK by TIC10 Signals Foxo3a Nuclear Translocation, TRAIL gene induction, and potent antitumor effects. Sci Transl Med 2013;5(171):171ra17.

61. Ishizawa J, Kojima K, Chachad D, et al. ATF4 induction through an atypical integrated stress response to ONC201 triggers p53-independent apoptosis in hematological malignancies. Sci Signal 2016;9(415):ra17.

62. Lu M, Xia L, Hoffman R. A novel combination of drugs which target both the intrinsic and extrinsic apoptotic pathways to eliminate myelofibrosis CD34+ cells. Blood 2019;134(Supplement_1):4201.

63. Ling T, Crispino JD, Zingariello M, et al. GATA1 insufficiencies in primary myelo-fibrosis and other hematopoietic disorders: consequences for therapy. Expert Rev Hematol 2018;11(3):169–84.

64. Chou JM, Li CY, Tefferi A. Bone marrow immunohistochemical studies of angio-genic cytokines and their receptors in myelofibrosis with myeloid metaplasia. Leuk Res 2003;27(6):499–504.

65. Zingariello M, Martelli F, Ciaffoni F, et al. Characterization of the TGF-β1 signaling abnormalities in the Gata1low mouse model of myelofibrosis. Blood 2013; 121(17):3345–63.

66. Varricchio L, Mascarenhas J, Migliaccio AR, et al. AVID200, a Potent Trap for TGF-β ligands inhibits TGF-β1 signaling in human myelofibrosis. Blood 2018; 132(Supplement 1):1791.

67. Verstovsek S, Manshouri T, Pilling D, et al. Role of neoplastic monocyte-derived fibrocytes in primary myelofibrosis. J Exp Med 2016;213(9):1723–40.

68. Verstovsek S, Hasserjian RP, Pozdnyakova O, et al. PRM-151 in myelofibrosis: efficacy and safety in an open label extension study. Blood 2018; 132(Supplement 1):686.

69. Verstovsek S, et al. A RANDOMIZED, DOUBLE BLIND PHASE 2 STUDY OF 3 DIFFERENT DOSES OF PRM-151 IN PATIENTS WITH MYELOFIBROSIS WHO WERE PREVIOUSLY TREATED WITH OR INELIGIBLE FOR RUXOLITINIB, in EHA24. 2019.

70. Marubayashi S, Koppikar P, Taldone T, et al. HSP90 is a therapeutic target in JAK2-dependent myeloproliferative neoplasms in mice and humans. J Clin Invest 2010;120(10):3578–93.

71. Gabriela SH, Somasundara A, Kleppe M, et al. Hsp90 inhibition disrupts JAK-STAT signaling and leads to reductions in splenomegaly in patients with myelo-proliferative neoplasms. Haematologica 2018;103(1):e5–9.

72. Speranza G, Anderson L, Chen AP, et al. First-in-human study of the epichaper-ome inhibitor PU-H71: clinical results and metabolic profile. Invest New Drugs 2018;36(2):230–9.

73. Pemmaraju N, Gundabolu K, Pettit K, et al. Phase 1b study of the epichaperome inhibitor PU-H71 administered orally with ruxolitinib continuation for the treat-ment of patients with myelofibrosis. Blood 2019;134(Supplement_1):4178.

74. Ataga KI, Kutlar A, Kanter J, et al. Crizanlizumab for the prevention of pain cri-ses in sickle cell disease. N Engl J Med 2016;376(5):429–39.

75. Bluteau D, Lordier L, Di Stefano A, et al. Regulation of megakaryocyte matura-tion and platelet formation. J Thromb Haemost 2009;7(Suppl 1):227–34.

76. Wen Q, Goldenson B, Silver SJ, et al. Identification of regulators of polyploidiza-tion presents therapeutic targets for treatment of AMKL. Cell 2012;150(3): 575–89.

77. Wen QJ, Yang Q, Goldenson B, et al. Targeting megakaryocytic-induced fibrosis in myeloproliferative neoplasms by AURKA inhibition. Nat Med 2015; 21(12):1473–80.

78. Gangat N, Marinaccio C, Swords R, et al. Aurora Kinase A inhibition provides clinical benefit, normalizes megakaryocytes, and reduces bone marrow fibrosis in patients with myelofibrosis: a phase I Trial. Clin Cancer Res 2019;25(16): 4898–906.

79. Doble BW, Woodgett JR. GSK-3: tricks of the trade for a multi-tasking kinase. J Cell Sci 2003;116(Pt 7):1175–86.

80. Jeffers A, Qin W, Owens S, et al. Glycogen synthase kinase-3β Inhibition with 9-ING-41 attenuates the progression of pulmonary fibrosis. Sci Rep 2019;9(1): 18925.

81. Wu X, Stenson M, Abeykoon J, et al. Targeting glycogen synthase kinase 3 for therapeutic benefit in lymphoma. Blood 2019;134(4):363–73.

82. Yan D, Pomicter AD, Tantravahi S, et al. Nuclear–cytoplasmic transport is a therapeutic target in myelofibrosis. Clin Cancer Res 2019;25(7):2323–35.

83. Fisher DAC, Miner CA, Engle EK, et al. Cytokine production in myelofibrosis exhibits differential responsiveness to JAK-STAT, MAP kinase, and NFκB signaling. Leukemia 2019;33(8):1978–95.

84. Testa U, Pelosi E, Frankel A, et al. CD 123 is a membrane biomarker and a therapeutic target in hematologic malignancies. Biomark Res 2014;2(1):4.

85. Pemmaraju N, Lane AA, Sweet KL, et al. Results of pivotal phase 2 clinical trial of tagraxofusp (SL-401) in patients with blastic plasmacytoid dendritic cell neoplasm (BPDCN). Blood 2018;132(Supplement 1):765.

86. Pemmaraju N, Gupta V, Ali H, et al. Results from a phase 1/2 clinical trial of tagraxofusp (SL-401) in patients with intermediate, or high risk, relapsed/refractory myelofibrosis. Blood 2019;134(Supplement_1):558.

87. Kiladjian J-J, Soret-Dulphy J, Resche-Rigon M, et al. Ruxopeg, a multi-center bayesian phase 1/2 adaptive randomized trial of the combination of ruxolitinib and pegylated interferon alpha 2a in patients with myeloproliferative neoplasm (MPN)-associated myelofibrosis. Blood 2018;132(Supplement 1):581.

88. Prestipino A, Emhardt AJ, Aumann K, et al. Oncogenic JAK2V617F causes PD-L1 expression, mediating immune escape in myeloproliferative neoplasms. Sci Transl Med 2018;10(429):eaam7729.

89. He Y, Cao J, Zhao C, et al. TIM-3, a promising target for cancer immunotherapy. Onco Targets Ther 2018;11:7005–9.

90. Spanoudakis E, Bazdiara I, Pantelidou D, et al. Dynamics of telomere's length and telomerase activity in Philadelphia chromosome negative myeloproliferative neoplasms. Leuk Res 2011;35(4):459–64.

91. Tefferi A, Lasho TL, Begna KH, et al. A Pilot Study of the Telomerase Inhibitor Imetelstat for Myelofibrosis. N Engl J Med 2015;373(10):908–19.

92. Baerlocher GM, Oppliger Leibundgut E, Ottmann OG, et al. Telomerase inhibitor imetelstat in patients with essential thrombocythemia. N Engl J Med 2015; 373(10):920–8.

93. Mascarenhas J, Komrokji RS, Cavo M, et al. Imetelstat Is effective treatment for patients with intermediate-2 or high-risk myelofibrosis who have relapsed on or are refractory to janus kinase inhibitor therapy: results of a phase 2 randomized study of two dose levels. Blood 2018;132(Supplement 1):685.

94. Mascarenhas J, et al. TELOMERASE ACTIVITY, TELOMERE LENGTH AND HTERT EXPRESSION CORRELATE WITH CLINICAL OUTCOMES IN HIGHER-RISK MYELOFIBROSIS (MF) RELAPSED/REFRACTORY (R/R) TO JANUS KINASE INHIBITOR TREATED WITH IMETELSTAT. 2020.

95. Mascarenhas J, Komrokji RS, Cavo M, et al. Potential Disease-Modifying Activity of Imetelstat Demonstrated By Reduction in Cytogenetically Abnormal Clones and Mutation Burden Leads to Clinical Benefits in Relapsed/Refractory Myelofibrosis Patients. Blood 2020;136(Supplement 1):39–40.

96. Mascarenhas J, Komrokji RS, Cavo M, et al. Correlation analyses of imetelstat exposure with pharmacodynamic effect, efficacy and safety in a phase 2 study in patients with higher-risk myelofibrosis refractory to janus kinase inhibitor

identified an optimal dosing regimen for phase 3 study. Blood 2020; 136(Supplement 1):33–4.

97. Geron Announces Plans for Imetelstat Phase 3 Clinical Trial in Myelofibrosis.
98. Mascarenhas J, Harrison C, Kiladjian J-J, et al. A Randomized Open-Label, Phase 3 Study to Evaluate Imetelstat Versus Best Available Therapy (BAT) in Patients with Intermediate-2 or High-Risk Myelofibrosis (MF) Refractory to Janus Kinase (JAK) Inhibitor. Blood 2020;136(Supplement 1):43–4.
99. Stegelmann F, Koschmieder S, Isfort S, et al. S1608 ruxolitinib plus pomalidomide in myelofibrosis with anemia: results from the mpnsg-0212 combination trial (NCT01644110). HemaSphere 2019;3(S1):740–1.
100. Rampal RK, Verstovsek S, Devlin SM, et al. Safety and Efficacy of Combined Ruxolitinib and Thalidomide in Patients with Myelofibrosis: A Phase II Study. Blood 2019;134(Supplement_1):4163.
101. Iancu-Rubin C, Mosoyan G, Wang J, et al. Stromal cell-mediated inhibition of erythropoiesis can be attenuated by Sotatercept (ACE-011), an activin receptor type II ligand trap. Exp Hematol 2013;41(2):155.e17.
102. Carrancio S, Markovics J, Wong P, et al. An activin receptor IIA ligand trap promotes erythropoiesis resulting in a rapid induction of red blood cells and haemoglobin. Br J Haematol 2014;165(6):870–82.
103. Bose P, Daver N, Pemmaraju N, et al. Sotatercept (ACE-011) alone and in combination with ruxolitinib in patients (pts) with myeloproliferative neoplasm (MPN)-associated myelofibrosis (MF) and anemia. Blood 2017;130(Supplement 1):255.
104. Gerds AT, Vannucchi AM, Passamonti F, et al. A Phase 2 Study of Luspatercept in Patients with Myelofibrosis-Associated Anemia. Blood 2019; 134(Supplement_1):557.
105. Palandri F, Breccia M, Bonifacio M, et al. Life after ruxolitinib: Reasons for discontinuation, impact of disease phase, and outcomes in 218 patients with myelofibrosis. Cancer 2019;126(6):1243–52.
106. Newberry KJ, Patel K, Masarova L, et al. Clonal evolution and outcomes in myelofibrosis after ruxolitinib discontinuation. Blood 2017;130(9):1125–31.

Quality of Life in Myeloproliferative Neoplasms

Symptoms and Management Implications

Ruben Mesa, MD[a,*], Jeanne Palmer, MD[b], Ryan Eckert, MS[a,c], Jennifer Huberty, PhD[a,c]

KEYWORDS

- Myeloproliferative neoplasm • Quality of life • Inflammation • Integrative medicine

KEY POINTS

- Myeloproliferative neoplasms can be associated with a number of different symptoms that can be quantified by using the myeloproliferative neoplasm symptom assessment form.
- The symptoms likely have a biologic basis and are related to inflammation generated from a dysregulated JAK-STAT pathway.
- Treatment for myeloproliferative neoplasms attempts to control counts, as well as decrease inflammation and symptom burden.
- There are an increasing data supporting a nonpharmacologic/integrative approach to managing the symptoms associated with myeloproliferative neoplasm, using activities such as yoga and meditation.

INTRODUCTION

The myeloproliferative neoplasms (MPN) are a family of interrelated disorders that include essential thrombocythemia (ET), polycythemia vera (PV), and myelofibrosis (MF). These disorders share biological underpinnings with somatic mutation-driven myeloproliferation, risk of thrombotic events, risk of hemorrhagic events, potential splenomegaly, possible cytopenias (either disease and/or therapy toxicity related), potential progression (from ET/PV to MF) or to acute myeloid leukemia (acute myeloid leukemia or MPN blast phase). Importantly, in addition to this range of burdens that patients with MPN can experience, they can also experience significant disease-related symptoms such as fatigue, vascular symptoms (headaches, difficulties with

[a] Mays Cancer Center, UT Health San Antonio MD Anderson, 7979 Wurzbach Road, San Antonio, TX 78229, USA; [b] Division of Hematology & Medical Oncology, Mayo Clinic, 5777 East Mayo boulevard, Phoenix, AZ, 85054, USA; [c] Arizona State University College of Health Solutions, 550 North 3rd Street, Phoenix, AZ 85004, USA
* Corresponding author.
E-mail address: mesar@uthscsa.edu

Hematol Oncol Clin N Am 35 (2021) 375–390
https://doi.org/10.1016/j.hoc.2020.12.006
0889-8588/21/© 2020 Elsevier Inc. All rights reserved.

concentration, complex migraines), splenomegaly-related symptoms (abdominal pain, abdominal fullness, early satiety), and constitutional symptoms (night sweats, weight loss).

Quality of life is a complex construct that can include many subjective constructs that are deeply individualized. Health-related quality of life narrows that focus and, for someone with an illness, can include disease-related symptoms, drug-related toxicities, the financial toxicity of health care, the impact on employment and activities of daily living, the impact on limiting desired activities, the stress of uncertainty, and fear of the future. In this article, we discuss MPN symptoms (biological underpinnings, accurate assessment), the impact of medical therapies on MPN symptoms, drivers of MPN health-related quality of life, stem cell transplantation and health-related quality of life, and nonpharmacologic strategies for improving health-related quality of life for patients with MPN.

MEASURING PATIENT-REPORTED OUTCOMES IN PATIENTS WITH MYELOPROLIFERATIVE NEOPLASMS

It has long been recognized by treating physicians and MPN patients alike that various symptoms were characteristic and typical of MPNs, such as pruritus, fatigue, and weight loss, but there has been little quantification of these symptoms before the early 2000s. In 2006, as a collaborative effort between patient groups (CMPN Education Foundation led by Joyce Niblack, JD) and our team, we conducted the first large-scale survey of patients with MPN, leveraging the outreach of an online MPN community, to quantify the types of symptoms, their prevalence, MPN features, comorbidities (measured by the Charlson Comorbidity Index), and demographics.[1] A total of 1179 patients with MPN (median age, 56 years; 41.4% men) completed the survey. Fatigue was demonstrated to be the most commonly reported symptom (80.7%). Additionally, quantification of the presence of other symptoms was demonstrated. Other symptoms reported by patients with MPN included pruritis (53%), night sweats (50%), bone pain (44%), fevers (14%), weight loss (13%), and spleen pain owing to splenomegaly (6%). Furthermore, the majority of patients reported a symptom-related restriction on their ability to participate in both social functions and physical activity. Although slightly less common, approximately 35% reported needing assistance with activities of daily living and approximately 11% reported an MPN-associated medical disability. The findings of this survey helped to quantify the presence of MPN-related symptoms, demonstrated the high prevalence and significant impact of fatigue for patients with MPN, and underscored the importance of health-related quality of life assessment in clinical trials owing to fatigue being a major contributor to poor health-related quality of life.

Patient-reported outcome forms for MPNs had not been developed before the phase I trial of ruxolitinib in MF, so when we observed dramatic and rapid improvement in MPN symptoms as a result of that therapy it was clear we needed a validated instrument for quantifying that benefit. We first interrogated existing patient-reported outcome instruments, and found none were adequate to capture the spectrum of symptoms relevant in MF (spleen-related symptoms, constitutional symptoms, etc). We leveraged our prior survey data to create the construct of the Myelofibrosis Symptom Assessment Form (MFSAF). In 2009,[2] we initially developed and validated the 20-item MFSAF among 24 patients with MF, of which items included the entire Brief Fatigue Inventory, splenomegaly-associated symptoms (eg, early satiety, abdominal pain, inactivity, cough), catabolic and proliferative symptoms (eg, night sweats, itching, bone pain, fever, weight loss), and overall quality of life. Patients rated the MFSAF as easy to understand and as addressing most of their symptoms. Additionally, the MFSAF performed well as compared with other instruments that assessed symptoms addressed in the MFSAF. Questions from the Memorial Symptom Assessment Scale and Brief Pain Inventory were all highly correlated with their MFSAF counterparts ($P<.01$).

In a 2011 trial of 87 patients with MF undergoing a phase II trial of the JAK1 and JAK2 inhibitor INCB018424,[3] we used a slightly modified set of questions for the MFSAF, including some exploratory items in addition to the original MFSAF items, which can be seen in **Table 1**. When assessing correlations between baseline disease features and MFSAF items, we found massive splenomegaly (>20 cm below the costal margin) to be positively associated with worse fatigue item scores ($P = .01$), a decreased ability to walk around and exercise ($P = .0001$), decreased ability to bend ($P = .03$), hindrance to perform daily activities ($P = .004$), and a worse quality of life ($P = .01$). Therapy with INCB018424 resulted in a rapid decrease in MF-associated symptoms, with 46% to 85% of patients experiencing improvement in each individual item assessed by the MFSAF. The greatest improvements were reported by patients experiencing abdominal discomfort, night sweats, pruritus, and an altered body image, as well as fever, and corresponded with improvements in the individual MF symptom scales as well as the patients' overall assessment of quality of life (see **Table 1**).

Table 1
Modified MFSAF administered serially to 87 patients with MF

Original MFSAF Items	Scale
General fatigue	(Absent) 0 1 2 3 4 5 6 7 8 9 10 (worst imaginable)
Abdominal pain (and discomfort)	(Absent) 0 1 2 3 4 5 6 7 8 9 10 (worst imaginable)
Inactivity (ability to move and walk around)	(Absent) 0 1 2 3 4 5 6 7 8 9 10 (worst imaginable)
Cough	(Absent) 0 1 2 3 4 5 6 7 8 9 10 (worst imaginable)
Night sweats	(Absent) 0 1 2 3 4 5 6 7 8 9 10 (worst imaginable)
Bone pain (diffuse not joint pain or arthritis)	(Absent) 0 1 2 3 4 5 6 7 8 9 10 (worst imaginable)
Fever (>100 °F)	(Absent) 0 1 2 3 4 5 6 7 8 9 10 (worst imaginable)
Change in appetite/unintentional weight loss in past 6 months	(Absent) 0 1 2 3 4 5 6 7 8 9 10 (worst imaginable)
Overall quality of life	(As good as it can be) 0 1 2 3 4 5 6 7 8 9 10 (as bad as it can be)

Exploratory Items	Scale
Ability to bend down including to tie shoes	(Absent) 0 1 2 3 4 5 6 7 8 9 10 (worst imaginable)
Altered bowel movement and/or difficult or painful urination	(Absent) 0 1 2 3 4 5 6 7 8 9 10 (worst imaginable)
Body image and hindrance to perform daily activities	(Absent) 0 1 2 3 4 5 6 7 8 9 10 (worst imaginable)
Difficulty sleeping	(Absent) 0 1 2 3 4 5 6 7 8 9 10 (worst imaginable)
Swelling of extremities (arms and legs)	(Absent) 0 1 2 3 4 5 6 7 8 9 10 (worst imaginable)

Circle the 1 number that best describes how much difficulty you have had with each of the following symptoms during the past week.

Subsequently, we developed the MFSAF 2.0 to support the COMFORT-1 trial, and this instrument was validated in the conduct of that trial.[4] This version specifically excluded fatigue out of deference to the US Food and Drug Administration, which at that point felt fatigue was too multifactorial to function as a metric for drug efficacy. Patients receiving ruxolitinib (n = 127) in this trial experienced improvements in individual MF-related symptoms, although patients receiving placebo (n = 100) experienced worsening (P<.001). The majority (91%) of ruxolitinib-treated patients designated as 50% or more Total Symptom Score (TSS) responders (≥50% TSS improvement) self-reported their condition as either much improved or very much improved on the Patient Global Impression of Change scale. These patients achieved significant improvements in the European Organization for Research and Treatment of Cancer Quality of Life Questionnaire-Core 30 functional domains and global health status and quality of life versus patients receiving placebo, who experienced worsening on these measures (P = .0135). Ruxolitinib-treated patients with a lesser degree of symptom improvement (<50% TSS responders) also achieved improvements over placebo on these measures. The degree of spleen volume reduction with ruxolitinib correlated with improvements in TSS, Patient Global Impression of Change, Patient Reported Outcomes Measurement Information System (PROMIS) Fatigue Scale, and EORTC Global Health Status/quality of life. Ruxolitinib-treated patients who achieved a 35% or greater decrease in spleen volume experienced the greatest improvements in these patient-reported outcomes.

Further refinements in language, collaboration with the PRO Institute and members of the Study Endpoints and Labeling Development team at the US Food and Drug Administration led to the final version of the MFSAF 4.0 (**Table 2**).[5] With a total of 7 items, the MFSAF 4.0 had a total possible score range of 0 to 70. Additionally, a 24-hour recall format was chosen because this format is the most likely to be used in a clinical trial. Subsequent efforts were undertaken to demonstrate that the results between these subtly evolved patient-reported outcomes are able to be compared (see **Table 2**).

Table 2
Items of the MFSAFv4.0 diary

Item	Scale
During the past 24 hours, how severe was your worst fatigue?	(Absent) 0 1 2 3 4 5 6 7 8 9 10 (worst imaginable)
During the past 24 hours, how severe were your worst night sweats?	(Absent) 0 1 2 3 4 5 6 7 8 9 10 (worst imaginable)
During the past 24 hours, how severe was your worst itching?	(Absent) 0 1 2 3 4 5 6 7 8 9 10 (worst imaginable)
During the past 24 hours, how severe was your worst abdominal discomfort?	(Absent) 0 1 2 3 4 5 6 7 8 9 10 (worst imaginable)
During the past 24 hours, how severe was your worst pain under your ribs on your left side?	(Absent) 0 1 2 3 4 5 6 7 8 9 10 (worst imaginable)
During the past 24 hours, what was the worst feeling of full ness you had after beginning to eat	(Absent) 0 1 2 3 4 5 6 7 8 9 10 (worst imaginable)
During the past 24 hours, how severe was your worst bone pain (no joint or arthritis pain)?	(Absent) 0 1 2 3 4 5 6 7 8 9 10 (worst imaginable)

Patients with ET and PV have overlapping symptoms with patients with MF, yet there can be additional symptoms present that are more prevalent with elevated counts. In an effort to be able to adequately capture the spectrum of symptoms across ET, PV, and MF we added and developed the MPN Symptom Assessment Form (MPN-SAF; total items = 10).[6] Modified from the 7-item MFSAF v4.0, we added 3 additional items to capture the wider range of symptomatology experienced by patients with MPN as a whole. In addition to the 7 questions within the MFSAF v4.0, we added 3 questions related to early satiety, inactivity, and concentration problems (**Table 3**).[7] We realized that certain symptoms might be reflected in more than 1 question in the MPN-SAF, so we analyzed the performance of each question and were able to refine to 10 core items. The MPN-SAF TSS (MPN-SAF TSS or MPN10 for simplicity) is the most rapid, easy to use, and validated instrument to assess MPN symptoms in clinical trials (see **Table 3**).[7]

BIOLOGY OF MYELOPROLIFERATIVE NEOPLASM SYMPTOMS AND INFLAMMATION, CYTOKINES, AND BIOLOGY

To better understand the biology of the symptom burden, it is important to understand the inflammatory milieu that is present in many patients with MPNs. JAK-STAT signaling is dysregulated in most MPNs, and STAT3 is closely tied to expression of immunomodulatory cytokines (IL-6, IL-10, and IL-17), growth factors (fibroblast growth factor and vascular endothelial growth factor), and matrix metalloproteinases.[8] However, the impact on the immune system is far greater than that explained by dysregulation in the JAK-STAT

Table 3
MPN-SAFTSS (ie, MPN10)

Item	Scale
Please rate your fatigue by circling the one number that best describes your worst level of fatigue during the past 24 hours.	(Absent) 0 1 2 3 4 5 6 7 8 9 10 (worst imaginable)
Circle the one number that describes how much difficulty you have had with each of the following symptoms during the past week:	
Filling up quickly when you eat (early satiety)	(Absent) 0 1 2 3 4 5 6 7 8 9 10 (worst imaginable)
Abdominal discomfort	(Absent) 0 1 2 3 4 5 6 7 8 9 10 (worst imaginable)
Inactivity	(Absent) 0 1 2 3 4 5 6 7 8 9 10 (worst imaginable)
Problems with concentration - compared with before the diagnosis	(Absent) 0 1 2 3 4 5 6 7 8 9 10 (worst imaginable)
Night sweats	(Absent) 0 1 2 3 4 5 6 7 8 9 10 (worst imaginable)
Itching (pruritus)	(Absent) 0 1 2 3 4 5 6 7 8 9 10 (worst imaginable)
Bone pain (diffuse, not joint pain or arthritis)	(Absent) 0 1 2 3 4 5 6 7 8 9 10 (worst imaginable)
Fever	(Absent) 0 1 2 3 4 5 6 7 8 9 10 (worst imaginable)
Unintentional weight loss in 1ast 6 months	(Absent) 0 1 2 3 4 5 6 7 8 9 10 (worst imaginable)

pathway. In one study evaluating patients with primary MF, IL-1β, IL-1RA, IL-2R, IL-6, IL-8, IL-10, IL-12, IL-13, IL-15, tumor necrosis factor (TNF)-α, granulocyte colony stimulating factor, IFN-α, MIP-1α, MIP-1β, hepatocyte growth factor, IP-10, MIG, MCP-1, and vascular endothelial growth factor were all found to be elevated in the peripheral blood.[9] Elevations in the following 6 factors were associated with decreased survival: IL-8 ($P<.001$), IL-2R ($P<.001$), IL-12 ($P = .009$), IL-15 ($P = .004$), IP-10 ($P = .01$), and MIP-1β ($P = .03$).[9] Increased levels of IL-8 or IL-2R were associated with the presence of constitutional symptoms, transfusion need, leukocytosis, and decreased survival.[9] An increase in inflammatory cytokines has also been described in PV and ET.[10,11] Interestingly, there is evidence that the inflammation may not only be a hallmark of disease, but drive the clonal progression of the disease.[12]

Connections between inflammation and quality of life are expected, because an inflammatory state often results in fevers, night sweats, muscle wasting, and decreased appetite in the setting of malignancy.[8] Specifically, in patients with MF in the COMFORT study, low ferritin was associated with itching and night sweats, a higher IL-1RA level was associated with a loss of appetite, and higher CD40 L, Pal1, and RANTES levels were associated with not sleeping well. Changes in these cytokines were noted with treatment of ruxolitinib and improvement in symptoms.[13] However, in the JAKARTA studies evaluating fedratinib, the clinical response was not correlated to cytokine levels.[14]

SYMPTOMS AND JAK INHIBITION

The introduction of JAK inhibitors has resulted in a marked improvement in the quality of life of patients with MPN. As outlined elsewhere in this article, the symptom benefits initially observed when treating patients with JAK inhibitors helped to drive the development of our current symptom scoring systems. This ultimately led to the response criteria proposed for MF, specifically a decrease in symptom burden as measured by the MPN-SAF by 50% and spleen volume reduction of 35%. Although the response criteria require a 50% decrease in the MPN-TSS, a meaningful benefit to the patient can be observed with a smaller decrease in the MPN-TSS. An analysis was done on the COMFORT1 study on relationship between Patient Global Impression of Change and in which 27 of 59 patients who had less than 50% reduction in TSS reported they felt very much improved or much improved.[4]

Ruxolitinib

The first JAK inhibitor studied was ruxolitinib, which was evaluated in the COMFORT-1 and COMFORT-2 studies. In addition to being important in establishing the critical impact of quality of life for patients as an end point for studies, the COMFORT-1 study in particular was instrumental in the development of MPN-SAF, as reviewed elsewhere in this article. Ruxolitinib has also been studied in patients with PV in the RESPONSE study.[15] The primary end point of this study was a composite of patients who achieved both hematocrit control and a spleen volume reduction of 35% or more.[15] However, patient-reported outcomes, including the MPN-SAF, were also collected. In patients treated with ruxolitinib, 49% of patients experienced a 50% decrease in the MPN-SAF score as compared with 5% of patients receiving standard therapy.[15]

Fedratinib

Fedratinib is another JAK inhibitor that was approved by the US Food and Drug Administration for MF in the fall of 2019. The JAKARTA-1 study[14] was the phase III study conducted in 94 centers worldwide. Patients were randomized to 1 of 3 groups: 400 mg/d, 500 mg/d, or placebo. A total of 289 patients were enrolled from December 2011 to September 2012, with 96, 97, and 96 patients randomly assigned to fedratinib 400 mg, 500 mg, and placebo, respectively. The symptom response at week 24 was 33 of 91 (36%), 31 of 91 (34%), and 6 of 85 (7%) in the 400-mg, 500-mg, and placebo groups, respectively. Improvement in symptom burden was noted within 4 weeks and durable until week 24.

Momelotinib

Momelotinib is a JAK1/2 inhibitor, as well as direct inhibition of the bone morphogenic protein receptor kinase activin A receptor, type I–mediated expression of hepcidin.[16] This not only provides JAK inhibition, it also has a beneficial impact on anemia. There were 2 studies to evaluate the efficacy of momelotinib, SIMPLIFY-1 and SIMPLIFY-2. SIMPLIFY-1 was a study for JAK inhibitor–naïve patients, and compared ruxolitinib with momelotinib. A reduction in MPN-SAF TSS was achieved in 28% of patients who received momelotinib and 42.2% of patients who received ruxolitinib, indicating less symptomatic improvement in patients who received momelotinib.[17] SIMPLIFY-2 was a randomized study of momelotinib versus best available therapy for patients who had inadequate response to ruxolitinib.[18] A reduction in a TSS of at least 50% was observed in 26% of patients receiving momelotinib compared with 6% of those receiving best available therapy, despite the fact that 80% in the best available therapy arm received ruxolitinib.

Pacritinib

PERSIST-1 was a study that compared pacritinib 400 mg/d with best available therapy (excluding ruxolitinib) in a 2:1 randomization. The study was stopped early owing to unexpected poor outcomes in PERSIST-2, so the median time of follow up was 23.2 months. A total of 327 patients were randomized in this study in a 2:1 fashion; 220 patients were assigned to pacritinib, and 107 to best available therapy; however, owing to the early study closure, only 168 in the pacritinib arm and 85 in the best available therapy arm were evaluable. At week 24, in the intention-to-treat population, a 50% decrease in the MPN-SAF was achieved in 19% in the pacritinib arm and 10% in the best available therapy arm, which was not statistically significant. The PERSIST-2 study was conducted in patients who had a platelet count of less than 100×10^9/L, approximately one-half the patients had been previously exposed to ruxolitinib. This study compared pacritinib 400 mg/d, pacritinib 200 mg twice daily, and best available therapy (which included ruxolitinib) in patients. A greater than 50% reduction in the MPN-SAF was appreciated in 25% of the pooled pacritinib cohort versus 14% in best available therapy cohort, which was not statistically significant. Despite these results, the benefit to these patients, who constitute a patient population in dire need of treatment options, may be present even in the absence of a 50% symptom decrease.

SYMPTOMS AND CYTOREDUCTION

The symptom burden in patients with MPNs is related to the inflammatory milieu; however, symptomatology can also be related to the higher blood counts. In patients with PV, cytoreduction is almost uniformly recommended, whether it be through therapeutic phlebotomy, hydroxyurea, or interferon. However, in ET and using the International Working Group for Myeloproliferative Neoplasms Research and Treatment criteria, not all patients will meet criteria for cytoreduction, because their risk of thrombotic events may be quite low.[19]

The symptom burden in PV can be quite severe.[6] There is evidence that control of hemoglobin may have an impact on the symptom burden. In a study of patients in the original MPN-SAF study, as well as CYTO-PV, patients who were receiving therapeutic phlebotomy were noted to have a higher symptom burden as compared with those who did not.[7] However, even those patients who have adequate cytoreduction may experience a significant symptom burden.[20] In 1 study, patients who had PV that was well-controlled based on blood counts and spleen size, were randomized to either continuation of hydroxyurea or ruxolitinib. Those patients who received ruxolitinib achieved better symptom control, suggesting that the symptom burden may be due to more than just blood counts.[20]

Some patients have a significant symptom burden with ET. Biologically, the symptom burden should decrease as the platelets decrease, especially in the setting of microvascular symptoms; however, there are fewer studies that demonstrate this benefit. It was best shown in a study comparing ruxolitinib versus best available therapy for ET. In this study, although both arms of the study sustained similar decreases in platelet counts, the patients in the ruxolitinib arm experienced greater improvement in their symptom burden.[21]

SYMPTOMS, QUALITY OF LIFE, AND ALLOGENIC STEM CELL TRANSPLANTATION

Allogeneic stem cell transplantation is a curative therapy for patients with MF. Owing to the high morbidity and mortality associated with this therapy, it is reserved for those with either Dynamic International Prognostic Scoring System intermediate 2 or high-risk disease, or those with other high-risk molecular markers. In a survey, we demonstrated that many patients did not want to proceed with transplantation owing to concerns over quality of life.[22] However, in a study done on patients with MF who proceeded with transplantation, it was found that, although there was a decrease in quality of life initially after transplantation, as would be expected, at 1 year 61% of patients reported an improved quality of life as compared with before undergoing transplantation.[23] Interestingly, MF-specific symptoms were significantly improved after transplantation.[23]

FATIGUE

Fatigue is debilitating for patients with MPNs and is challenging to treat effectively. The causes of fatigue are frequently multifactorial, related to both physical conditions, such as the illness itself, inflammation, or medications, in addition to emotional and psychological factors. In a survey done on patients with MPN, the average severity of fatigue as measured by 24-hour Brief Fatigue Inventory was 6.2 of 10. It was noted that fatigue negatively impacted multiple aspects of life and greatly limited daily activities.[24] In this study, there was a higher prevalence of mood disorders that likely contributed to the fatigue, in addition to the effects of the MPN.[24] There are many ways of dealing with fatigue, including pharmacologic as well as nonpharmacologic methods. There is increasing evidence that a sedentary lifestyle increases fatigue[24,25] and that physical activity may improve fatigue as well as quality of life.[25] This factor is reviewed more comprehensively in the section reviewing nonpharmacologic strategies for managing MPN symptoms.

SYMPTOMS AND DRUGS IN THE MYELOPROLIFERATIVE NEOPLASM PIPELINE

As reviewed elsewhere in this volume, there are many new therapeutic options for patients with MPNs. It is an exciting time, and many novel therapeutics are being tested that not only control blood counts and symptoms, but may also impact the biology of the disease. In MF, where the symptom burden is most severe, there are several approaches to address unmet needs. There are 2 primary unmet needs for those patients with a high symptom burden. One group that has a severe unmet need is those patients who have failed ruxolitinib. This status is associated with clonal progression of the disease and a poor survival rate.[26] The response to ruxolitinib can be salvaged by addition of a novel agent. One example is adding navitoclax, which binds to the proteins in the B-cell lymphoma-2 family. In this group, MPN-TSS improved 20% as compared with baseline.[27] Another example is addition of a PI3Kδ inhibitor such as parsaclisib or umbralisib. A study recently presented at European Haematology Congress adding parsaclisib to ruxolitinib in patients with inadequate response to single agent ruxolitinib showed a median improvement of MPN-TSS of 14.0% to 51.6% in treated patients, depending on the dosing strategy.[28] In a study adding umbralisib to ruxolitinib, a median improvement of 35% was noted in the MPN-TSS.[29] Another significant unmet need is in patients with thrombocytopenia or anemia. Some of the novel JAK inhibitors, as described elsewhere in this article, address this unmet need. These drugs do not seem to induce severe myelosuppression and the dose can be adjusted to provide enough JAK inhibition to ameliorate symptoms.

NONSYMPTOM DRIVERS OF QUALITY OF LIFE IN PATIENTS WITH MYELOPROLIFERATIVE NEOPLASMS

Quality of life is related to more than just physical symptoms of disease. Quality of life can also be impacted by psychological distress associated with the diagnosis, as well as the impact that the MPN diagnosis can have a patient's work and social life. The MPN Landmark Survey had several aims, one of which, discussed in the next section, was to identify treatment goals. Another aim sought to understand the impact MPNs have on a person's daily life, including finances, ability to work, and relationships with others. Patients with MF, PV, and ET, expressed that their condition caused emotional hardship in 33%, 14%, and 23% of patients, respectively, and 34%, 29%, and 26% of patients reported that they had felt worried or anxious about the disease. One-quarter of patients (26%) reported that their MPN interfered with daily activities. Further, patients with MPN felt their disease had a high impact on their family or social life (26%). One-half of the patients who responded to this survey were employed at the time of the survey; however, in patients with a high symptom burden, there were a higher percentage who voluntarily left their job or were let go, took early retirement, took a lower paying job, or received disability. Patients also reported that they missed 4.8, 3.3, or 2.6 hours of work in the last 7 days in MF, PV, and ET, respectively.

DIFFERENCES IN TREATMENT GOALS BETWEEN PATIENTS WITH MYELOPROLIFERATIVE NEOPLASMS AND PROVIDERS

In 2017, we published an article that described the findings of our MPN Landmark Survey that had 813 MPN respondents and 457 hematologist/oncologist respondents who treated patients with MPNs.[30] These findings highlighted some of the disparities in symptom perceptions and treatment goals between patients and providers. For example, most physician respondents reported that their typical symptom assessments included a prognostic risk classification as well as an inquiry into specific symptoms that patients are most important to manage. However, patients report far less recollection of specific prognostic assessment use and inquiry into specific symptoms. Treatment goals also differed between providers and patients. Patients with MPN reported that to slow or delay the progression of their condition was their most important goal, whereas physicians reported symptom improvement and the prevention of vascular or thrombotic events to be most important in their treatment goals for patients. Highlighting some of these disparities in perceptions and treatment goals, more than one-third of patient respondents with MPN were not very satisfied with their physician's overall management and communication. These misaligned perceptions and goals likely affect patient–provider satisfaction and success, and these findings highlight some important areas of care and patient education that can be addressed for better patient–provider communication.

QUALITY OF LIFE AND SYMPTOMS IMPACT ON TREATMENT GUIDELINES

In light of the differences in perceptions and goals, the assessment of quality of life and symptom burden is critical when pursuing treatment for MPNs. The current National Comprehensive Cancer Network guidelines highlight the importance of evaluating symptom burden; in fact, in the decision trees for choosing therapy, symptom burden is a consideration.[31] For both ET and PV, symptomatic disease is an indication for treatment along with other factors, such as thrombotic or hemorrhagic events. In many cases, the degree of symptom burden helps to guide the therapy chosen; for example, in those patients with debilitating symptoms, JAK inhibition is a suitable choice.[15,20,21]

NONPHARMACOLOGIC STRATEGIES FOR MANAGING SYMPTOMS OF MYELOPROLIFERATIVE NEOPLASMS

It has long been recognized that there are many possible nonpharmacologic approaches and interventions that can be used to help alleviate the symptoms of chronic disease, including malignancies. Historically, the majority of research in nonpharmacologic interventions (ie, cognitive [meditation, education, etc] and/or physical [yoga, exercise, dietary interventions]) have been conducted in breast cancer survivors. The literature for these approaches has been limited in hematologic malignancies and nonexistent for aiding patients with MPN. We formed the MPN quality of life study group (www.mpnqol.org/) as a multidisciplinary research team to bring scientific rigor to the study and application of these methods. In 2015 and 2016, we conducted a feasibility study investigating the acceptability, practicality, demand, and preliminary effects of an online-streamed yoga intervention on patients with MPN.[32] Patients with MPN were recruited nationally using internet-based strategies (eg, social media, forums, email) and by reaching out to organizational and foundation partners (eg, the MPN Research Foundation). Enrolled participants were asked to complete 12 weeks of online-streamed yoga via Udaya.com. Participants were asked to complete 60 min/wk of online yoga, but were able to participate in additional yoga videos provided each week if they wanted to do more than the prescribed minimum of 60 min/wk. A total of 55 patients with MPN were enrolled at baseline and 38 completed the intervention. Of those, 68% (n = 21/28) were satisfied or very satisfied with online yoga, 75% (n = 23/31) felt it was helpful for coping with MPN-related symptoms, 75% (n = 23/31) felt safe while participating in online yoga, and 82% (n = 25/31) would recommend online yoga to other patients with MPN. Weekly self-reported yoga participation averaged approximately 50 min/wk, with 37% of participants achieving a 12-week average of 60 min/wk or more. Additionally, there were significant pre–post (ie, week 0 to week 12) changes in self-reported total symptom burden and fatigue (measured with the MPN-SAF TSS) as well as anxiety, depression and sleep disturbance (measured with National Institutes of Health PROMIS). Feasibility measures were defined according to Bowen and colleagues[33] for this study. Although a priori benchmarks for demand were not met owing to fewer than 70% of participants achieving a 12-week self-reported yoga participation average of 60 min/wk or more, benchmarks were met for acceptability, practicality, and preliminary effects, demonstrating the feasibility of online yoga for patients with MPN.

In a follow-up pilot study conducted in 2016 and 2017, we investigated the effects of an online-streamed yoga intervention as compared with a wait-list control group in patients with MPN.[34] Similar to our feasibility work, patients with MPN were recruited nationally using internet-based strategies (eg, social media, forums, email) and by reaching out to organizational and foundation partners (eg, the MPN Research Foundation). Eligible and consenting participants were randomly assigned to 12 weeks of online-streamed yoga via Udaya.com (the same 12-week prescription as in feasibility study described elsewhere in this article) or a 12-week wait-list control group. In addition, we remotely gathered blood draws (through Quest Diagnostics) for inflammatory biomarkers (ie, TNF-α, IL-1, IL-6, and IL-8), which were assessed at baseline and after the intervention (week 12). A total of 62 patients with MPN were enrolled at baseline and 48 completed the intervention (online yoga = 27; control group = 21). Self-reported yoga participation was a bit higher than in our prior feasibility study at approximately 56 min/wk with 48% (n = 13/27) averaging at least 60 min/wk as prescribed. Small to moderate effect sizes were seen from the yoga intervention at the midpoint (week 7), after the intervention (week 12), and at follow-up (week 16) for sleep disturbance (d = −0.26 to −0.61), pain intensity (d = −0.34 to −0.51), anxiety (d = −0.27 to −0.37), and depression (d = −0.53 to −0.78) as assessed with the National Institutes of Health PROMIS as well as a decrease in TNF-α from baseline to after the intervention (−1.3 ± 1.5 pg/mL).

Based on findings from our online yoga research with patients with MPN, in which participants reported that the mindfulness component of yoga was helpful for their fatigue, we conducted a smartphone-based meditation app feasibility trial in patients with MPN in 2017 and 2018.[35] Again, patients with MPN were recruited nationally using internet-based strategies (eg, social media, forums, email) and by reaching out to organizational and foundation partners (eg, the MPN Research Foundation). The aim of this study was to examine the feasibility of 2 different consumer-based meditation smartphone apps in patients with MPN and to examine the limited efficacy of smartphone-based meditation on symptoms compared with an educational control group. Eligible and consented patients were enrolled into 1 of 4 groups, 2 of which received varying orders of 2 consumer-based apps (10% Happier meditation app and Calm meditation app) and 2 that received one of the apps alone for the second 4 weeks of the 8-week intervention after an educational, fatigue management handout control condition. Participants were asked to perform 10 min/d of meditation, regardless of the app and the order in which they received the apps. Feasibility outcomes were measured at weeks 5 and 9 with an investigator-developed survey. The feasibility outcomes were defined by Bowen and colleagues[33] and included acceptability, demand, and limited efficacy for depression, anxiety, pain intensity, sleep disturbance, sexual function, quality of life, and global health via the National Institutes of Health PROMIS, as well as total symptom burden via the MPN-SAF TSS. A total of 128 patients with MPN were enrolled across all 4 groups, with 73.4% of patients (n = 94/128) completing the intervention. Of the participants who completed the 10% Happier app, 61% (n = 46/76) enjoyed it, 66% (n = 50/76) were satisfied with the content, and 77% (n = 59/76) would recommend to others. Of those who completed the Calm app, 83% (n = 56/68) enjoyed it, 84% (n = 57/68) were satisfied with the content, and 97% (n = 66/68) would recommend to others. Of those who completed the educational control, 91% (n = 56/61) read it, 87% (n = 53/61) enjoyed it, and 71% (n = 43/61) learned something. Participants who completed the 10% Happier app averaged 31 ± 33 min/wk; patients completing the Calm app averaged 71 ± 74 min/wk. The 10% Happier app participants saw small effects on anxiety ($P<.001$; d = -0.43), depression ($P = .02$; d = -0.38), sleep disturbance ($P = .01$; d = -0.40), total symptom burden ($P = .13$; d = -0.27), and fatigue ($P = .06$; d = -0.30), and moderate effects on physical health ($P<.001$; d = 0.52). The Calm app participants saw small effects on anxiety ($P = .29$; d = -0.22), depression ($P = .09$; d = -0.29), sleep disturbance ($P = .002$; d = -0.47), physical health ($P = .005$; d = 0.44), total symptom burden ($P = .13$; d = -0.27), and fatigue ($P = .13$; d = -0.27). Educational control participants (n = 61) did not have effects on any patient-reported outcomes, except for a moderate effect on physical health ($P<.001$; d = 0.77) (**Table 4**).

Through the last 5 years of our nonpharmacologic work with patients with MPN, we have demonstrated the feasibility and preliminary effects of delivering online-streamed yoga and meditation via a smartphone app to patients with MPN (see **Table 4** for a summary of outcomes across our prior work). Additionally, there is evidence of preliminary effects of online-streamed yoga on a variety of physical and psychological outcomes, particularly for improving anxiety, depression, and sleep disturbance; we saw these outcomes improve in both our feasibility and pilot work. Elevated inflammation is of particular concern for patients with MPN, and we also demonstrated preliminarily reductions in TNF-α after 12 weeks of 60 min/wk of online-streamed yoga. Furthermore, qualitative data gathered from both our feasibility and pilot work[36] reflected some of what we saw quantitatively in that participants most frequently self-reported improvements in sleep, decreases in fatigue, and decreases in stress. The convenience of doing online yoga at home was also by far the most commonly reported benefit of doing yoga remotely. Finally, smartphone-based meditation seems to have preliminary effects on a range of physical and psychological symptoms overlapping with much of the improvements we saw in our online-streamed yoga work, including improvements in total symptom burden, fatigue, anxiety, depression, sleep disturbance, and physical health. Similar to the qualitative work in our online yoga studies, qualitative data also revealed that participants in the meditation app study

Table 4
Summary of nonpharmacologic study outcomes

| Study | Outcomes | |
	Feasibility	Preliminary Effects
2015/2016 Online Yoga Feasibility Study	Demonstrated Acceptability and practicality of delivering online- streamed yoga to patients with MPN	↓ Total symptom burden ↓ Fatigue ↓ Anxiety ↓ Depression ↓ Sleep disturbance
2016/2017 Online Yoga Pilot Study	N/A	↓ Pain intensity ↓ Sleep disturbance ↓ Anxiety ↓ Depression ↓ TNF-α
2017/2018 Meditation App Feasibility Study	The Calm app was more feasible to deliver to patients with MPN when compared with the 10% Happier app	↓ Total symptom burden ↓ Fatigue ↓ Anxiety ↓ Depression ↓ Sleep disturbance ↓ Physical health

reported improvements in sleep, decreases in fatigue, and improvements in overall mental health most frequently.[37] This line of research has shed some light on the potential usefulness of nonpharmacologic, mindfulness-based strategies for improving a range of outcomes among patients with MPN; however, questions remain, including the following.

1. What are the unique components of these mindfulness-based strategies that have specific effects on MPN symptoms or outcomes? (Is it the meditation and mindfulness aspect of yoga driving changes? Is the physical movement of yoga driving changes? What components of meditation drive the changes we have seen?)
2. What are the true effects of online yoga or smartphone-based meditation on patients with MPN in larger powered trials?
3. What is the dose–response relationship between online yoga and smartphone-based meditation on MPN patient symptoms? What is the minimum effective "dose" with regards to how much time is spent participating in the activity, and how many weeks the activity is done regularly?
4. What are the long-term, latent effects of these nonpharmacologic approaches on outcomes?

Further work is underway to answer these questions and to better understand the true effects of these mindfulness-based strategies on MPN symptoms and quality of life-related outcomes.

SUMMARY

The MPNs have been a model for the identification of disease-associated symptoms, development of validated instruments of patient-reported outcomes to quantify those symptoms, and understanding of how those symptoms impact quality of life. Further research in the linkages of disease-associated biology and the biological underpinnings of these symptoms has been impactful and may lead to therapeutic advances. Subsequent inclusion of symptomatic improvement in the process of drug approvals (ruxolitinib and fedratinib) and the vast majority of drugs in the development pipeline should act as a model for other hematologic malignancies. Finally, significant evidence is developing that various nonpharmacologic interventions can aid in decreasing MPN associated symptoms and that various modalities can be combined to develop improvement in MPN patient quality of life.

CLINICS CARE POINTS

- It is important for providers to assess MPN symptom burden and quality of life at each interaction they have with their patients in the clinic.
- Providers should ask patients what the goals of their treatment are in order to better align themselves with the goals and needs of the patients they work with.
- When considering treatment for MPN patients to reduce or manage symptom burden, know that there are both pharmacologic and nonpharmacologic treatments and modalities available and for providers to consider.

ACKNOWLEDGMENTS

The authors acknowledge the tremendous partnership with MPN patients (special note of Joyce Niblack, Antje Hjerpe, Zhen Senyak, Robert Rosen, David Alexander), the CMPN Education Foundation, The MPN Research Foundation, MPN Voice, and

MPN Forum, which made all of these efforts possible with the goal of decreasing the burden on MPN disease.

DISCLOSURE

Authors have nothing to disclose.

REFERENCES

1. Mesa RA, Niblack J, Wadleigh M, et al. The burden of fatigue and quality of life in myeloproliferative disorders (MPDs). Cancer 2007;109(1):68–76.
2. Mesa RA, Schwager S, Radia D, et al. The Myelofibrosis Symptom Assessment Form (MFSAF): an evidence-based brief inventory to measure quality of life and symptomatic response to treatment in myelofibrosis. Leuk Res 2009;33(9): 1199–203.
3. Mesa RA, Kantarjian H, Tefferi A, et al. Evaluating the serial use of the Myelofibrosis Symptom Assessment Form for measuring symptomatic improvement: performance in 87 myelofibrosis patients on a JAK1 and JAK2 inhibitor (INCB018424) clinical trial. Cancer 2011;117(21):4869–77.
4. Mesa RA, Gotlib J, Gupta V, et al. Effect of ruxolitinib therapy on myelofibrosis-related symptoms and other patient-reported outcomes in COMFORT-I: a randomized, double-blind, placebo-controlled trial. J Clin Oncol 2013;31(10): 1285–92.
5. Gwaltney C, Paty J, Kwitkowski VE, et al. Development of a harmonized patient-reported outcome questionnaire to assess myelofibrosis symptoms in clinical trials. Leuk Res 2017;59:26–31.
6. Emanuel RM, Dueck AC, Geyer HL, et al. Myeloproliferative neoplasm (MPN) symptom assessment form total symptom score: prospective international assessment of an abbreviated symptom burden scoring system among patients with MPNs. J Clin Oncol 2012;30(33):4098–103.
7. Scherber RM, Geyer HL, Dueck AC, et al. The potential role of hematocrit control on symptom burden among polycythemia vera patients: insights from the CYTO-PV and MPN-SAF patient cohorts. Leuk Lymphoma 2017;58(6):1481–7.
8. Geyer HL, Dueck AC, Scherber RM, et al. Impact of inflammation on myeloproliferative neoplasm symptom development. Mediators Inflamm 2015;2015:284706.
9. Tefferi A, Vaidya R, Caramazza D, et al. Circulating Interleukin (IL)-8, IL-2R, IL-12, and IL-15 levels are independently prognostic in primary myelofibrosis: a comprehensive cytokine profiling study. J Clin Oncol 2011;29(10):1356–63.
10. Pourcelot E, Trocme C, Mondet J, et al. Cytokine profiles in polycythemia vera and essential thrombocythemia patients: clinical implications. Exp Hematol 2014;42(5):360–8.
11. Vaidya R, Gangat N, Jimma T, et al. Plasma cytokines in polycythemia vera: phenotypic correlates, prognostic relevance, and comparison with myelofibrosis. Am J Hematol 2012;87(11):1003–5.
12. Hasselbalch HC. Perspectives on chronic inflammation in essential thrombocythemia, polycythemia vera, and myelofibrosis: is chronic inflammation a trigger and driver of clonal evolution and development of accelerated atherosclerosis and second cancer? Blood 2012;119(14):3219–25.
13. Squires M, Harrison CN, Barosi G, et al. The relationship between cytokine levels and symptoms in patients (Pts) with myelofibrosis (MF) from COMFORT-II, a Phase 3 Study of Ruxolitinib (RUX) Vs Best Available Therapy (BAT). Blood 2013;122(21):4070.

14. Pardanani A, Harrison C, Cortes JE, et al. Safety and efficacy of fedratinib in patients with primary or secondary myelofibrosis: a randomized clinical trial. JAMA Oncol 2015;1(5):643–51.
15. Vannucchi AM, Kiladjian JJ, Griesshammer M, et al. Ruxolitinib versus standard therapy for the treatment of polycythemia vera. N Engl J Med 2015;372(5): 426–35.
16. Asshoff M, Petzer V, Warr MR, et al. Momelotinib inhibits ACVR1/ALK2, decreases hepcidin production, and ameliorates anemia of chronic disease in rodents. Blood 2017;129(13):1823–30.
17. Mesa RA, Kiladjian JJ, Catalano JV, et al. SIMPLIFY-1: a phase III randomized trial of momelotinib versus ruxolitinib in janus kinase inhibitor-naïve patients with myelofibrosis. J Clin Oncol 2017;35(34):3844–50.
18. Harrison CN, Vannucchi AM, Platzbecker U, et al. Momelotinib versus best available therapy in patients with myelofibrosis previously treated with ruxolitinib (SIMPLIFY 2): a randomised, open-label, phase 3 trial. Lancet Haematol 2018; 5(2):e73–81.
19. Barbui T, Thiele J, Carobbio A, et al. Disease characteristics and clinical outcome in young adults with essential thrombocythemia versus early/prefibrotic primary myelofibrosis. Blood 2012;120(3):569–71.
20. Mesa R, Verstovsek S, Kiladjian J-J, et al. Changes in quality of life and disease-related symptoms in patients with polycythemia vera receiving ruxolitinib or standard therapy. Eur J Haematol 2016;97(2):192–200.
21. Harrison CN, Mead AJ, Panchal A, et al. Ruxolitinib vs best available therapy for ET intolerant or resistant to hydroxycarbamide. Blood 2017;130(17):1889–97.
22. Palmer J, Scherber R, Girardo M, et al. Patient perspectives regarding allogeneic bone marrow transplantation in myelofibrosis. Biol Blood Marrow Transplant 2019; 25(2):398–402.
23. Palmer J, Kosiorek HE, Wolschke C, et al. Assessment of quality of life following allogeneic stem cell transplant for myelofibrosis. Biol Blood Marrow Transplant 2019;25(11):2267–73.
24. Scherber RM, Kosiorek HE, Senyak Z, et al. Comprehensively understanding fatigue in patients with myeloproliferative neoplasms. Cancer 2016;122(3):477–85.
25. Tolstrup Larsen R, Tang LH, Brochmann N, et al. Associations between fatigue, physical activity, and QoL in patients with myeloproliferative neoplasms. Eur J Haematol 2018;100(6):550–9.
26. Newberry KJ, Patel K, Masarova L, et al. Clonal evolution and outcomes in myelofibrosis after ruxolitinib discontinuation. Blood 2017;130(9):1125–31.
27. Harrison CN, Garcia JS, Mesa RA, et al. Results from a phase 2 study of navitoclax in combination with ruxolitinib in patients with primary or secondary myelofibrosis. Blood 2019;134(Supplement_1):671.
28. Yacoub A, Wang ES, Rampal RK, et al. Novel therapies and pitfalls in MPN. Paper presented at: European Hematology Association Annual Conference. Virtual, November 26, 2020.
29. Moyo T, Palmer J, Huang Y. Resurrecting response to ruxolitinib: a phase I study testing the combination of ruxolitinib and the PI3K delta inhibitor umbralisib in ruxolitinib-experienced myelofibrosis. HemaSphere 2018;2:19–20.
30. Mesa RA, Miller CB, Thyne M, et al. Differences in treatment goals and perception of symptom burden between patients with myeloproliferative neoplasms (MPNs) and hematologists/oncologists in the United States: findings from the MPN Landmark survey. Cancer 2017;123(3):449–58.

31. Network NCC. Myeloproliferative Neoplasm, Version 3/2019. 2020. Available at: https://www.nccn.org/professionals/physician_gls/pdf/mpn.pdf. Accessed October 20, 2020.

32. Huberty J, Eckert R, Gowin K, et al. Feasibility study of online yoga for symptom management in patients with myeloproliferative neoplasms. Haematologica 2017; 102(10):e384–8.

33. Bowen DJ, Kreuter M, Spring B, et al. How we design feasibility studies. Am J Prev Med 2009;36(5):452–7.

34. Huberty J, Eckert R, Dueck A, et al. Online yoga in myeloproliferative neoplasm patients: results of a randomized pilot trial to inform future research. BMC Complement Altern Med 2019;19(1):121.

35. Huberty J, Eckert R, Larkey L, et al. Smartphone-based meditation for myeloproliferative neoplasm patients: feasibility study to inform future trials. JMIR Form Res 2019;3(2):e12662.

36. Huberty J, Eckert R, Larkey L, et al. Perceptions of myeloproliferative neoplasm patients participating in an online yoga intervention: a qualitative study. Integr Cancer Ther 2018;17(4):1150–62.

37. Huberty J, Eckert R, Larkey L, et al. Experiences of using a consumer-based mobile meditation app to improve fatigue in myeloproliferative patients: qualitative study. JMIR Cancer 2019;5(2):e14292.

Application of Stem Cell Therapy in Myelofibrosis

Marta B. Davidson, PhD, MD, FRCPC[a], Vikas Gupta, MD, FRCP, FRCPath[b],*

KEYWORDS

- Myelofibrosis • Risk-stratification • Allogeneic • Stem cell • Ruxolitinib

KEY POINTS

- Hematopoietic stem cell transplantation (HCT) requires careful patient selection based on disease-, patient-, and transplant-related factors.
- Genetic information may further optimize disease prognostication and patient selection for HCT.
- In an era of JAK inhibitors, the optimal timing of HCT needs careful consideration.

BACKGROUND

Myelofibrosis (MF) belongs to a group of clonal stem cell disorders known as the *BCR-ABL*-negative myeloproliferative neoplasms (MPN). MF can occur as a primary bone marrow disorder (primary myelofibrosis [PMF]) or evolve from a preceding MPN such as polycythemia vera (PV) or essential thrombocytosis (ET), also known as post-PV-MF or post-ET-MF, respectively. Aberrant cell signaling through the *JAK2-STAT3/5* pathway is at the center of MF pathogenesis, driven by mutually exclusive somatic mutations in the Janus Kinase 2 (*JAK2*), calreticulin (*CALR*), or the thrombopoietin receptor (*MPL*) in most patients with MF.[1,2] MF biology is further influenced by altered gene expression promoted by somatic mutations in genes regulating DNA methylation (*TET2, DNMT3A, IDH1/IDH2*), histone modification (*ASXL1, EZH2*), and RNA splicing (*SF3B1, U2AF1, ZRSR2, SRSF2*). It is also well established that proinflammatory, profibrotic, and proangiogenic cytokines are overexpressed in patients with MF.[3] This altered cytokine milieu contributes to the characteristic clinical manifestations of MF, including constitutional symptoms, cardiovascular events, and disease progression. MF is the most aggressive of the MPNs and carries a significant risk of premature death and transformation to acute leukemia.

[a] Division of Medical Oncology and Hematology, University Health Network, Princess Margaret Cancer Centre, 700 University 6W091, Toronto, Ontario M5G 1Z5, Canada; [b] Department of Medicine, Princess Margaret Cancer Centre, Suite 5-303C, 610-University Avenue, University of Toronto, Toronto, Ontario M5G 2M9, Canada
* Corresponding author.
E-mail address: vikas.gupta@uhn.ca

Hematol Oncol Clin N Am 35 (2021) 391–407
https://doi.org/10.1016/j.hoc.2020.12.004   **hemonc.theclinics.com**

Allogeneic hematopoietic stem cell transplantation (HCT) is the only potentially curative treatment option for patients with MF at present. HCT, however, can be associated with significant morbidity and mortality. Appropriate patient selection is therefore paramount to minimize the risk-to-benefit ratio. It is important to note that no randomized controlled trials have compared HCT with non-transplant treatment strategies, and recommendations guiding transplant decisions are largely based on retrospective analyses and expert opinion. The decision to proceed with HCT needs to be individualized for each patient and take into consideration disease characteristics and prognosis, patient fitness and preferences, and transplant logistics including available donor type. Here we review the most critical questions in the management of patients with chronic-phase MF with HCT: who, when, and how.

Trends in Allogeneic Stem Cell Transplantation for Myelofibrosis

The last decade ushered in targeted therapy for MF with Food and Drug Administration (FDA) approval of JAK inhibitors (JAKi), namely ruxolitinib (2011), and fedratinib (2019). Although effective at decreasing symptom burden, JAKi do not have long-term disease-modifying capability. Accordingly, HCT remains a valid treatment modality in MF, and its use has continuously increased over the last 2 decades as indicated by registry data from the Center for International Blood and Marrow Transplant Research (CIBMTR) (**Fig. 1**A). In 2018, the number of patients with MF undergoing HCT more than doubled compared with 2011. HCT for older patients with MF has also steadily increased (**Fig. 1**B). Transplantation of older individuals has undoubtedly been facilitated by use of reduced intensity conditioning (RIC), which has been gaining popularity (**Fig. 1**D). Peripheral blood remains the predominant stem cell source among MF HCT recipients. The use of unrelated donors (URD) has also been increasing among patients with MF (**Fig. 1**C). Although there has been a small increase in the use of haploidentical donors in recent years, the use of alternative donors (AD; haploidentical, umbilical cord blood [UCB]) in general remains low in MF (see **Fig. 1**C).

Patient Selection for Allogeneic Stem Cell Transplantation

Consideration of disease-associated factors and hematopoietic stem cell transplantation outcomes

The course of MF can be quite variable, ranging from an indolent disorder with survival of more than a decade to a rapidly progressive disease with death occurring within months. The early identification of patients at risk for poor outcomes and therefore those in whom the risks of HCT may be warranted is critical. To that end, the prognostic value of clinical factors associated with MF has been systematically interrogated to generate predictive models that facilitate such identification (**Fig. 2**). Further, recent progress in our understanding of the mutational landscape of MF has advanced these models through the inclusion of novel molecularly defined risk factors. In this section, we review the major risk stratification tools for MF with a focus on novel scoring systems, how they can be used to guide transplant decisions, as well as their limitations.

Conventional risk stratification. In 1996, Dupriez and colleagues published the Lille score, which became the first broadly adopted MF prognostic scoring system. The Lille score, based only on hemoglobin (Hb) and white blood cell count, stratifies patients into 1 of 3 risk categories according to survival.[4] Cervantes and colleagues[5] (1998) subsequently proposed risk stratification according to 3 factors, namely anemia (Hb <100 g/L), circulating blasts greater than or equal to 1%, and constitutional

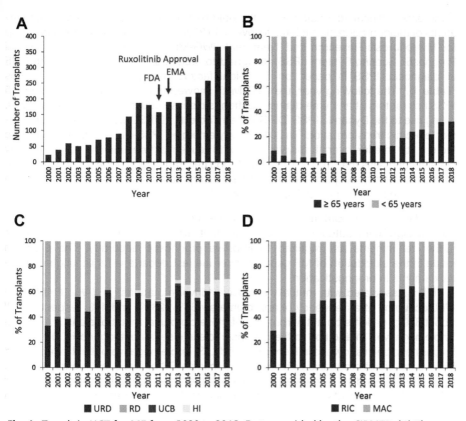

Fig. 1. Trends in HCT for MF from 2000 to 2018. Data provided by the CIBMTR. (*A*) The number of HCTs carried out by year. Timing of ruxolitinib approval by the FDA and the European Medicines Agency (EMA) is indicated. (*B*) The percentage of HCT recipients by age group: younger than 65 years and 65 years or older. (*C*) The percentage of HCT by donor type: related (RD), unrelated (URD), haploidentical (HI), and umbilical cord blood (UCB). (*D*) The percentage of HCT by conditioning regimen: myeloablative conditioning (MAC), reduced intensity conditioning (RIC). The data presented here are preliminary and were obtained from the Coordinating Center of the Center for International Blood and Marrow Transplant Research. The analysis has not been reviewed or approved by the Statistical or Scientific Committees of the CIBMTR.

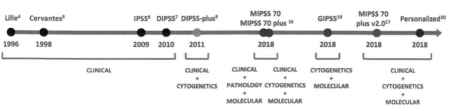

Fig. 2. Evolution of risk stratification for myelofibrosis. Timeline of risk score publication and their components.

symptoms, delineating 3 risk groups. It would be over a decade before the next iterations of major prognostic systems followed. In 2009, the international Working Group for Myelofibrosis Research and Treatment (IWG-MRT) developed the International Prognostic Scoring System (IPSS) designed to predict survival in patients with PMF at diagnosis. IPSS is based on 5 clinical factors and delineates 4 risk groups (**Table 1**).[6] The following year, the IWG-MRT showed that acquisition of the same 5 IPSS risk factors at any time during a patient's disease course also predicts survival, giving rise to the Dynamic IPSS (DIPSS) (see **Table 1**).[7] DIPSS was also shown to predict leukemic transformation.[8] In 2011, newly emerging IPSS-independent prognostic factors for inferior overall survival (OS) and leukemia free survival (LFS), namely platelet count less than 100×10^9/L, red blood cell transfusion dependence, and "unfavorable karyotype" (see **Table 1**), were incorporated into the DIPSS model to generate the more refined DIPSS-plus score.[9]

Molecular risk stratification. Conventional risk models are powerful predictive tools, but the significant outcome heterogeneity that exists within risk groups suggests further refinements are required to improve prognostic accuracy. The progress made in the elucidation of MF genetics over the last decade is facilitating such advancements in prognostication.

PMF is associated with mutually exclusive "driver mutations" in *JAK2*, *CALR*, and *MPL* occurring at a frequency of approximately 65%, 23%, and 4%, respectively.[10] About 8% of patients do not harbor any of these canonical mutations and are termed "triple negative." In addition to their intrinsic role in disease pathogenesis, driver mutations have been shown to influence OS and LFS. Triple-negative patients were found to have the worst prognosis with a reported median OS of just over 3 years, followed by *JAK2V617F* and *MPL*-mutated patients with predicted survivals of about 9 years.[10] *CALR*-mutated patients with MF were found to have the best prognosis with a

Table 1
Modern risk stratification models based on clinical and laboratory parameters

Risk Factor	Prognostic Scoring Models for Myelofibrosis (Points)		
	IPSS	DIPSS	DIPSS-Plus[b]
Hemoglobin (g/L)	<100 (1)	<100 (2)	DIPSS risk level:
WBC (x 10⁹/L)	>25 (1)	>25 (1)	Low (0)
Age (years)	>65 (1)	>65 (1)	Intermediate-1 (1)
Peripheral blast count (%)	≥1% (1)	≥1% (1)	Intermediate-2 (2)
Constitutional Symptoms	Yes (1)	Yes (1)	High (3)
Platelet Count (x 10⁹/L)			<100 (1)
Transfusion-dependence			Yes (1)
Karyotype[a]			Unfavorable (1)
Risk Group	**Points (Median OS, Years)**		
Low	0 (11.3)	0 (Not reached)	0 (15.4)
Intermediate 1	1 (7.9)	1–2 (14.2)	1 (6.5)
Intermediate 2	2 (4)	3–4 (4.0)	2–3 (2.9)
High	≥3 (2.3)	≥5 (1.5)	≥4 (1.3)

Abbreviation: WBC, white blood cell count.
[a] Unfavorable karyotype: complex karyotype or sole or 2 abnormalities that include +8, −7/7q-, i(17q), −5/5q-, 12p-, inv (3), or 11q23 rearrangement.
[b] Calculation of DIPSS-plus score should begin with the calculation of DIPSS risk score. Points are assigned according to risk category as indicated. Additional points should be assigned for the indicated DIPSS-independent variables.

reported median OS of 17.7 years. The survival advantage conferred by *CALR* mutation was later shown to be restricted to type 1 or type 1–like mutations.[11,12]

Approximately 80% of the patients with PMF harbor additional mutations in genes known to be recurrently mutated in myeloid malignancies, some with prognostic implications.[13] Mutations in transcriptional and epigenetic regulators including *ASXL1*, *SRSF2*, *IDH1/2*, and *EZH2* confer increased risk of mortality and leukemic transformation.[14] Further, increasing numbers of mutations are also deleterious; patients with 2 or more high molecular risk (HMR) mutations are predicted to have a median survival of 2.3 years, whereas those with one or none had predicted survivals of 7 and 12.3 years, respectively.[15]

Guglielmelli and colleagues[16] (2018) integrated mutational data with clinical and histologic risk factors into the Mutation-Enhanced International Prognostic Scoring System (MIPSS70) for transplant-age patients ($\leq$70 year). MIPSS70 delineates 3 risk categories (see **Table 2**). MIPSS70-plus (Karyotype-enhanced MIPSS70), described in the same publication, also incorporated a 2-tiered cytogenetic risk variable, adding a "very high-risk" category (see **Table 2**). The next iteration of the "mutation-enhanced" systems was MIPSS70+ version 2.0 (MIPSS70+ v2.0), which incorporated a new HMR mutation in the *U2AF* gene, sex- and severity-adjusted hemoglobin thresholds, and the revised 3-tiered cytogenetic risk stratification[17,18] (see **Table 2**). This model further defined a "very low-risk" category (see **Table 2**). The Genetics-Inspired Prognostic Scoring System (GIPSS) is a simplified scoring system based solely on cytogenetic and mutational data that also robustly risk stratifies patients with MF.[19] These genetic-based models have not yet been validated for "dynamic" use.

Grinfeld and colleagues (2018) sequenced the coding regions of 69 genes among 2035 patients with MPN including 309 patients with primary and secondary MF. The genomic data were combined with clinical variables to derive a personalized multistage predictive model (https://www.sanger.ac.uk/science/tools/progmod/progmod). The investigators identified 8 genomic subgroups with distinct clinical phenotypes, risk of leukemic transformation, and event-free survival.[20] This model captures the prognostic significance of *TP53* mutations, not included in other risk systems. Mutations in *TP53*, known to be deleterious across all malignancies, were shown to confer an especially poor prognosis with high risk of leukemic transformation and a median OS of 2.4 years. In addition, mutations in epigenetic regulators, spliceosome machinery, and RAS pathway were found to be strongly associated with accelerated-phase MPNs. The model outperformed IPSS and DIPSS, but it is unknown how it compares with other mutation-based risk models.

Risk stratification for secondary myelofibrosis. In clinical practice, the above-described models are frequently applied to secondary MF (SMF), although they were derived from PMF cohorts and may have poorer prognostic accuracy in SMF.[21,22] Accordingly, MYSEC-PM (Myelofibrosis Secondary to PV and ET—Prognostic Model) was developed based on the characteristics among patients with SMF.[23] It is important to note that MYSEC-PM heavily weighs age, such that the high-risk group is primarily composed of patients aged 70 years or older, raising the concern that this may decrease the sensitivity of the scoring system to other high-risk features.[24] Moreover, important prognostic factors such as cytogenetics were not included in the model due to insufficient numbers of patients with available data. To-date, enrollment in clinical trials for patients with both PMF and SMF continues to be based on traditional scoring systems, which we continue to apply to SMF in our practice (see **Table 1; Table 2**).

Table 2
Molecular risk stratification models

Risk Factor	Prognostic Scoring Models for Myelofibrosis (Points)		
	MIPSS 70	MIPSS70 plus	MIPSS70-plus v2.0
Online Calculator	http://www.mipss70 score.it		http://www.mipss70 score.it
Hemoglobin (g/L)	<100 (1)	<100 (1)	Moderate[a] (1) Severe[b] (2)
WBC (x 10⁹/L)	>25 (2)	–	–
Peripheral blast count	≥2% (1)	≥2% (1)	≥2% (1)
Constitutional Symptoms	Yes (1)	Yes (1)	Yes (2)
Platelet Count (x 10⁹/L)	<100 (2)	–	–
BM fibrosis grade	≥2 (1)	–	–
Presence of HMR[c] mutation	Present (1)	Present (1)	Present (2)
≥2 HMR mutations	Present (2)	Present (2)	Present (3)
CALR type 1/like mutation	Absent (1)	Absent (2)	Absent (2)
Karyotype			
Unfavorable	–	Present[d] (3)	Present[e] (3)
Very High-Risk (VHR)	–	–	Present[f] (4)
Number of Risk Tiers	3	4	5

Risk Group	Points (Median OS, Years)		
Very low	–	–	0 (Not reached)
Low	0–1 (Not reached)	0–2 (Not reached)	1–2(16.4)
Intermediate	2–4 (6.3)	3 (24.2)	3–4 (7.7)
High	≥5 (3.1)	4–6 (10.4)	5–8 (4.1)
Very High	–	≥7 (3.9)	≥9 (1.8)

[a] Moderate anemia: hemoglobin 80 to 99 g/L in women; 90 to 109 g/L in men
[b] Severe anemia: hemoglobin less than 80 g/L in women and less than 90 g/L in men.
[c] In MIPSS70 and MIPSS70-plus, high molecular risk (HMR) mutations include *ASXL1, EZH2, SRSF2,* and *IDH1/2*; MIPSS70-plus v2.0 HMR also includes mutated *U2AF1.*
[d] Any abnormal karyotype other than normal karyotype or sole abnormalities of 20q2, 13q2, +8, chromosome 1 translocation/duplication, -Y, or sex chromosome abnormality other than -Y.[16]
[e] Sole abnormality of +8, 7q-, sole translocations not involving chromosome 1. Two abnormalities not including a VHR abnormality. Monosomal karyotype without a VHR abnormality. Sole abnormalities not otherwise classified.
[f] Single/multiple abnormalities of −7, i(17q), inv(3)/3q21, 12p–/12p11.2, 11q–/11q23, or other autosomal trisomies not including +8/+9.

Although the above-described models are useful for identifying patients in whom disease risk may call for HCT, it is important to recognize that they were not designed to predict outcomes following HCT. Several studies, however, have shown that post-HCT survival correlates with DIPSS,[25] DIPSS-plus,[26,27] and MIPSS70+v2.0[28] risk categories. By contrast, a recent study by the European Blood and Marrow Transplantation Group (EBMT) of 2916 transplanted patients with MF found no association between DIPSS category and survival.[29] To directly address prognosis after HCT, scoring systems incorporating transplant-specific factors have been designed, of which the most recent is the Myelofibrosis Transplant Scoring System that integrates clinical, cytogenetic, molecular, and transplant-related information.[30]

It is currently unclear which risk model is optimal for prognostication in MF. Each model has its inherent advantages and limitations. We favor models that incorporate cytogenetic and mutation data due to their enhanced discriminative power over those that rely solely on clinical features. In settings where such data are unavailable, DIPSS remains a reasonable predictive tool. Further, at follow-up we continue to apply DIPSS and DIPSS-plus to identify changes in risk category. In any case, it is incumbent on the clinician to recognize the inherent limitations of the prognostic systems they are using to avoid pitfalls. No model is entirely comprehensive, and important prognostic variables have been included or excluded based on statistical significance in any single analysis. Moreover, these models have never been prospectively validated nor are they based on patients treated with JAKi therapy, which may influence outcomes.[31] One must also recognize that in certain situations, patients may fall into different risk categories between the different systems (**Box 1**). Such discrepancies complicate patient selection for HCT and underscore the need to comprehensively consider disease-, patient-, and transplant-specific factors in transplant decisions.

Transplant outcomes in comparative studies. There are no randomized trials comparing HCT with non-HCT treatment strategies in MF. The comparative studies that do exist are few and retrospective. During the pre-ruxolitinib era, the benefit of HCT for higher risk MF was demonstrated in a matched analysis of patients with PMF younger than 65 years, treated with HCT versus non-HCT approaches.[32] Patients with DIPSS intermediate-2 or high-risk disease had superior survival following HCT, whereas the risk of HCT outweighed any benefit in low-risk patients. The benefit among intermediate-1 patients was equivocal. More recently, a long-term OS advantage was observed for patients with intermediate-1 MF or higher who underwent HCT over patients treated with a non-HCT therapy; however, this was at the cost of inferior survival in the first year following HCT due to the upfront treatment-related risk.[33] Although some patients with intermediate-1 disease do benefit from HCT, appropriate patient selection and timing are critical given the high risk of complications. Prospective trials are needed to evaluate the benefit of HCT compared with other therapeutic

---

Box 1
Variability in risk stratification between prognostic scoring systems

Case Presentation

59-year-old female with JAK2 V617F-mutated post-ET MF. The patient has no constitutional symptoms and no splenomegaly. Hemoglobin is 118 g/L, WBC 26.2 × 10⁹/L, platelets 962 × 10⁹/L, and 3% circulating blasts. Bone marrow biopsy revealed MF-2 fibrosis. Cytogenetic analysis yielded only 4 metaphases, which showed a normal female karyotype. NGS revealed a pathogenic *TP53* variant and no HMR mutations. The patient has been intolerant of cytoreduction with hydroxyurea and anagrelide due to side-effects. She is otherwise healthy and fit. A haploidentical donor has been identified. Her prognostic risk scores are as follows:

Prognostic System	Risk Group
IPSS	Intermediate-2
DIPSS	Intermediate-1
DIPSS-plus	N/A
MIPSS70	High
MIPSS70-plus v2.0	N/A
Personalized MPN	Median OS 2.4 y

Should this patient undergo HCT?

The various prognostic models estimate a median OS for this patient in the range of 2.4 to 7.9 years. Given the presence of *TP53* mutation, greater than 2% circulating blasts, and a high MIPSS70 risk score, we referred the patient for HCT.

modalities. To this end, a pan-Canadian study will be prospectively evaluating outcomes among transplant-eligible high-risk patients with MF treated with either upfront HCT or best available therapy (NCT04217356).

Consideration of patient-related factors

Age, performance status, and comorbidities. In addition to disease-based indications, patient-specific factors need to be considered in transplant decisions. With a median age at diagnosis in the seventh decade, the MF population naturally comprises an older group. Age is considered an independent risk factor for inferior HCT outcomes,[34–38] and 70 years is generally considered the upper age limit for HCT although this varies across institutions. However, successful HCTs have been performed in well-selected older patients; we therefore caution against the use of age alone as an arbiter for HCT referral. Performance status (PS) and comorbidities are also important predictors of HCT outcomes.[26,39,40] Poor PS may be due to MF or non-MF factors, and these should be carefully evaluated and optimized whenever possible. JAKi therapy can ameliorate constitutional symptoms and possibly improve PS.[41] "Wholistic" approaches such as a comprehensive geriatric assessment or the recently described frailty index may also be informative regarding fitness for HCT.[42–45]

Patient preference. Not all patients may find the risks of HCT acceptable even in the setting of optimal disease-based indications, donor, and candidate status. A retrospective analysis at our center found that 50% (38/71) of patients with an optimal donor did not undergo HCT, primarily due to patient preference (30/38).[46] Such patients may choose to pursue other treatment options including JAKi therapy or clinical trials. Close follow-up is required in these situations to detect early signs of treatment failure or disease progression, at which time patients may be more willing to consider HCT.

CURRENT EXPERT GUIDANCE

The poor survival predicted by conventional risk models and the apparent benefit of HCT in higher-risk patients form the basis for the current European and North American guidelines for HCT in patients with MF (**Table 3**). Briefly, patients with a projected survival of less than 5 years should be evaluated for HCT, and those deemed fit should be offered HCT as a potential curative treatment.[47,48] By contrast, low-risk patients should be managed with non-HCT strategies, whereas decisions regarding HCT need to be individualized in intermediate-1–risk patients based on additional high-risk features.

Timing of Hematopoietic Stem Cell Transplantation

The optimal timing of HCT is a matter of debate. The probability of a successful HCT significantly declines once patients progress to acute leukemia.[49] With passage of time, patients may also acquire other complications that compromise or even prohibit successful HCT including advancing age, worsening PS, and development of MF and non-MF–related comorbidities. Conversely, if performed too early, HCT may significantly compromise quality of life due to treatment-related morbidity, especially among patients who were asymptomatic or responding to JAKi, making the timing of transplant a challenging decision (**Box 2**).

Hematopoietic stem cell transplantation in the era of JAK inhibitors

Several studies indicate that patients who respond to ruxolitinib therapy have improved survival after HCT compared with nonresponders or those who lose response,[50,51] suggesting HCT should be pursued at the time of optimal JAKi response. However, it is

Table 3
Expert guidance regarding hematopoietic stem cell transplantation in myelofibrosis

Risk Group	NCCN 2017[48]	EBMT/ELN 2015[47]
Low Intermediate-1	Should consider HCT if: • Refractory transfusion-dependent anemia • Circulating blasts >2% • Adverse cytogenetics • *CALR* negative and *ASXL1* mutated Evaluation for HCT recommended in: • Thrombocytopenia • Complex cytogenetics	Monitor for disease progression Consider if age <65 y and: • Refractory, transfusion-dependent anemia • PB blasts >2% • Adverse cytogenetics • Triple negative • *ASXL1* mutated

Intermediate-2
High
	Recommended in all fit patients;
	   fitness is based on age, PS,
	   comorbidities, psychosocial status,
	   patient preference,
	   availability of caregiver
		All younger than 70 y
		   should be considered

Abbreviations: EBMT, European Blood and Marrow Transplantation Group; ELN, European Leuke-miaNet; NCCN, National Comprehensive Cancer Network.

unclear whether the improved HCT outcomes are directly due to JAKi or merely reflect an inherently more favorable disease biology in these patients. The benefit of early over delayed HCT in the setting of JAKi therapy merits prospective evaluation.

Peri-HCT ruxolitinib has also garnered interest for its immunomodulatory effect to potentially ameliorate graft versus host disease (GVHD). Although results have been mixed with respect to benefit, the rates of acute and chronic GVHD among ruxolitinib-treated patients with MF seem similar to historical rates.[50–54]

Concerns about the safety of ruxolitinib in the peri-HCT setting have been raised. Serious adverse events were observed in the JAK-ALLO trial including cardiogenic shock and tumor lysis syndrome, necessitating a temporary suspension of the trial.[55] It is speculated that the sudden cessation of JAKi may have contributed to these adverse events due to rebound cytokine flare. However, the results of several studies

---

Box 2
Timing of HCT in patients treated with JAKi

Case Presentation

66-year-old male diagnosed with *CALR* (type1)-mutated Post-ET MF 2 years earlier. The patient developed symptomatic splenomegaly and was therefore started on Ruxolitinib with excellent spleen response (65% reduction). Currently his hematologic parameters are: Hemoglobin 97 g/L, WBC 8.4×10^9/L, platelets 411×10^9/L, and 2% circulating blasts. Normal male karyotype. No HMR on NGS. He remains asymptomatic at this time. Should this patient proceed to HCT?

Risk Score	Risk Group
IPSS	High
DIPSS	Intermediate-2
DIPSS-plus	Intermediate-2
MIPSS70	Intermediate
MIPSS70-plus v2.0	Low

Given the lower risk disease predicted by molecular risk scores taken together with the patient's ongoing response to JAKi and his preference, HCT has been deferred for now.

have shown that cessation of ruxolitinib close to the time of conditioning and/or a gradual taper allows for the safe use of ruxolitinib before HCT.[41,50,51,53,56]

In summary, several retrospective and prospective studies have shown no adverse impact on transplant outcomes with the use of pre-HCT JAKi. However, evidence for a clear benefit of pre-HCT JAKi is also lacking. In our practice, we use JAKi therapy before HCT in patients with symptomatic splenomegaly and/or constitutional symptoms with the aim of improving this symptom burden before HCT, as described in the MPD-RC114 trial.[56]

How to Transplant

In addition to the many factors outlined thus far, the success of HCT in MF depends on HCT strategies that must be carefully selected to balance the risk of transplant-related toxicities, graft failure, and disease relapse.

Donor type and stem cell source

Generally, allografts other than those from matched-sibling donors (MSD) have been associated with inferior outcomes in MF, including shorter OS and increased nonrelapse mortality (NRM), with mismatched unrelated donors having the worst outcomes.[27,57–59] Importantly, however, some studies have found no differences in outcomes between MSD and well-matched URD.[25,37,51] Given the advancing age of most of the patients with MF, suitable MSDs are not available in a significant proportion of patients, thus URDs continue to be readily used in MF (see **Fig. 1**C). In recent years, advancements in preparative regimens, GVHD prophylaxis, and graft manipulation have allowed for increasing use of AD, including haploidentical allografts, with improving outcomes.[60,61] Although the use of AD in MF has increased in the last several years (see **Fig. 1**C), it still comprises only a small fraction of HCTs. Experience with UCB allografts in MF remains limited, with use often reserved for transformed disease.[62] Data thus far suggest engraftment with UCB may be inferior to other stem cell sources.[63]

Data from the CIBMTR reveal that peripheral blood is the source of stem cells in most of the HCT in MF (CIBMTR personal communication). There is limited data regarding outcomes according to stem cell sources in MF.

Conditioning intensity

The optimal conditioning regimen for HCT in MF is unknown. Historically, 5-year survival rates following HCT with conventional myeloablative conditioning (MAC) have ranged from 30% to 60%.[36,40,58] MAC has been associated with significant toxicity and treatment-related mortality especially among older patients.[34,58,64] Accordingly, the use of RIC has gained traction in MF HCT (see **Fig. 1**D). Prospective studies of RIC in patients with MF have shown 5-year OS rates greater than 60%, with particularly favorable outcomes in younger patients.[36,37,59] There are no prospective trials comparing MAC and RIC; however, in retrospective studies, outcomes, including survival, treatment-related toxicities, and relapse are generally similar, even with RIC cohorts largely comprising older patients. A study by the Nordic cooperative group actually showed a survival advantage for RIC after adjusting for age (5-year OS MAC vs RIC; 49% vs 59%).[36] A more recent retrospective study by the EBMT, involving 2224 patients with MF, again showed no difference in OS and NRM between MAC and RIC but did show a nonsignificant trend toward relapse with RIC, suggesting MAC may be more appropriate for younger patients who are more likely to tolerate it.[65]

Role of splenectomy before hematopoietic stem cell transplantation

More than 50% of patients with MF will develop splenomegaly during the course of their disease. Massive splenomegaly is associated with inferior HCT outcomes including increased engraftment failure and mortality, in some studies.[38,66] Data on the role of splenectomy before HCT are inconsistent, with some studies showing benefit and some showing potential harm. More rapid engraftment has been shown in splenectomized patients both retrospectively[67] and prospectively.[37] However, both EBMT and CIBMTR registry data suggest no OS advantage for splenectomy.[40,65] Contradictory data exist regarding post-HCT relapse in splenectomized patients.[37,67] Elective splenectomy among patients with MF has been associated with perioperative complications as high as 30%, of which thrombosis and bleeding comprise a significant proportion.[68] Taken together, there are no data at present to support routine pre-HCT splenectomy for massive splenomegaly. At our center, decisions regarding pre-HCT splenectomy are individualized and restricted to JAKi-refractory patients with massive splenomegaly.

Approach

The Princess Margaret Hospital approach to hematopoietic stem cell transplantation in patients with myelofibrosis

We begin selection of patients for HCT with an assessment of disease-risk, preferably using tools that incorporate cytogenetic and mutation data, if available. We refer all "fit" and agreeable patients with high-risk or very high-risk disease by comprehensive risk models or those with *TP53* mutations for consideration of upfront HCT (**Fig. 3,**

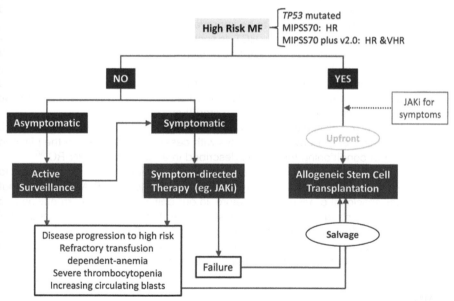

Fig. 3. The Princess Margaret Hospital approach to HCT in patients with MF. Patients with higher risk MF are referred for upfront HCT. Symptomatic patients with non–high-risk MF should be treated with symptom-directed therapies such as JAKi. Those who are asymptomatic should be monitored for symptom development and disease progression. Patients who fail ruxolitinib due to either intolerance, lack of efficacy, or loss of response should then be referred for transplant. Patients who develop other high-risk features such as refractory transfusion-dependent anemia, severe thrombocytopenia, or increasing circulating blast count should also be referred for HCT. HR, high risk; VHR, very high risk.

Table 4
The Princess Margaret Cancer Center approach to patient selection for upfront hematopoietic stem cell transplantation

Cohort	Median Survival	Comments
TP53 mutated MF	2.4 y[20]	*TP53*-mutated patients are considered high risk irrespective of other risk factors.
MIPSS70-plus v2.0 very high risk	1.8 y[17]	If cytogenetic results are available, in *TP53* wild-type patients, risk stratification will be done using MIPSS70-plus v2.0.
MIPSS70 High risk	3.1 y[16]	If valid cytogenetic results are not available, then in *TP53* wild-type patients, risk stratification will be done according to MIPSS70.

Table 4). We consider *TP53* mutations high risk due to the poor expected survival in these patients[20] and the lack of efficacy of HCT once these patients transform to acute leukemia.[69]

We observe patients with intermediate-risk disease closely for development of other high-risk features and/or progressive disease including those who fail JAKi therapy owing to the subsequent poor survival in these patients, consistent with Canadian consensus guidelines.[70]

At our institution, we initiate JAKi therapy in HCT-eligible patients who are symptomatic while concurrently initiating a donor search and referring to HCT. We have detailed discussions with patients regarding early versus delayed HCT. As outlined earlier, post-HCT outcomes seem to be improved in ruxolitinib responders. However, some patients choose to forgo early HCT. In such patients we monitor for signs of ruxolitinib failure and progressive disease and reopen the HCT discussion at that time. It is important to remember that JAKi are not disease modifying and that eventually more than half of patients discontinue JAKi therapy either due to loss of response or due to intolerance.[31] The window of opportunity for cure with HCT must therefore not be missed while pursuing these symptom-directed therapies.

For patients on ruxolitinib who are undergoing HCT, once HCT plans are confirmed, we initiate a taper of JAKi over 4 to 5 days with cessation 1 day before the planned date of start of conditioning therapy as described in a study from MPN-RC.[56]

Although the anticlonal activity of tyrosine kinase inhibitors has been shown to reduce relapse in the post-HCT setting for Philadelphia-positive B-ALL, JAKi do not have similar anticlonal properties. Therefore, in our opinion, there is currently no role for JAKi for prevention of MF relapse post-HCT. Potential uses of JAKi post-HCT include steroid-refractory GVHD, for which ruxolitinib has FDA approval. Further, the use of JAKi can be considered in patients who have relapsed MF post-HCT and who develop symptomatic splenomegaly and/or constitutional symptoms.

SUMMARY

MF is the most aggressive of the *BCR-ABL* negative MPNs. HCT remains the only potentially curative treatment option at this time. Given the potential for significant treatment-related morbidity and mortality, HCT candidates must be chosen carefully with consideration of disease-, patient-, and transplant-related factors. Patients with high-risk disease have the most to gain from HCT. Several risk stratification tools exist, and ones that include cytogenetic and mutational data in addition to clinical factors likely have the most accurate predictive accuracy. Patient fitness for HCT including age, PS, comorbidities, frailty, and preferences also need to be considered. Transplant strategy then needs to be chosen based on patient factors and available donor type. Furthermore, the timing of transplant needs to be considered. Some patients may benefit from initiation of JAKi therapy before transplant. Lastly, lower risk patients with MF should be closely followed over time for disease progression and assessment for HCT eligibility.

CLINICS CARE POINTS

- Fit patients with MF with high-risk disease can potentially benefit from HCT.
- In low-risk MF, the harms of HCT outweigh the benefit.
- HCT decisions in intermediate-risk patients must be individualized.

DISCLAIMER

The views expressed in this article are that of the authors and do not reflect the position of the Center for International Blood and Marrow Transplant Research.

DISCLOSURES

M.B. Davidson has nothing to disclose. V. Gupta: Research funding through Institution: Incyte, Novartis; Advisory board: Novartis, Celgene, Sierra Oncology, Pfizer.

REFERENCES

1. Klampfl T, Gisslinger H, Harutyunyan AS, et al. Somatic mutations of calreticulin in myeloproliferative neoplasms. N Engl J Med 2013;369(25):2379–90.
2. Nangalia J, Massie CE, Baxter EJ, et al. Somatic CALR mutations in myeloproliferative neoplasms with nonmutated JAK2. N Engl J Med 2013;369(25):2391–405.
3. Gangat N, Tefferi A. Myelofibrosis biology and contemporary management. Br J Haematol 2020;191(2):152–70.
4. Dupriez B, Morel P, Demory JL, et al. Prognostic factors in agnogenic myeloid metaplasia: a report on 195 cases with a new scoring system. Blood 1996; 88(3):1013–8.
5. Cervantes F, Barosi G, Demory JL, et al. Myelofibrosis with myeloid metaplasia in young individuals: disease characteristics, prognostic factors and identification of risk groups. Br J Haematol 1998;102(3):684–90.
6. Cervantes F, Dupriez B, Pereira A, et al. New prognostic scoring system for primary myelofibrosis based on a study of the International Working Group for Myelofibrosis Research and Treatment. Blood 2009;113(13):2895–901.
7. Passamonti F, Cervantes F, Vannucchi AM, et al. A dynamic prognostic model to predict survival in primary myelofibrosis: a study by the IWG-MRT (International Working Group for Myeloproliferative Neoplasms Research and Treatment). Blood 2010;115(9):1703–8.
8. Passamonti F, Cervantes F, Vannucchi AM, et al. Dynamic international prognostic scoring system (DIPSS) predicts progression to acute myeloid leukemia in primary myelofibrosis. Blood 2010;116(15):2857–8.
9. Gangat N, Caramazza D, Vaidya R, et al. DIPSS plus: a refined dynamic international prognostic scoring system for primary myelofibrosis that incorporates

prognostic information from karyotype, platelet count, and transfusion status. J Clin Oncol 2011;29(4):392–7.

10. Rumi E, Pietra D, Pascutto C, et al. Clinical effect of driver mutations of JAK2, CALR, or MPL in primary myelofibrosis. Blood 2014;124(7):1062–9.

11. Tefferi A, Nicolosi M, Mudireddy M, et al. Driver mutations and prognosis in primary myelofibrosis: Mayo-Careggi MPN alliance study of 1,095 patients. Am J Hematol 2018;93(3):348–55.

12. Guglielmelli P, Rotunno G, Fanelli T, et al. Validation of the differential prognostic impact of type 1/type 1-like versus type 2/type 2-like CALR mutations in myelofibrosis. Blood Cancer J 2015;5:e360.

13. Tefferi A, Lasho TL, Finke CM, et al. Targeted deep sequencing in primary myelofibrosis. Blood Adv 2016;1(2):105–11.

14. Vannucchi AM, Lasho TL, Guglielmelli P, et al. Mutations and prognosis in primary myelofibrosis. Leukemia 2013;27(9):1861–9.

15. Guglielmelli P, Lasho TL, Rotunno G, et al. The number of prognostically detrimental mutations and prognosis in primary myelofibrosis: an international study of 797 patients. Leukemia 2014;28(9):1804–10.

16. Guglielmelli P, Lasho TL, Rotunno G, et al. MIPSS70: mutation-enhanced international prognostic score system for transplantation-age patients with primary myelofibrosis. J Clin Oncol 2018;36(4):310–8.

17. Tefferi A, Guglielmelli P, Lasho TL, et al. MIPSS70+ Version 2.0: Mutation and Karyotype-Enhanced International Prognostic Scoring System for Primary Myelofibrosis. J Clin Oncol 2018;36(17):1769–70.

18. Tefferi A, Nicolosi M, Mudireddy M, et al. Revised cytogenetic risk stratification in primary myelofibrosis: analysis based on 1002 informative patients. Leukemia 2018;32(5):1189–99.

19. Tefferi A, Guglielmelli P, Nicolosi M, et al. GIPSS: genetically inspired prognostic scoring system for primary myelofibrosis. Leukemia 2018;32(7):1631–42.

20. Grinfeld J, Nangalia J, Baxter EJ, et al. Classification and personalized prognosis in myeloproliferative neoplasms. N Engl J Med 2018;379(15):1416–30.

21. Gowin K, Coakley M, Kosiorek H, et al. Discrepancies of applying primary myelofibrosis prognostic scores for patients with post polycythemia vera/essential thrombocytosis myelofibrosis. Haematologica 2016;101(10):e405–6.

22. Hernandez-Boluda JC, Pereira A, Gomez M, et al. The international prognostic scoring system does not accurately discriminate different risk categories in patients with post-essential thrombocythemia and post-polycythemia vera myelofibrosis. Haematologica 2014;99(4):e55–7.

23. Passamonti F, Giorgino T, Mora B, et al. A clinical-molecular prognostic model to predict survival in patients with post polycythemia vera and post essential thrombocythemia myelofibrosis. Leukemia 2017;31(12):2726–31.

24. Hernandez-Boluda JC, Pereira A, Correa JG, et al. Performance of the myelofibrosis secondary to PV and ET-prognostic model (MYSEC-PM) in a series of 262 patients from the Spanish registry of myelofibrosis. Leukemia 2018;32(2):553–5.

25. Scott BL, Gooley TA, Sorror ML, et al. The dynamic international prognostic scoring system for myelofibrosis predicts outcomes after hematopoietic cell transplantation. Blood 2012;119(11):2657–64.

26. Samuelson Bannow BT, Salit RB, Storer BE, et al. Hematopoietic cell transplantation for myelofibrosis: the dynamic international prognostic scoring system plus risk predicts post-transplant outcomes. Biol Blood Marrow Transplant 2018; 24(2):386–92.

27. Gupta V, Malone AK, Hari PN, et al. Reduced-intensity hematopoietic cell transplantation for patients with primary myelofibrosis: a cohort analysis from the center for international blood and marrow transplant research. Biol Blood Marrow Transplant 2014;20(1):89–97.
28. Ali H, Aldoss I, Yang D, et al. MIPSS70+ v2.0 predicts long-term survival in myelofibrosis after allogeneic HCT with the Flu/Mel conditioning regimen. Blood Adv 2019;3(1):83–95.
29. Hernandez-Boluda JC, Pereira A, Kroger N, et al. Determinants of survival in myelofibrosis patients undergoing allogeneic hematopoietic cell transplantation. Leukemia 2020. https://doi.org/10.1038/s41375-020-0815-z.
30. Gagelmann N, Ditschkowski M, Bogdanov R, et al. Comprehensive clinical-molecular transplant scoring system for myelofibrosis undergoing stem cell transplantation. Blood 2019;133(20):2233–42.
31. Verstovsek S, Mesa RA, Gotlib J, et al. Long-term treatment with ruxolitinib for patients with myelofibrosis: 5-year update from the randomized, double-blind, placebo-controlled, phase 3 COMFORT-I trial. J Hematol Oncol 2017;10(1):55.
32. Kroger N, Giorgino T, Scott BL, et al. Impact of allogeneic stem cell transplantation on survival of patients less than 65 years of age with primary myelofibrosis. Blood 2015;125(21):3347–50 [quiz 3364].
33. Gowin K, Ballen K, Ahn KW, et al. Survival following allogeneic transplant in patients with myelofibrosis. Blood Adv 2020;4(9):1965–73.
34. Guardiola P, Anderson JE, Bandini G, et al. Allogeneic stem cell transplantation for agnogenic myeloid metaplasia: a European group for blood and marrow transplantation, societe francaise de greffe de moelle, gruppo italiano per il trapianto del midollo osseo, and fred hutchinson cancer research center collaborative study. Blood 1999;93(9):2831–8.
35. Nivison-Smith I, Dodds AJ, Butler J, et al. Allogeneic hematopoietic cell transplantation for chronic myelofibrosis in Australia and New Zealand: older recipients receiving myeloablative conditioning at increased mortality risk. Biol Blood Marrow Transplant 2012;18(2):302–8.
36. Abelsson J, Merup M, Birgegard G, et al. The outcome of allo-HSCT for 92 patients with myelofibrosis in the Nordic countries. Bone Marrow Transplant 2012; 47(3):380–6.
37. Kroger N, Holler E, Kobbe G, et al. Allogeneic stem cell transplantation after reduced-intensity conditioning in patients with myelofibrosis: a prospective, multicenter study of the Chronic Leukemia Working Party of the European Group for Blood and Marrow Transplantation. Blood 2009;114(26):5264–70.
38. Alchalby H, Yunus DR, Zabelina T, et al. Risk models predicting survival after reduced-intensity transplantation for myelofibrosis. Br J Haematol 2012;157(1): 75–85.
39. Sorror ML, Maris MB, Storb R, et al. Hematopoietic cell transplantation (HCT)-specific comorbidity index: a new tool for risk assessment before allogeneic HCT. Blood 2005;106(8):2912–9.
40. Ballen KK, Shrestha S, Sobocinski KA, et al. Outcome of transplantation for myelofibrosis. Biol Blood Marrow Transplant 2010;16(3):358–67.
41. Jaekel N, Behre G, Behning A, et al. Allogeneic hematopoietic cell transplantation for myelofibrosis in patients pretreated with the JAK1 and JAK2 inhibitor ruxolitinib. Bone Marrow Transplant 2014;49(2):179–84.
42. Mohile SG, Dale W, Somerfield MR, et al. Practical Assessment and Management of Vulnerabilities in Older Patients Receiving Chemotherapy: ASCO Guideline for Geriatric Oncology. J Clin Oncol 2018;36(22):2326–47.

43. Muffly LS, Kocherginsky M, Stock W, et al. Geriatric assessment to predict survival in older allogeneic hematopoietic cell transplantation recipients. Haematologica 2014;99(8):1373–9.

44. Aniket Bankar SA, Elliot Smith, Dongyang Yang, et al. Prevalence and Impact of Frailty on Outcomes in Myelofibrosis. Paper presented at: 12th International Congress on Myeloproliferative Neoplasms. New York, October 24–25, 2019.

45. Salas MQ, Atenafu EG, Bascom O, et al. Pilot study on frailty and functionality on routine clinical assessment in allogeneichematopoietic cell transplantation to predict outcomes. Blood 2019;134(Supplement_1):380.

46. Smith E, Lu L, Viswabandya A, et al Factors influencing selection of upfront hematopoietic stem cell transplantation versus best available non-transplant therapy in Myelofibrosis. Paper presented at: 12th International congress on myeloproliferative neoplasms. New York, October 24-25, 2019.

47. Kroger NM, Deeg JH, Olavarria E, et al. Indication and management of allogeneic stem cell transplantation in primary myelofibrosis: a consensus process by an EBMT/ELN international working group. Leukemia 2015;29(11):2126–33.

48. Mesa R, Jamieson C, Bhatia R, et al. Myeloproliferative neoplasms, version 2.2017, NCCN clinical practice guidelines in oncology. J Natl Compr Canc Netw 2016;14(12):1572–611.

49. Ciurea SO, de Lima M, Giralt S, et al. Allogeneic stem cell transplantation for myelofibrosis with leukemic transformation. Biol Blood Marrow Transplant 2010; 16(4):555–9.

50. Stubig T, Alchalby H, Ditschkowski M, et al. JAK inhibition with ruxolitinib as pretreatment for allogeneic stem cell transplantation in primary or post-ET/PV myelofibrosis. Leukemia 2014;28(8):1736–8.

51. Shanavas M, Popat U, Michaelis LC, et al. Outcomes of allogeneic hematopoietic cell transplantation in patients with myelofibrosis with prior exposure to janus kinase 1/2 inhibitors. Biol Blood Marrow Transplant 2016;22(3):432–40.

52. Kroger N, Shahnaz Syed Abd Kadir S, Zabelina T, et al. Peritransplantation ruxolitinib prevents acute graft-versus-host disease in patients with myelofibrosis undergoing allogenic stem cell transplantation. Biol Blood Marrow Transplant 2018; 24(10):2152–6.

53. Salit RB, Scott BL, Stevens EA, et al. Pre-hematopoietic cell transplant Ruxolitinib in patients with primary and secondary myelofibrosis. Bone Marrow Transplant 2020;55(1):70–6.

54. Shahnaz Syed Abd Kadir S, Christopeit M, Wulf G, et al. Impact of ruxolitinib pretreatment on outcomes after allogeneic stem cell transplantation in patients with myelofibrosis. Eur J Haematol 2018;101(3):305–17.

55. Robin M, Francois S, Huynh A, et al. Ruxolitinib before allogeneic hematopoietic stem cell transplantation (HSCT) In patients with myelofibrosis : a preliminary descriptive report of the JAK ALLO study, a Phase II trial sponsored by goelams-FIM in collaboration with the sfgmtc. Blood 2013; 122(21):306.

56. Gupta V, Kosiorek HE, Mead A, et al. Ruxolitinib therapy followed by reduced-intensity conditioning for hematopoietic cell transplantation for myelofibrosis: myeloproliferative disorders research consortium 114 study. Biol Blood Marrow Transplant 2019;25(2):256–64.

57. Rondelli D, Goldberg JD, Isola L, et al. MPD-RC 101 prospective study of reduced-intensity allogeneic hematopoietic stem cell transplantation in patients with myelofibrosis. Blood 2014;124(7):1183–91.

58. Patriarca F, Bacigalupo A, Sperotto A, et al. Allogeneic hematopoietic stem cell transplantation in myelofibrosis: the 20-year experience of the Gruppo Italiano Trapianto di Midollo Osseo (GITMO). Haematologica 2008;93(10):1514–22.
59. Mannina D, Zabelina T, Wolschke C, et al. Reduced intensity allogeneic stem cell transplantation for younger patients with myelofibrosis. Br J Haematol 2019; 186(3):484–9.
60. Luznik L, O'Donnell PV, Symons HJ, et al. HLA-haploidentical bone marrow transplantation for hematologic malignancies using nonmyeloablative conditioning and high-dose, posttransplantation cyclophosphamide. Biol Blood Marrow Transplant 2008;14(6):641–50.
61. Bregante S, Dominietto A, Ghiso A, et al. Improved outcome of alternative donor transplantations in patients with myelofibrosis: from unrelated to haploidentical family donors. Biol Blood Marrow Transplant 2016;22(2):324–9.
62. Takagi S, Ota Y, Uchida N, et al. Successful engraftment after reduced-intensity umbilical cord blood transplantation for myelofibrosis. Blood 2010;116(4): 649–52.
63. Murata M, Nishida T, Taniguchi S, et al. Allogeneic transplantation for primary myelofibrosis with BM, peripheral blood or umbilical cord blood: an analysis of the JSHCT. Bone Marrow Transplant 2014;49(3):355–60.
64. Daly A, Song K, Nevill T, et al. Stem cell transplantation for myelofibrosis: a report from two Canadian centers. Bone Marrow Transplant 2003;32(1):35–40.
65. McLornan D, Szydlo R, Koster L, et al. Myeloablative and reduced-intensity conditioned allogeneic hematopoietic stem cell transplantation in myelofibrosis: a retrospective study by the chronic malignancies working party of the european society for blood and marrow transplantation. Biol Blood Marrow Transplant 2019; 25(11):2167–71.
66. Bacigalupo A, Soraru M, Dominietto A, et al. Allogeneic hemopoietic SCT for patients with primary myelofibrosis: a predictive transplant score based on transfusion requirement, spleen size and donor type. Bone Marrow Transplant 2010; 45(3):458–63.
67. Robin M, Esperou H, de Latour RP, et al. Splenectomy after allogeneic haematopoietic stem cell transplantation in patients with primary myelofibrosis. Br J Haematol 2010;150(6):721–4.
68. Mesa RA, Nagorney DS, Schwager S, et al. Palliative goals, patient selection, and perioperative platelet management: outcomes and lessons from 3 decades of splenectomy for myelofibrosis with myeloid metaplasia at the Mayo Clinic. Cancer 2006;107(2):361–70.
69. Gupta V, Kennedy, J., Capo-Chichi, J., et al Impact of Genetic Mutations on the Outcomes of Allogeneic Hematopoietic Cell Transplantation in Patients with Acute Myeloid Leukemia with Antecedent Myeloproliferative Neoplasm. Paper presented at: Transplantation and Cellular Therapy Meetings; February 19, 2020, 2020; Orlando, Florida.
70. Gupta V, Cerquozzi S, Foltz L, et al. Patterns of ruxolitinib therapy failure and its management in myelofibrosis: perspectives of the canadian myeloproliferative neoplasm group. JCO Oncol Pract 2020. https://doi.org/10.1200/JOP.19.00506.

Immunotherapy and Immunomodulation in Myeloproliferative Neoplasms

Naveen Pemmaraju, MD[a],*, Natalie C. Chen, MD, PhD[b],
Srdan Verstovsek, MD, PhD[c]

KEYWORDS

• MPN • Immunotherapy • JAK-STAT • Interferon ICI • IMiD

KEY POINTS

• Myeloproliferative neoplasms are characterized by chronic inflammation.
• Various agents with immunomodulating and immunosuppressive properties, including interferon-based approaches, immunomodulatory drugs, corticosteroids, and JAK inhibitors, have been used with varying degrees of success in treating different myeloproliferative neoplasms.
• New combinations of these agents will likely augment their therapeutic potential.

INTRODUCTION

Myeloproliferative neoplasms (MPNs) are characterized by increased clonal expansion of peripheral blood cells of the myeloid lineage and classical *BCR-ABL*–negative MPNs include polycythemia vera (PV), essential thrombocythemia (ET), and myelofibrosis (MF).[1] Although the 3 conditions have distinct presentations, they are unified by abnormal cytokine signaling, malignant clonal expansion, and varying levels of bone marrow inflammation and fibrosis.[2] Compared with healthy controls, patients with MF had significant elevation in approximately 20 cytokines, of which increased levels of IL-8, IL-2R, IL12, IL-15, and IFN-γ–inducible protein 10 were all associated with inferior survival.[3] Tumor necrosis factor (TNF)-α has been previously shown to promote leukemic progression by inducing failure of normal hematopoiesis and is elevated in patients with MPNs.[2,4] Interestingly, Fleischman and colleagues[5] showed that TNF-α selectively promotes the growth of *JAK2V617F*-positive MPN cells over

Funding: This research is supported in part by the MD Anderson Cancer Center Support Grant P30 CA016672 and the SagerStrong Foundation.
[a] Department of Leukemia, The University of Texas MD Anderson Cancer Center, 1515 Holcombe Boulevard #3000, Houston, TX 77030, USA; [b] Department of Internal Medicine, The University of Texas School of Health Sciences at Houston, 6431 Fannin, MSB 1.150, Houston, TX 77030, USA; [c] Department of Leukemia, The University of Texas MD Anderson Cancer Center, 1515 Holcombe Boulevard #428, Houston, TX 77030, USA
* Corresponding author.
E-mail address: npemmaraju@mdanderson.org

controls, which could contribute to clonal expansion of mutant copies during MPN progression.

Although the precise primary oncologic events underlying MPN pathogenesis remain to be clarified, the most studied association has been with various driver mutations.[6] Genetic sequencing, clonal analysis, and protein expression showed that tyrosine kinase JAK2V617F mutation occurs in 95% of patients with PV and 50% to 60% of patients with ET and MF, leading to hyperactive Janus Kinase and Signal Transducer and Activator of Transcription proteins (JAK-STAT) signaling pathways downstream of erythropoietin receptor and thrombopoietin receptor (MPL).[7–10] Additionally, activating mutation in MPL and inactivating mutations in LNK or c-CBL (both are negative regulators of JAK-STAT pathways) have all been detected at low frequencies in MPNs contributing to increased JAK-STAT signaling.[11–13] Finally, somatic mutations in calreticulin (CALR) are found in 60% to 80% of patients who do not have JAK2 or MPL mutations.[14–16] CALR is an endoplasmic reticulum resident chaperone protein and mutant CALR C-terminus has been shown to drive pathogenesis of MPNs, likely through binding with MPL, leading to the activation of JAK-STAT signaling.[17,18] CALR mutation has also been linked to aberrant superoxide reduction pathway contributing to DNA damage in MPN cells.[19,20] Finally, mutations in epigenetic regulators, including TET2, DNMT3A, IDH1/2, EZH2, and ASXL1 have also been identified in patients who have MPNs with or without JAK2 mutations.[21–25]

The management of MPNs is highly individualized and constantly evolving. The cornerstone treatment for higher risk patients with PV and ET include thrombotic risk reduction using aspirin as well as cytoreduction with hydroxyurea (HU) or IFN-based therapy.[26,27] HU is associated with significant side effects and 24% of patients with PV or ET develop resistance requiring second-line therapy.[28] Interferon is also frequently used as a frontline therapy with new formulations showing an improved toxicity profile in recent clinical trials.[29] Furthermore, the JAK1/2 inhibitor ruxolitinib is approved in both intermediate- to high-risk MF, as well as advanced PV after HU intolerance or failure.[30–34]

Ongoing research efforts are dedicated to improving the efficacy and safety of established treatment modalities as well as characterizing novel therapeutic approaches, many of which target the immune system and are examined in this review (**Fig. 1**).

INTERFERON-α

The interferons are a class of naturally occurring cytokines with diverse activities, including modulating both innate and adaptive immunities, promoting apoptotic pathways, and regulating cell differentiation and angiogenesis.[35] Clinically, IFN-α treatment effectively controls not only myeloid proliferation, but also constitutional symptoms and has been hypothesized to modify disease at MPN the genomic level.[36–38] Despite its effectiveness, the use of IFN has been historically limited in many studies owing to its toxicities with frequent discontinuation owing to treatment-related adverse events.[35] A polyethyleneglycol tail was later added to the cytokine to prolong its half-life and increase drug stability, with the goal of decreasing the administration frequency and associated toxicities. Clinical trials have yielded positive results for this pegylated form.

For instance, the pegylated IFN-α2a (PEG) was shown to result in complete response (CR) rate of 70% in patients with PV and 76% in patients ET, with excellent tolerability at 90 μg weekly in a phase II study.[39] In a follow-up analysis by the same

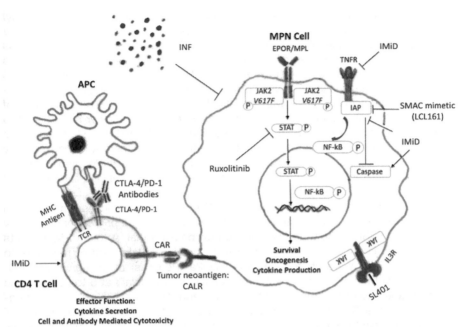

Fig. 1. Immunomodulating agents in MPN treatment. APC, antigen-presenting cell; CTLA-1, cytotoxic T lymphocyte-associated antigen 4; EPOR, erythropoietin receptor; IAP, inhibitor of apoptosis; IMiD, immunomodulatory drugs; MPL, thrombopoietin receptor; PD-1, programmed death 1; SMAC, mitochondrial protein second mitochondrial activator of caspase. Immunotherapeutic agents used or investigated in treating MPNs are labeled in *red*.

group, complete hematologic response was observed in 76% and 77% of patients with PV and ET, respectively, by 42 months. Additionally, 18% of patients with PV and 17% of patients with ET had undetectable levels of *JAK2V617F*. Further genetic profiling demonstrated that patients with mutations other than JAK2V617F such as *TET2* have lower response rates although the underlying mechanism remains to be clarified.[40]

In the more recent Myeloproliferative Disorders Research Consortium (MPD-RC)-111 study, Yacoub and colleagues[41] demonstrated that PEG could also be effective among patients with HU refractory or intolerant ET and PV. By the 12th month of study, ET patients had overall response rate of 69.2% and CR of 43.1%. For the PV cohort, the overall response rate was 60% and 22% of patients achieved a CR. Clinically, patients with a CR also had improved MPN-related symptom scores. Subgroup analyses performed for patients with different driver mutation profiles including JAK2V617F, *CALR*, *MPL*, and triple negative showed that patients with *CALR* mutation had higher CR rates than non-*CALR* mutated patients (56% vs 28%), although the difference did not reach statistical significance. Finally, patients with a CR also had reduced JAK2V617F variant allele.[41] In a related trial comparing HU and PEG for treatment-naïve patients with a high risk for ET or PV, the CR rates were similar for HU and PEG at 12 and 24 months. Moreover, PEG caused a higher rate of grade 3 and 4 toxicities compared with HU.[42] A longer follow-up analysis on the relative effectiveness and adverse side effects of PEG compared with HU for ET and PV in this study population would be of interest.

The PROUD-PV and its extension, the CONTINUATION-PV studies showed that, although ropeginterferon-α2b (ROPeg) was not statistically superior to HU for PV at

12 months, its effectiveness increased overtime.[43] In this randomized, phase III study, 257 patients in Europe with early stage PV were assigned 1:1 to either the HU (500 mg/d) or ROPeg (subcutaneously every 2 weeks at 100 μg) to assess whether ROPeg is noninferior to HU. At the end of 12 months, a CR with a normal spleen size was achieved in 21% and 28% of the ROPeg and HU groups, respectively. However, ROPeg (53% patients had a CR with normal spleen size) showed improved effectiveness compared with HU (46%) with statistical significance ($P = .012$) by the end of 36 months. It is also important to note that ROPeg caused a lower rate of serious treatment-related adverse events compared with HU. Overall, the study suggests that ROPeg is noninferior compared with the standard of care therapy for both efficacy and safety among patients with early stage PV. Interestingly, ROPeg and HU treatments have different toxicity profiles, which makes ROPeg a valuable alternative for patients who were intolerant of HU.[43]

To further minimize toxicity and improve effectiveness, combination therapy with PEG and ruxolitinib has been studied for patients with PV and primary or secondary MF in the COMBI study, which is a single-arm phase II trial. A total of 50 patients were enrolled in the study, 46 of whom were previously intolerant or refractory to PEG-IFNα2. They were started on PEG-IFNα2a (Pegasys) at 45 μg/wk or PEG-IFNα2b (PegIntron) at 35 μg/wk subcutaneously and ruxolitinib at 5 to 20 mg twice a day. At the end of the 2-year treatment, 9% and 31% and 28% and 44% of patients reached a CR or partial response (based on the 2013 ELN and IWG-MRT response criteria) for PV and MF, respectively. Furthermore, MPN symptom scores, peripheral blood counts, and *JAK2* mutation burden all decreased with treatment.[44,45] The most frequent hematologic adverse events included anemia, thrombocytopenia, and leukopenia, and the most frequent nonhematologic adverse event was upper airway infection. This study demonstrated that combination therapy with low-dose PEG-IFNα2 and ruxolitinib could be an effective alternative treatment for patients who could not tolerate or had failed standard dose PEG-IFNα2 single therapy.[30,45] These results were corroborated by the preliminary results of RUXOPEG, an ongoing phase I/II clinical trial examining the safety profile and effectiveness of a ruxolitinib–INF-α combination for patients with MPN-associated MF. By 6 months of treatment, spleen size, blood counts, and the JAK2V617F allele mutation burden had all decreased. Additionally, no dose-limiting toxicities were observed with ruxolitinib 15 mg 2 times per day and IFN-α at 135 μg/wk.[46] Long-term follow-up studies comparing the combination therapy with current first-line therapies will be valuable.

IMMUNOMODULATORY DRUGS

Immunomodulatory drugs refer to thalidomide and its analogues (lenalidomide and pomalidomide), which are glutamic acid derivatives originally recognized for their antiangiogenic and anti-inflammatory properties through inhibition of TNF-α production in the management of multiple myeloma.[47,48] Over time, studies revealed the multifaceted functions of immunomodulatory drugs in cancer treatment, which can be categorized as (1) a direct antitumor effect by promoting apoptotic signaling,[49–51] (2) regulation of the tumor microenvironment, including angiogenesis, cytokine production, and cellular adhesion and migration,[52–54] and (3) immune modulation including costimulation of T cells, natural killer cells leading to their proliferation and activation as well as suppression of T regulatory (Treg) cell expansion.[55–57] Clinical trials have demonstrated the effectiveness of thalidomide as single-agent therapy in the treatment of MF with myeloid metaplasia.[58,59] To improve its efficacy and minimize toxicity, subsequent studies examined combination therapy with a tapering dose of prednisone, which resulted in further improvement in cytopenia and splenomegaly at lower doses that were more tolerable.[60,61] Lenalidomide– and pomalidomide-prednisone–based combinations also demonstrated good response rates for patients with MF in subsequent clinical trials with limitations.[62–65] Although a pomalidomide plus prednisone regimen resulted in improved anemia in 40% of patients with MF with good tolerability at 0.5 mg/d of pomalidomide, a significant number of patients withdrew from the study owing to a lack of response.[66,67] This limited response was similarly demonstrated in the RESUME trial, in which pomalidomide at 0.5 mg/d did not yield significant increases in the percentage of patients achieving red blood cell transfusion independence compared with placebo.[68] Furthermore, single-agent pomalidomide at doses of greater than 2.5 mg/d resulted in significant bone marrow suppression in the majority of patients with MF enrolled in a subsequent dose-finding study, which limits its therapeutic potential.[69] Additionally, immunomodulatory drugs have also been studied in combination with other agents including cyclophosphamide, TNF-alpha inhibitor etanercept, as well as ruxolitinib.[70,71] The first clinical trial testing the feasibility, efficacy, and safety of a ruxolitinib–lenalidomide combination was terminated early owing to treatment failure and significant toxicities.[72] Thus far in the ongoing study, the thalidomide–ruxolitinib combination has yielded improved thrombocytopenia, as well as a decrease in spleen size and symptom burden with good tolerability in an ongoing phase II study for patients with MF.[73]

IMMUNE CHECKPOINT INHIBITORS

Immune responses to foreign and self-antigens are delicately regulated by a 2-signal model.[74] Currently, hundreds of on-going clinical trials are examining the role of immune checkpoint inhibitors (ICIs) in diverse malignancies.[75] Although ICIs have revolutionized the therapeutic paradigm for solid tumors, their roles in the management of myeloid malignancies remain to be clarified.[76] Aberrant immune checkpoint pathways have been implicated in the development of B-cell malignancies,[77] multiple myeloma,[78] large T-cell lymphoma,[77] mantle cell lymphoma,[79] Hodgkin lymphoma,[80] and T-cell leukemia,[81] as well as acute myeloid leukemia (AML),[82] among others. Specifically, studies suggest that increased programmed death (PD) ligand 1/2 expressions are correlated with a worse prognosis, lower responsiveness to hypomethylating agents, and an increased risk of relapse in AML.[83–87] Additionally, CTLA-4 was found to be highly expressed in blast cells from bone marrow samples of patients with AML and CTLA-4 inhibition has been shown to have antileukemic effects in murine models for myeloid leukemia.[88–90] Multiple clinical trials examining the efficacy and safety of anti-PD1 and CTLA-4 antibodies for AML and myelodysplastic syndrome have yielded promising early results.[91] Although studies suggest that ICIs are associated with significant immune-related adverse events, including colitis, dermatitis, myositis, and transaminitis at therapeutic doses,[92–94] the majority of them fortunately responded to therapy[95]

Although the results from clinical trials for myelodysplastic syndrome and AML suggest a possible role for ICIs in myeloid disorder management either as a single agent or in combination with the standard of care regimens, our understanding of ICIs in the treatment of MPNs remains limited. Although 1 study examining the role of PD-1 inhibitor (nivolumab) in patients with MF was terminated early owing to a lack of response (clinicaltrials.gov), other active clinical trials are evaluating the role of PD-1 (pembrolizumab), programmed death ligand 1 (durvalumab), and PD-1 (nivolumab) plus CTLA4 (ipilimumab) blockade in patients with MF (clinicaltrials.gov).[27,96]

CELL-MEDIATED IMMUNOTHERAPY AND CHIMERIC ANTIGEN RECEPTOR-MODIFIED T CELLS

In addition to overcoming immune suppression by ICIs, one can also promote immune surveillance of tumor cells through boosting the numbers and function effector cells.[97] As one of the earliest attempts at augmenting cellular immune compartments, hematopoietic stem cell transplant (HSCT) was first shown have antileukemic effect, leading to clinical remission among patients with leukemia in 1980.[98] HSCT significantly decreased the relapse rates of many hematologic malignancies and remains the only known curative treatment for MF to date.[99–101] Various immune cells including T cells, natural killer cells, and macrophages were identified to be the major mediators for this graft-versus-tumor effect.[102–104] Building on this knowledge, donor leukocyte infusion was successfully used as therapy for patients with recurrent chronic myeloid leukemia in 1988 and later in AML and acute lymphoblastic leukemia.[105,106]

In addition to directly contributing to tumor cell killing, donor T cells could also attack host tissues causing graft-versus-host-disease (GVHD).[106] GVHD occurs in approximately 30% to 70% of allogeneic HSCT recipients and causes significant morbidity and mortality in those affected.[107,108] As the frontline therapy for GVHD, glucocorticoid is only effective in half the patients who develop GVHD.[109,110] For patients with underlying malignant and nonmalignant hematologic diseases complicated by glucocorticoid-refractory GVHD, ruxolitinib was recently shown to yield significantly higher overall response rates and a longer median failure-free survival compared with controls in a phase III clinical trial.[32] This established a third US Food and Drug Administration approval for ruxolitinib, following approval for intermediate- and high-risk MF and advanced PV.

Allogeneic HSCT and donor leukocyte infusion can be considered the original personalized immunotherapy for cancer treatment, which inspired the subsequent development of adoptive cellular therapy to further minimize GVHD by developing effector cells that target specific tumor antigens.[111] T cells could be genetically engineered to express chimeric antigen receptors (CARs) that recognize specific tumor antigens. Carl June and colleagues demonstrated that infusion of CAR-modified T cells (CAR-Ts) expressing receptor for B-cell antigen CD19 coupled with costimulatory receptor CD137 led to CR in a patient with refractory chronic lymphocytic leukemia and the response persisted for at least 10 months after treatment.[112] Since then, much advancement has been made in the field. The role of CAR-T therapy in the management of myeloid malignancies, more specifically MPNs, represents an unexplored and exciting topic for future investigations. Genetic studies identified many mutations including *JAK2* and *CALR* that can drive the pathogenesis of MPNs as discussed elsewhere in this article and are therefore candidates for CAR-T antigenic targets. Additionally, those mutations are tumor specific and entirely absent from the human genome. Therefore, they are known as neoantigens, which are more likely to be immunogenic and can generate robust effector responses required for killing tumor cells.[113,114] Specifically, Holmstrom and colleagues[115] showed that JAK2V617F-specific CD8$^+$ cytotoxic T lymphocytes can recognize and kill cell lines with the JAK2V617F mutation in vivo.

The same group were able to culture CD4$^+$ T cells that specifically recognized patient-derived *CALR* mutant cells. Upon interaction with target cells, those CD4$^+$ T cells become activated, leading to cytotoxic effects likely through downstream activation of CD8$^+$ T cells and natural killer cells, which could be abrogated by PD-1/CTLA-4 signaling.[116,117] Additionally, mutant *CALR* was shown to be secreted to interact with *MPL* receptors on neighboring cells leading to suppressed phagocytosis of cancer cells by dendritic cells.[118,119] This paracrine immunosuppressive effect makes targeting *CALR* a potentially attractive adjuvant to ICIs and antibody-dependent cell-mediated cytotoxicity approaches such as anti-CD47 monoclonal antibodies.[120] CD47 signaling promotes the downregulation of leukemic cell phagocytosis by immune cells, contributing to a worse prognosis. Anti-CD47 monoclonal antibodies are under active clinical investigations for hematologic malignancies treatment likely via increased phagocytosis of cancer cells[121–124] (Clinicaltrials.gov). To conclude, CALR is an ideal neoantigen candidate for cell-based immunotherapy, including CAR-T therapy, in MPN.[125]

Despite the promising results of these early studies, patients can relapse after CAR-T therapy because some of the tumor cells can lose the targeted antigen, which can be particularly problematic for myeloid malignancies owing to the significant antigenic variability and evolution that occurs over time.[126] As a result, the coadministration of several CAR-Ts or CAR-T–expressing multiple antigens such as both JAK2V617F and CALR simultaneously, can be used to prevent tumor antigen escape in MPN.[127,128]

RUXOLITINIB: FIRST-IN-CLASS JAK INHIBITOR, WITH A FOCUS ON IMMUNOMODULATORY PROPERTIES

JAK inhibition represents the modern backbone of MF management in addition to HSCT in appropriate patients.[129] The first approved JAK inhibitor, ruxolitinib, was established in the well-known COMFORT 1 and 2 studies, with follow-up studies confirming its long-term clinical benefit. The emerging story for the field of JAK inhibitors has been the understanding of their class effect in terms of immunosuppressive and immunomodulatory effects. Of interest, the administration of JAK inhibitors has been proposed to have both deleterious and beneficial effects on the development of infections and lymphoma. Further studies are required to clarify the conflicting roles of JAK inhibitors in the disease courses of various conditions.

Although Porpaczy and colleagues[130] alerted the increased incidence of aggressive C-MYC rearranged B-cell lymphoma in patients with MF treated with JAK inhibitor, a larger retrospective review of 2583 patients with MPNs by Pemmaraju and colleagues[131] did not show a significant association between the development of lymphomas and JAK inhibitor use,[132] which was corroborated by subsequent studies from other groups.[133,134] Finally, lymphoma was not reported as adverse events in patients on JAK inhibitors from the COMFORT1, COMFORT-II, and JUMP trials during long-term follow-up.[135–137] In fact, ruxolitinib has actually been shown to be effective in treating subcutaneous panniculitis-like T-cell lymphoma, likely through the inhibition of cytokine secretion.[138]

Given its known anti-inflammatory effects, ruxolitinib has been extended to treat other conditions with aberrant immune activations including GVHD, as discussed elsewhere in this article, hemophagocytic lymphohistiocytosis and novel coronavirus disease-2019 (COVID-19) infection. A pilot trial demonstrated that ruxolitinib treatment resulted in resolution of cytopenia as well as improved markers of inflammation and immune cell activation in patients with hemophagocytic lymphohistiocytosis.[139] The immunomodulatory property of ruxolitinib can be a double-edged sword in the era of the COVID-19 pandemic. On the one hand, the use of ruxolitinib in treating MPNs needs to be carefully monitored given its immune suppressive properties and potential association with opportunistic infections including tuberculosis, cryptococcal infection, and hepatitis B virus reactivation, especially considering that patients with MPNs are at high risk for COVID-19 complications owing to older age and myelosuppression at baseline.[140,141] At the same time, JAK inhibitors could also be effective in the treatment of COVD-19 infection as an immunosuppressant. Studies showed that the course of COVID-19 infection is characterized by fulminant proinflammatory cytokine release with multiorgan damage similar to that observed in hemophagocytic lymphohistiocytosis and a JAK inhibitor has been proposed as a potential therapy for COVID-19 cytokine release syndrome.[142,143] Fedratinib effectively suppressed TH17 signature cytokines, which are increased during COVID-19 infection, in a murine cell culture model.[144] In a pilot study on patients with moderate COVID-19 pneumonia, 2 weeks of treatment with baricitinib at 4 mg/d resulted in fewer intensive care unit admissions as well as an improved discharge rate, with no significant adverse events compared with the standard of care therapy with lopinavir, ritonavir, and hydroxychloroquine.[145] After treatment with ruxolitinib for a median duration of 9 days, 12 of 14 patients achieved significant decrease in their COVID-19 inflammation score and 11 patients had sustained clinical improvement. Four active clinical trials are planned to examine the efficacy and safety of ruxolitinib in the treatment of COVID-19 infection (NCT04330495, NCT04348071, NCT04340232, and NCT04477993).

FUTURE DIRECTIONS: MPNs, INFLAMMATION, AND NOVEL AGENTS WITH IMMUNE-MODULATING FEATURES

Recent studies have identified several novel agents that could also control MPN progression through regulating immune responses such as molecules that modulate the inhibitor of apoptosis (IAP) signaling pathways.[146] IAP family members are a diverse group of proteins including cellular (c)-IAP and c-IAP2.[147] Originally, IAPs were found to suppress cellular apoptosis through inhibition of caspase activation.[148,149] Studies later showed that c-IAPs regulate nuclear factor-κB signaling through interaction with TNF receptor-associated factor proteins within the TNF receptor complex.[150,151] IAP can be inhibited by the mitochondrial protein second mitochondrial activator of caspase (SMAC) endogenously and SMAC mimetics (SMACs) have been used in cancer management including myeloid leukemia initially because it disinhibits the apoptosis pathway.[152–154] Subsequently, preclinical and clinical studies demonstrated that IAP antagonism also promoted tumor death through its immunologic modulatory roles.[146] SMACs have been shown to augment proliferation of cytotoxic CD8 T cells and antitumor cytokine production in vaccination and T-cell activation murine models.[155,156] When combined with ICIs in murine models for melanoma, SMAC coadministration yields improved cytotoxic T-cell activities and fewer immunosuppressive T cells mediated by type I INF and TNF-α signaling.[157] LCL161 is an SMAC that binds with high affinity to cIAP1 and was previously shown to have significant antitumor effect in a preclinical mouse model and patients with relapsed or refractory myeloma mediated by TNF-α signaling.[158,159] Importantly, LCL161 also selectively induced cell death in cell line and murine models of JAK2V617F-driven MPNs over wild-type controls in a JAK-STAT and nuclear factor-κB activation–dependent manner.[160] In a phase II clinical trial by Pemmaraju and colleagues[161] examining the safety and efficacy of LCL161 in patients with primary MF or post-PV/ET MF, objective responses based on both clinical improvements and cytogenetic remission were observed in approximately 30% of patients, supporting a role of LCL161 in MPN treatment. Considering that TNF-α signaling is central to MPN pathogenesis, the therapeutic effect of LCL161 on MPN could be mediated by the TNF-α pathway.[162]

Tagraxofusp-ezrs (SL401) is an immunotoxin that consists of a recombinant protein consisted of IL-3 fused to diphtheria toxin directed at the IL-3 receptor (CD123).[163] CD123 has been shown to be expressed at high levels in AML, myelodysplastic syndrome, chronic myeloid leukemia, acute lymphoblastic leukemia, blastic plasmacytoid dendritic-cell neoplasm and MPN and, therefore, has been targeted in the treatment of various cancers.[164] Having demonstrated effectiveness of SL401 in blastic plasmacytoid dendritic-cell neoplasm previously and attaining approval from the US Food and Drug Administration as the first CD123 targeted agent and first agent approved for blastic plasmacytoid dendritic-cell neoplasm,[165] Pemmaraju and colleagues[166] are currently performing a phase I/II clinical trial on SL-401 in patients with intermediate or relapsed or refractory MF, who failed or are intolerant of JAK inhibitors. Early results from this trial suggest that SL-401 treatment can be efficacious at doses associated with manageable treatment-related adverse events for MF. Additionally, preclinical studies (cells lines and patient samples) demonstrated synergistic effects of SL401 with HMA and ruxolitinib in the treatment of chronic myelomonocytic leukemia and MPNs, respectively,[167,168] which could be explored in future clinical trials.

As the most severe stage of the MPN disease progression, MF has poor prognosis owing to lack of effective treatments.[169] Activation of JAK-STAT pathway and associated excess production of profibrotic cytokine and growth factor contributes to the development of MF.[170] Additionally, fibrocytes and megakaryocytes have been identified as the major source of this altered milieu contributing to bone marrow fibrosis.[171,172] Verstovsek and colleagues[172] demonstrated that bone marrow samples from patients with MF contain abundance of neoplastic fibrocytes that produce collagen, fibronectin and growth factor β, which are known to promote tissue fibrosis.[173] Treatments with fibrocyte inhibitor pentraxin-2 delays the progression of bone marrow fibrosis contributing to improved survival of MF murine models.[172] Finally, the recombinant human pentraxin-2 molecule has been shown to have good tolerability and yielded improvements in bone marrow fibrosis, blood counts, and spleen size in patients with either primary or secondary MF at a median follow-up of 31 months.[174,175] Megakaryocytes are precursors to platelets and are known to facilitate bone marrow fibrosis through chemokine production.[171,176] Furthermore, small molecules that induce megakaryocyte apoptosis such as the AURKA inhibitor MLN8237 have been shown to decrease MF disease burden in preclinical and early clinical studies,[176,177] which further confirms impaired megakaryocyte differentiation as a therapeutic target for MF. The first in-depth single-cell proteomic analysis of MF megakaryocytes progenitors by Psaila and colleagues[178] identified genes that are associated with MF phenotype development during megakaryopoiesis and hence are potential molecular targets. Specifically, they demonstrated that the surface marker G6B is expressed at significantly higher level in mutant clone MF megakaryocytes compared with wild type and is therefore a potential target for immunotherapy.[178]

Finally, Treg cells are also a viable target for treating MPN. Tregs are T cells that express the transcription factor forkhead box P3 and they play important immune modulatory roles by promoting immune self-tolerance.[179] MPN is characterized by a chronic proinflammatory microenvironment associated with deregulated JAK-STAT signaling[180] and recent studies suggest that Treg population is decreased in patients with MPN compared with healthy controls.[181] Additionally, Treg can redifferentiate to acquire a proinflammatory profile facilitating the activation of antitumoral effector T cells, which has been postulated to synergize with JAK inhibition in treating MPNs.[181,182] The feasibility, safety, and efficacy of Treg infusion in treating hematologic malignancies is being actively investigated in an ongoing clinical trial by Kadia and colleagues.[183] Targeting Treg signaling represents a promising therapeutic avenue to be investigated in MPN management.

DISCUSSION

The link between cancer and chronic inflammation was proposed by Virchow as early as the nineteenth century and this concept has been solidified by an enlarging body of scientific evidence ever since that time.[184] Epidemiologic, molecular, and clinical studies all suggest that deregulated immune activation is not only central to the development of MPNs, but can also lead to an increased prevalence of comorbidities, including cardiovascular disease, thromboembolic complications, autoimmune diseases, and secondary cancers among others.[185,186] As a result, therapeutic interventions that dampen immune activation including JAK inhibitor, steroids, IFN-α and immunomodulatory drug has been used judiciously in the management of MPNs (see **Fig. 1**). At the same time, tumor cells can develop the ability to escape immune mediated cytotoxicity as a survival mechanism and therapies directed at promoting antigen specific T-cell activation including ICI and CAR-T are under active investigation (see **Fig. 1**). From nonspecific immune suppression to personalized, antigen specific immune modulation, the field of immunotherapy has made significant progress and further research will enable us to better harness the immune system in the treatment of MPN.

CLINICS CARE POINTS

- Immunomodulatory therapy in treatment of patients with MPNs have historically included various classes of agents including interferons and IMiDs.
- For patients with myelofibrosis (MF) who are intolerant or have failed standard therapies including JAK inhibitors, novel approaches including clinical trials should be considered; several new classes of drugs aiming to target the immune micro-environment, apoptosis/cell death pathways, and a host of other immunomodulatory mechanisms, alone or in combination with other agents are being actively investigated at this time.

DECLARATION OF INTEREST

N. Pemmaraju: Consulting/honorarium: Celgene; Stemline; Incyte; Novartis; Mustang-Bio; Roche Diagnostics, LFB, Pacylex. Research funding/clinical trials support: Stemline; Novartis; Abbvie; Samus; Cellectis; Plexxikon; Daiichi-Sankyo; Affymetrix, SagerStrong Foundation N.C. Chen: None S. Verstovsek: Consulting: Constellation; Pragmatist; Sierra; Incyte; Novartis; Celgene; Research funding/clinical trials support: Incyte Corporation; Roche; NS Pharma; Celgene; Gilead; Promedior; CTI BioPharma Corp.; Genentech; Blueprint Medicines Corp.; Novartis; Sierra Oncology; Pharma Essentia; Astrazeneca; Ital Pharma; Protagonist Therapeutics.

REFERENCES

1. Campbell PJ, Green AR. The myeloproliferative disorders. N Engl J Med 2006; 355(23):2452–66.
2. Tefferi A. Pathogenesis of myelofibrosis with myeloid metaplasia. J Clin Oncol 2005;23(33):8520–30.
3. Tefferi A, Vaidya R, Caramazza D, et al. Circulating interleukin (IL)-8, IL-2R, IL-12, and IL-15 levels are independently prognostic in primary myelofibrosis: a comprehensive cytokine profiling study. J Clin Oncol 2011;29(10):1356–63.
4. Beyne-Rauzy O, Recher C, Dastugue N, et al. Tumor necrosis factor alpha induces senescence and chromosomal instability in human leukemic cells. Oncogene 2004;23(45):7507–16.

5. Fleischman AG, Aichberger KJ, Luty SB, et al. TNFalpha facilitates clonal expansion of JAK2V617F positive cells in myeloproliferative neoplasms. Blood 2011;118(24):6392–8.
6. Levine RL, Gilliland DG. Myeloproliferative disorders. Blood 2008;112(6):2190–8.
7. Baxter EJ, Scott LM, Campbell PJ, et al. Acquired mutation of the tyrosine kinase JAK2 in human myeloproliferative disorders. Lancet 2005;365(9464):1054–61.
8. James C, Ugo V, Le Couedic JP, et al. A unique clonal JAK2 mutation leading to constitutive signalling causes polycythaemia vera. Nature 2005;434(7037):1144–8.
9. Kralovics R, Passamonti F, Buser AS, et al. A gain-of-function mutation of JAK2 in myeloproliferative disorders. N Engl J Med 2005;352(17):1779–90.
10. Levine RL, Wadleigh M, Cools J, et al. Activating mutation in the tyrosine kinase JAK2 in polycythemia vera, essential thrombocythemia, and myeloid metaplasia with myelofibrosis. Cancer Cell 2005;7(4):387–97.
11. Pikman Y, Lee BH, Mercher T, et al. MPLW515L is a novel somatic activating mutation in myelofibrosis with myeloid metaplasia. PLoS Med 2006;3(7):e270.
12. Oh ST, Simonds EF, Jones C, et al. Novel mutations in the inhibitory adaptor protein LNK drive JAK-STAT signaling in patients with myeloproliferative neoplasms. Blood 2010;116(6):988–92.
13. Sanada M, Suzuki T, Shih LY, et al. Gain-of-function of mutated C-CBL tumour suppressor in myeloid neoplasms. Nature 2009;460(7257):904–8.
14. Klampfl T, Gisslinger H, Harutyunyan AS, et al. Somatic mutations of calreticulin in myeloproliferative neoplasms. N Engl J Med 2013;369(25):2379–90.
15. Nangalia J, Massie CE, Baxter EJ, et al. Somatic CALR mutations in myeloproliferative neoplasms with nonmutated JAK2. N Engl J Med 2013;369(25):2391–405.
16. Lekovic D, Gotic M, Skoda R, et al. Bone marrow microvessel density and plasma angiogenic factors in myeloproliferative neoplasms: clinicopathological and molecular correlations. Ann Hematol 2017;96(3):393–404.
17. Elf S, Abdelfattah NS, Baral AJ, et al. Defining the requirements for the pathogenic interaction between mutant calreticulin and MPL in MPN. Blood 2018;131(7):782–6.
18. Elf S, Abdelfattah NS, Chen E, et al. Mutant calreticulin requires both its mutant C-terminus and the thrombopoietin receptor for oncogenic transformation. Cancer Discov 2016;6(4):368–81.
19. Theocharides AP, Lundberg P, Lakkaraju AK, et al. Homozygous calreticulin mutations in patients with myelofibrosis lead to acquired myeloperoxidase deficiency. Blood 2016;127(25):3253–9.
20. Nieborowska-Skorska M, Maifrede S, Dasgupta Y, et al. Ruxolitinib-induced defects in DNA repair cause sensitivity to PARP inhibitors in myeloproliferative neoplasms. Blood 2017;130(26):2848–59.
21. Delhommeau F, Dupont S, Della Valle V, et al. Mutation in TET2 in myeloid cancers. N Engl J Med 2009;360(22):2289–301.
22. Tefferi A, Lasho TL, Abdel-Wahab O, et al. IDH1 and IDH2 mutation studies in 1473 patients with chronic-, fibrotic- or blast-phase essential thrombocythemia, polycythemia vera or myelofibrosis. Leukemia 2010;24(7):1302–9.
23. Abdel-Wahab O, Pardanani A, Rampal R, et al. DNMT3A mutational analysis in primary myelofibrosis, chronic myelomonocytic leukemia and advanced phases of myeloproliferative neoplasms. Leukemia 2011;25(7):1219–20.

24. Ernst T, Chase AJ, Score J, et al. Inactivating mutations of the histone methyl-transferase gene EZH2 in myeloid disorders. Nat Genet 2010;42(8):722–6.

25. Carbuccia N, Murati A, Trouplin V, et al. Mutations of ASXL1 gene in myeloproliferative neoplasms. Leukemia 2009;23(11):2183–6.

26. Barbui T, Barosi G, Birgegard G, et al. Philadelphia-negative classical myeloproliferative neoplasms: critical concepts and management recommendations from European LeukemiaNet. J Clin Oncol 2011;29(6):761–70.

27. Masarova L, Bose P, Verstovsek S. The Rationale for Immunotherapy in Myeloproliferative Neoplasms. Curr Hematol Malig Rep 2019;14(4):310–27.

28. Alvarez-Larran A, Pereira A, Cervantes F, et al. Assessment and prognostic value of the European LeukemiaNet criteria for clinicohematologic response, resistance, and intolerance to hydroxyurea in polycythemia vera. Blood 2012; 119(6):1363–9.

29. Sever M, Newberry KJ, Verstovsek S. Therapeutic options for patients with polycythemia vera and essential thrombocythemia refractory/resistant to hydroxyurea. Leuk Lymphoma 2014;55(12):2685–90.

30. Vannucchi AM, Kiladjian JJ, Griesshammer M, et al. Ruxolitinib versus standard therapy for the treatment of polycythemia vera. N Engl J Med 2015;372(5): 426–35.

31. Harrison C, Kiladjian JJ, Al-Ali HK, et al. JAK inhibition with ruxolitinib versus best available therapy for myelofibrosis. N Engl J Med 2012;366(9):787–98.

32. Zeiser R, von Bubnoff N, Butler J, et al. Ruxolitinib for glucocorticoid-refractory acute graft-versus-host disease. N Engl J Med 2020;382(19):1800–10.

33. Santos FP, Verstovsek S. Breakthroughs in myeloproliferative neoplasms. Hematology 2012;17(Suppl 1):S55–8.

34. Verstovsek S, Mesa RA, Gotlib J, et al. A double-blind, placebo-controlled trial of ruxolitinib for myelofibrosis. N Engl J Med 2012;366(9):799–807.

35. Kiladjian JJ, Chomienne C, Fenaux P. Interferon-alpha therapy in bcr-abl-negative myeloproliferative neoplasms. Leukemia 2008;22(11):1990–8.

36. Giles FJ, Singer CR, Gray AG, et al. Alpha-interferon therapy for essential thrombocythaemia. Lancet 1988;2(8602):70–2.

37. Cacciola E, Giustolisi R, Guglielmo P, et al. Recombinant interferon alpha in the treatment of polycythemia vera. Blood 1991;77(12):2790–1.

38. Kiladjian JJ, Cassinat B, Turlure P, et al. High molecular response rate of polycythemia vera patients treated with pegylated interferon alpha-2a. Blood 2006;108(6):2037–40.

39. Quintas-Cardama A, Kantarjian H, Manshouri T, et al. Pegylated interferon alfa-2a yields high rates of hematologic and molecular response in patients with advanced essential thrombocythemia and polycythemia vera. J Clin Oncol 2009;27(32):5418–24.

40. Quintas-Cardama A, Abdel-Wahab O, Manshouri T, et al. Molecular analysis of patients with polycythemia vera or essential thrombocythemia receiving pegylated interferon alpha-2a. Blood 2013;122(6):893–901.

41. Yacoub A, Mascarenhas J, Kosiorek H, et al. Pegylated interferon alfa-2a for polycythemia vera or essential thrombocythemia resistant or intolerant to hydroxyurea. Blood 2019;134(18):1498–509.

42. Mascarenhas J, Kosiorek HE, Prchal JT, et al. Results of the Myeloproliferative Neoplasms- Research Consortium (MPN-RC) 112 randomized trial of pegylated interferon alfa-2a(PEG) versus hydroxyurea (HU) therapy for the treatment of high risk polycythemia vera (PV) and high risk essential thrombocythemia (ET) [abstract]. Blood 2018;132(Suppl 1). Abstract 577.

43. Gisslinger H, Klade C, Georgiev P, et al. Ropeginterferon alfa-2b versus standard therapy for polycythaemia vera (PROUD-PV and CONTINUATION-PV): a randomised, non-inferiority, phase 3 trial and its extension study. Lancet Haematol 2020;7(3):e196–208.

44. Anders Lindholm Sørensen SUM, Trine AK, Mads EB, et al. Ruxolitinib and interferon-a2 combination therapy for patients with polycythemia vera or myelofibrosis: a phase II study. Haematologica 2020;105:xxx.

45. Passamonti F, Griesshammer M, Palandri F, et al. Ruxolitinib for the treatment of inadequately controlled polycythaemia vera without splenomegaly (RESPONSE-2): a randomised, open-label, phase 3b study. Lancet Oncol 2017;18(1):88–99.

46. Kiladjian J-J, Soret-Dulphy J, Resche-Rigon M, et al. Ruxopeg, a multi-center Bayesian phase 1/2 adaptive randomized trial of the combination of ruxolitinib and pegylated interferon alpha 2a in patients with myeloproliferative neoplasm (MPN)-associated myelofibrosis. Blood 2018;132(Suppl 1):581.

47. van Rhee F, Dhodapkar M, Shaughnessy JD Jr, et al. First thalidomide clinical trial in multiple myeloma: a decade. Blood 2008;112(4):1035–8.

48. D'Amato RJ, Loughnan MS, Flynn E, et al. Thalidomide is an inhibitor of angiogenesis. Proc Natl Acad Sci U S A 1994;91(9):4082–5.

49. Mitsiades N, Mitsiades CS, Poulaki V, et al. Apoptotic signaling induced by immunomodulatory thalidomide analogs in human multiple myeloma cells: therapeutic implications. Blood 2002;99(12):4525–30.

50. Hideshima T, Chauhan D, Shima Y, et al. Thalidomide and its analogs overcome drug resistance of human multiple myeloma cells to conventional therapy. Blood 2000;96(9):2943–50.

51. Hideshima T, Cottini F, Nozawa Y, et al. p53-related protein kinase confers poor prognosis and represents a novel therapeutic target in multiple myeloma. Blood 2017;129(10):1308–19.

52. Corral LG, Haslett PA, Muller GW, et al. Differential cytokine modulation and T cell activation by two distinct classes of thalidomide analogues that are potent inhibitors of TNF-alpha. J Immunol 1999;163(1):380–6.

53. Mileshkin L, Honemann D, Gambell P, et al. Patients with multiple myeloma treated with thalidomide: evaluation of clinical parameters, cytokines, angiogenic markers, mast cells and marrow CD57+ cytotoxic T cells as predictors of outcome. Haematologica 2007;92(8):1075–82.

54. Geitz H, Handt S, Zwingenberger K. Thalidomide selectively modulates the density of cell surface molecules involved in the adhesion cascade. Immunopharmacology 1996;31(2–3):213–21.

55. Dredge K, Marriott JB, Todryk SM, et al. Protective antitumor immunity induced by a costimulatory thalidomide analog in conjunction with whole tumor cell vaccination is mediated by increased Th1-type immunity. J Immunol 2002; 168(10):4914–9.

56. Davies FE, Raje N, Hideshima T, et al. Thalidomide and immunomodulatory derivatives augment natural killer cell cytotoxicity in multiple myeloma. Blood 2001; 98(1):210–6.

57. LeBlanc R, Hideshima T, Catley LP, et al. Immunomodulatory drug costimulates T cells via the B7-CD28 pathway. Blood 2004;103(5):1787–90.

58. Elliott MA, Mesa RA, Li CY, et al. Thalidomide treatment in myelofibrosis with myeloid metaplasia. Br J Haematol 2002;117(2):288–96.

59. Marchetti M, Barosi G, Balestri F, et al. Low-dose thalidomide ameliorates cytopenias and splenomegaly in myelofibrosis with myeloid metaplasia: a phase II trial. J Clin Oncol 2004;22(3):424–31.

60. Mesa RA, Steensma DP, Pardanani A, et al. A phase 2 trial of combination low-dose thalidomide and prednisone for the treatment of myelofibrosis with myeloid metaplasia. Blood 2003;101(7):2534–41.

61. Thapaliya P, Tefferi A, Pardanani A, et al. International working group for myelofibrosis research and treatment response assessment and long-term follow-up of 50 myelofibrosis patients treated with thalidomide-prednisone based regimens. Am J Hematol 2011;86(1):96–8.

62. Mesa RA, Yao X, Cripe LD, et al. Lenalidomide and prednisone for myelofibrosis: Eastern Cooperative Oncology Group (ECOG) phase 2 trial E4903. Blood 2010;116(22):4436–8.

63. Chihara D, Masarova L, Newberry KJ, et al. Long-term results of a phase II trial of lenalidomide plus prednisone therapy for patients with myelofibrosis. Leuk Res 2016;48:1–5.

64. Daver N, Shastri A, Kadia T, et al. Phase II study of pomalidomide in combination with prednisone in patients with myelofibrosis and significant anemia. Leuk Res 2014;38(9):1126–9.

65. Begna KH, Pardanani A, Mesa R, et al. Long-term outcome of pomalidomide therapy in myelofibrosis. Am J Hematol 2012;87(1):66–8.

66. Tefferi A, Verstovsek S, Barosi G, et al. Pomalidomide is active in the treatment of anemia associated with myelofibrosis. J Clin Oncol 2009;27(27):4563–9.

67. Tefferi A, Verstovsek S, Barosi G, et al. Pomalidomide therapy in anemic patients with myelofibrosis: results from a phase-2 randomized multicenter study. Blood 2008;112(11):663.

68. Tefferi A, Al-Ali HK, Barosi G, et al. A randomized study of pomalidomide vs placebo in persons with myeloproliferative neoplasm-associated myelofibrosis and RBC-transfusion dependence. Leukemia 2017;31(4):896–902.

69. Mesa RA, Pardanani AD, Hussein K, et al. Phase 1/2 dose finding study of pomalidomide in myelofibrosis. Blood 2009;114(22):2911.

70. Garcia-Sanz R, Gonzalez-Porras JR, Hernandez JM, et al. The oral combination of thalidomide, cyclophosphamide and dexamethasone (ThaCyDex) is effective in relapsed/refractory multiple myeloma. Leukemia 2004;18(4):856–63.

71. Steensma DP, Mesa RA, Li CY, et al. Etanercept, a soluble tumor necrosis factor receptor, palliates constitutional symptoms in patients with myelofibrosis with myeloid metaplasia: results of a pilot study. Blood 2002;99(6):2252–4.

72. Daver N, Cortes J, Newberry K, et al. Ruxolitinib in combination with lenalidomide as therapy for patients with myelofibrosis. Haematologica 2015;100(8): 1058–63.

73. Rampal RK, Verstovsek S, Devlin SM, et al. Safety and efficacy of combined ruxolitinib and thalidomide in patients with myelofibrosis: a phase II study. Blood 2019;134(Supplement_1):4163.

74. Lafferty KJ, Cunningham AJ. A new analysis of allogeneic interactions. Aust J Exp Biol Med Sci 1975;53(1):27–42.

75. Daver N, Garcia-Manero G, Basu S, et al. Efficacy, safety, and biomarkers of response to azacitidine and nivolumab in relapsed/refractory acute myeloid leukemia: a nonrandomized, open-label, phase II study. Cancer Discov 2019;9(3): 370–83.

76. Bewersdorf JP, Stahl M, Zeidan AM. Immune checkpoint-based therapy in myeloid malignancies: a promise yet to be fulfilled. Expert Rev Anticancer Ther 2019;19(5):393–404.

77. Brown JA, Dorfman DM, Ma FR, et al. Blockade of programmed death-1 ligands on dendritic cells enhances T cell activation and cytokine production. J Immunol 2003;170(3):1257–66.

78. Liu J, Hamrouni A, Wolowiec D, et al. Plasma cells from multiple myeloma patients express B7-H1 (PD-L1) and increase expression after stimulation with IFN-{gamma} and TLR ligands via a MyD88-, TRAF6-, and MEK-dependent pathway. Blood 2007;110(1):296–304.

79. Rosenwald A, Wright G, Leroy K, et al. Molecular diagnosis of primary mediastinal B cell lymphoma identifies a clinically favorable subgroup of diffuse large B cell lymphoma related to Hodgkin lymphoma. J Exp Med 2003;198(6):851–62.

80. Chemnitz JM, Eggle D, Driesen J, et al. RNA fingerprints provide direct evidence for the inhibitory role of TGFbeta and PD-1 on CD4+ T cells in Hodgkin lymphoma. Blood 2007;110(9):3226–33.

81. Shimauchi T, Kabashima K, Nakashima D, et al. Augmented expression of programmed death-1 in both neoplastic and non-neoplastic CD4+ T-cells in adult T-cell leukemia/lymphoma. Int J Cancer 2007;121(12):2585–90.

82. Zhou Q, Munger ME, Highfill SL, et al. Program death-1 signaling and regulatory T cells collaborate to resist the function of adoptively transferred cytotoxic T lymphocytes in advanced acute myeloid leukemia. Blood 2010;116(14):2484–93.

83. Yang H, Bueso-Ramos C, DiNardo C, et al. Expression of PD-L1, PD-L2, PD-1 and CTLA4 in myelodysplastic syndromes is enhanced by treatment with hypomethylating agents. Leukemia 2014;28(6):1280–8.

84. Szczepanski MJ, Szajnik M, Czystowska M, et al. Increased frequency and suppression by regulatory T cells in patients with acute myelogenous leukemia. Clin Cancer Res 2009;15(10):3325–32.

85. Shenghui Z, Yixiang H, Jianbo W, et al. Elevated frequencies of CD4(+) CD25(+) CD127lo regulatory T cells is associated to poor prognosis in patients with acute myeloid leukemia. Int J Cancer 2011;129(6):1373–81.

86. Le Dieu R, Taussig DC, Ramsay AG, et al. Peripheral blood T cells in acute myeloid leukemia (AML) patients at diagnosis have abnormal phenotype and genotype and form defective immune synapses with AML blasts. Blood 2009; 114(18):3909–16.

87. Schnorfeil FM, Lichtenegger FS, Emmerig K, et al. T cells are functionally not impaired in AML: increased PD-1 expression is only seen at time of relapse and correlates with a shift towards the memory T cell compartment. J Hematol Oncol 2015;8:93.

88. Laurent S, Palmisano GL, Martelli AM, et al. CTLA-4 expressed by chemoresistant, as well as untreated, myeloid leukaemia cells can be targeted with ligands to induce apoptosis. Br J Haematol 2007;136(4):597–608.

89. Fevery S, Billiau AD, Sprangers B, et al. CTLA-4 blockade in murine bone marrow chimeras induces a host-derived antileukemic effect without graft-versus-host disease. Leukemia 2007;21(7):1451–9.

90. LaBelle JL, Hanke CA, Blazar BR, et al. Negative effect of CTLA-4 on induction of T-cell immunity in vivo to B7-1+, but not B7-2+, murine myelogenous leukemia. Blood 2002;99(6):2146–53.

91. Stahl M, Goldberg AD. Immune checkpoint inhibitors in acute myeloid leukemia: novel combinations and therapeutic targets. Curr Oncol Rep 2019;21(4):37.

92. Zeidan AM, Knaus HA, Robinson TM, et al. A multi-center phase I Trial of ipilimumab in patients with myelodysplastic syndromes following hypomethylating agent failure. Clin Cancer Res 2018;24(15):3519–27.

93. Davids MS, Kim HT, Bachireddy P, et al. Ipilimumab for patients with relapse after allogeneic transplantation. N Engl J Med 2016;375(2):143–53.

94. Berger R, Rotem-Yehudar R, Slama G, et al. Phase I safety and pharmacokinetic study of CT-011, a humanized antibody interacting with PD-1, in patients with advanced hematologic malignancies. Clin Cancer Res 2008;14(10):3044–51.

95. Assi R, Kantargian H, Daver NG, et al. Results of a phase 2, open-label study of Idarubicin (I), Cytarabine (A) and Nivolumab (Nivo) in patients with newly diagnosed acute myeloid leukemia (AML) and High-risk myelodysplastic syndrome (MDS). Blood 2018;132(Suppl 1):905 [Abstract].

96. Masarova L, Verstovsek S, Kantarjian H, et al. Immunotherapy based approaches in myelofibrosis. Expert Rev Hematol 2017;10(10):903–14.

97. Bachireddy P, Burkhardt UE, Rajasagi M, et al. Haematological malignancies: at the forefront of immunotherapeutic innovation. Nat Rev Cancer 2015;15(4):201–15.

98. Hansen JA, Clift RA, Thomas ED, et al. Transplantation of marrow from an unrelated donor to a patient with acute leukemia. N Engl J Med 1980;303(10):565–7.

99. Ciurea SO, de Lima M, Giralt S, et al. Allogeneic stem cell transplantation for myelofibrosis with leukemic transformation. Biol Blood Marrow Transplant 2010;16(4):555–9.

100. Popat UR, Mehta RS, Bassett R, et al. Fludarabine with a higher versus lower dose of myeloablative timed-sequential busulfan in older patients and patients with comorbidities: an open-label, non-stratified, randomised phase 2 trial. Lancet Haematol 2018;5(11):e532–42.

101. Mehta RS, Bassett R, Olson A, et al. Myeloablative conditioning using timed-sequential busulfan plus fludarabine in older patients with acute myeloid leukemia: long-term results of a prospective phase II clinical trial. Haematologica 2019;104(12):e555–7.

102. Weiden PL, Flournoy N, Thomas ED, et al. Antileukemic effect of graft-versus-host disease in human recipients of allogeneic-marrow grafts. N Engl J Med 1979;300(19):1068–73.

103. Korngold R, Sprent J. Lethal graft-versus-host disease after bone marrow transplantation across minor histocompatibility barriers in mice. Prevention by removing mature T cells from marrow. J Exp Med 1978;148(6):1687–98.

104. Ruggeri L, Capanni M, Urbani E, et al. Effectiveness of donor natural killer cell alloreactivity in mismatched hematopoietic transplants. Science 2002;295(5562):2097–100.

105. Kolb HJ, Mittermuller J, Clemm C, et al. Donor leukocyte transfusions for treatment of recurrent chronic myelogenous leukemia in marrow transplant patients. Blood 1990;76(12):2462–5.

106. Collins RH Jr, Shpilberg O, Drobyski WR, et al. Donor leukocyte infusions in 140 patients with relapsed malignancy after allogeneic bone marrow transplantation. J Clin Oncol 1997;15(2):433–44.

107. Lee SJ, Klein JP, Barrett AJ, et al. Severity of chronic graft-versus-host disease: association with treatment-related mortality and relapse. Blood 2002;100(2):406–14.

108. Flowers ME, Inamoto Y, Carpenter PA, et al. Comparative analysis of risk factors for acute graft-versus-host disease and for chronic graft-versus-host disease according to National Institutes of Health consensus criteria. Blood 2011;117(11):3214–9.

109. Garnett C, Apperley JF, Pavlu J. Treatment and management of graft-versus-host disease: improving response and survival. Ther Adv Hematol 2013;4(6): 366–78.

110. Chao N. Finally, a successful randomized trial for GVHD. N Engl J Med 2020; 382(19):1853–4.

111. Jenq RR, van den Brink MR. Allogeneic haematopoietic stem cell transplantation: individualized stem cell and immune therapy of cancer. Nat Rev Cancer 2010;10(3):213–21.

112. Porter DL, Levine BL, Kalos M, et al. Chimeric antigen receptor-modified T cells in chronic lymphoid leukemia. N Engl J Med 2011;365(8):725–33.

113. Gilboa E. The makings of a tumor rejection antigen. Immunity 1999;11(3): 263–70.

114. Schumacher TN, Schreiber RD. Neoantigens in cancer immunotherapy. Science 2015;348(6230):69–74.

115. Holmstrom MO, Hjortso MD, Ahmad SM, et al. The JAK2V617F mutation is a target for specific T cells in the JAK2V617F-positive myeloproliferative neoplasms. Leukemia 2017;31(2):495–8.

116. Holmstrom MO, Martinenaite E, Ahmad SM, et al. The calreticulin (CALR) exon 9 mutations are promising targets for cancer immune therapy. Leukemia 2018; 32(2):429–37.

117. Cimen Bozkus C, Roudko V, Finnigan JP, et al. Immune checkpoint blockade enhances shared neoantigen-induced T-cell immunity directed against mutated calreticulin in myeloproliferative neoplasms. Cancer Discov 2019;9(9): 1192–207.

118. Pecquet Ch BT Cl, Roy A, Vertenoeil G, et al. Secreted mutant calreticulins as rogue cytokines trigger thrombopoietin receptor activation specifically in CALR mutated cells: perspectives for MPN therapy. Blood 2018;132:4 [Abstract].

119. Liu P, Zhao L, Loos F, et al. Immunosuppression by mutated calreticulin released from malignant cells. Mol Cell 2020;77(4):748–760 e749.

120. Laengle J, Kabiljo J, Hunter L, et al. Histone deacetylase inhibitors valproic acid and vorinostat enhance trastuzumab-mediated antibody-dependent cell-mediated phagocytosis. J Immunother Cancer 2020;8(1):e000195.

121. Huang Y, Ma Y, Gao P, et al. Targeting CD47: the achievements and concerns of current studies on cancer immunotherapy. J Thorac Dis 2017;9(2):E168–74.

122. Majeti R, Chao MP, Alizadeh AA, et al. CD47 is an adverse prognostic factor and therapeutic antibody target on human acute myeloid leukemia stem cells. Cell 2009;138(2):286–99.

123. Jaiswal S, Jamieson CH, Pang WW, et al. CD47 is upregulated on circulating hematopoietic stem cells and leukemia cells to avoid phagocytosis. Cell 2009; 138(2):271–85.

124. Rinaldi CR, Boasman K, Simmonds M. Expression of CD47 and CALR in myeloproliferative neoplasms and myelodysplastic syndrome: potential new therapeutical targets. J Clin Oncol 2020;38(15_suppl):7557.

125. How J, Hobbs GS, Mullally A. Mutant calreticulin in myeloproliferative neoplasms. Blood 2019;134(25):2242–8.

126. Rashidi A, Walter RB. Antigen-specific immunotherapy for acute myeloid leukemia: where are we now, and where do we go from here? Expert Rev Hematol 2016;9(4):335–50.

127. Ruella M, Barrett DM, Kenderian SS, et al. Dual CD19 and CD123 targeting prevents antigen-loss relapses after CD19-directed immunotherapies. J Clin Invest 2016;126(10):3814–26.
128. Zah E, Lin MY, Silva-Benedict A, et al. T cells expressing CD19/CD20 bispecific chimeric antigen receptors prevent antigen escape by malignant B cells. Cancer Immunol Res 2016;4(6):498–508.
129. Gupta V, Hari P, Hoffman R. Allogeneic hematopoietic cell transplantation for myelofibrosis in the era of JAK inhibitors. Blood 2012;120(7):1367–79.
130. Porpaczy E, Tripolt S, Hoelbl-Kovacic A, et al. Aggressive B-cell lymphomas in patients with myelofibrosis receiving JAK1/2 inhibitor therapy. Blood 2018; 132(7):694–706.
131. Pemmaraju N, Kantarjian H, Nastoupil L, et al. Characteristics of patients with myeloproliferative neoplasms with lymphoma, with or without JAK inhibitor therapy. Blood 2019;133(21):2348–51.
132. Rumi E, Zibellini S. JAK inhibitors and risk of B-cell lymphomas. Blood 2019; 133(21):2251–3.
133. Rumi E, Zibellini S, Boveri E, et al. Ruxolitinib treatment and risk of B-cell lymphomas in myeloproliferative neoplasms. Am J Hematol 2019;94(7):E185–8.
134. Maffioli M, Giorgino T, Mora B, et al. Second primary malignancies in ruxolitinib-treated myelofibrosis: real-world evidence from 219 consecutive patients. Blood Adv 2019;3(21):3196–200.
135. Verstovsek S, Mesa RA, Gotlib J, et al. Long-term treatment with ruxolitinib for patients with myelofibrosis: 5-year update from the randomized, double-blind, placebo-controlled, phase 3 COMFORT-I trial. J Hematol Oncol 2017;10(1):55.
136. Harrison CN, Vannucchi AM, Kiladjian JJ, et al. Long-term findings from COMFORT-II, a phase 3 study of ruxolitinib vs best available therapy for myelofibrosis. Leukemia 2016;30(8):1701–7.
137. Al-Ali HK, Griesshammer M, le Coutre P, et al. Safety and efficacy of ruxolitinib in an open-label, multicenter, single-arm phase 3b expanded-access study in patients with myelofibrosis: a snapshot of 1144 patients in the JUMP trial. Haematologica 2016;101(9):1065–73.
138. Levy R, Fusaro M, Guerin F, et al. Efficacy of ruxolitinib in subcutaneous panniculitis-like T-cell lymphoma and hemophagocytic lymphohistiocytosis. Blood Adv 2020;4(7):1383–7.
139. Ahmed A, Merrill SA, Alsawah F, et al. Ruxolitinib in adult patients with secondary haemophagocytic lymphohistiocytosis: an open-label, single-centre, pilot trial. Lancet Haematol 2019;6(12):e630–7.
140. Paul S, Rausch CR, Jain N, et al. Treating leukemia in the time of COVID-19. Acta Haematol 2020;1–13. https://doi.org/10.1159/000508199.
141. Dioverti MV, Abu Saleh OM, Tande AJ. Infectious complications in patients on treatment with Ruxolitinib: case report and review of the literature. Infect Dis (Lond) 2018;50(5):381–7.
142. Mehta P, McAuley DF, Brown M, et al. COVID-19: consider cytokine storm syndromes and immunosuppression. Lancet 2020;395(10229):1033–4.
143. Richardson P, Griffin I, Tucker C, et al. Baricitinib as potential treatment for 2019-nCoV acute respiratory disease. Lancet 2020;395(10223):e30–1.
144. Wu D, Yang XO. TH17 responses in cytokine storm of COVID-19: an emerging target of JAK2 inhibitor Fedratinib. J Microbiol Immunol Infect 2020;53(3): 368–70.
145. Cantini F, Niccoli L, Matarrese D, et al. Baricitinib therapy in COVID-19: a pilot study on safety and clinical impact. J Infect 2020;81(2):318–56.

146. Dougan SK, Dougan M. Regulation of innate and adaptive antitumor immunity by IAP antagonists. Immunotherapy 2018;10(9):787–96.
147. Dynek JN, Vucic D. Antagonists of IAP proteins as cancer therapeutics. Cancer Lett 2013;332(2):206–14.
148. Crook NE, Clem RJ, Miller LK. An apoptosis-inhibiting baculovirus gene with a zinc finger-like motif. J Virol 1993;67(4):2168–74.
149. Riedl SJ, Renatus M, Schwarzenbacher R, et al. Structural basis for the inhibition of caspase-3 by XIAP. Cell 2001;104(5):791–800.
150. Vince JE, Wong WW, Khan N, et al. IAP antagonists target cIAP1 to induce TNFalpha-dependent apoptosis. Cell 2007;131(4):682–93.
151. Varfolomeev E, Blankenship JW, Wayson SM, et al. IAP antagonists induce autoubiquitination of c-IAPs, NF-kappaB activation, and TNFalpha-dependent apoptosis. Cell 2007;131(4):669–81.
152. Boddu P, Carter BZ, Verstovsek S, et al. SMAC mimetics as potential cancer therapeutics in myeloid malignancies. Br J Haematol 2019;185(2):219–31.
153. Infante JR, Dees EC, Olszanski AJ, et al. Phase I dose-escalation study of LCL161, an oral inhibitor of apoptosis proteins inhibitor, in patients with advanced solid tumors. J Clin Oncol 2014;32(28):3103–10.
154. Carter BZ, Mak PY, Mak DH, et al. Synergistic targeting of AML stem/progenitor cells with IAP antagonist birinapant and demethylating agents. J Natl Cancer Inst 2014;106(2):djt440.
155. Dougan M, Dougan S, Slisz J, et al. IAP inhibitors enhance co-stimulation to promote tumor immunity. J Exp Med 2010;207(10):2195–206.
156. Clancy-Thompson E, Ali L, Bruck PT, et al. IAP antagonists enhance cytokine production from mouse and human iNKT cells. Cancer Immunol Res 2018; 6(1):25–35.
157. Beug ST, Beauregard CE, Healy C, et al. Smac mimetics synergize with immune checkpoint inhibitors to promote tumour immunity against glioblastoma. Nat Commun 2017;8:14278.
158. Gyrd-Hansen M, Meier P. IAPs: from caspase inhibitors to modulators of NF-kappaB, inflammation and cancer. Nat Rev Cancer 2010;10(8):561–74.
159. Chesi M, Mirza NN, Garbitt VM, et al. IAP antagonists induce anti-tumor immunity in multiple myeloma. Nat Med 2016;22(12):1411–20.
160. Craver BM, Nguyen TK, Nguyen J, et al. The SMAC mimetic LCL-161 selectively targets JAK2(V617F) mutant cells. Exp Hematol Oncol 2020;9:1.
161. Pemmaraju N, Carter BZ, Kantarjian HM, et al. Results for Phase II clinical trial of LCL161, a SMAC mimetic, in patients with primary myelofibrosis (PMF), post-polycythemia vera myelofibrosis (post-PV MF) or post-essential thrombocytosis myelofibrosis (post-ET MF). Blood 2016;128(22):3105.
162. Heaton WL, Senina AV, Pomicter AD, et al. Autocrine TNF signaling favors malignant cells in myelofibrosis in a Tnfr2-dependent fashion. Leukemia 2018; 32(11):2399–411.
163. Frankel AE, Ramage J, Kiser M, et al. Characterization of diphtheria fusion proteins targeted to the human interleukin-3 receptor. Protein Eng 2000;13(8): 575–81.
164. Economides MP, McCue D, Lane AA, et al. Tagraxofusp, the first CD123-targeted therapy and first targeted treatment for blastic plasmacytoid dendritic cell neoplasm. Expert Rev Clin Pharmacol 2019;12(10):941–6.
165. Pemmaraju N, Lane AA, Sweet KL, et al. Tagraxofusp in blastic plasmacytoid dendritic-cell neoplasm. N Engl J Med 2019;380(17):1628–37.

166. Pemmaraju N, Gupta V, Ali H, et al. Results from a Phase 1/2 clinical trial of ta-graxofusp (SL-401) in Patients with Intermediate, or High Risk, Relapsed/Re-fractory Myelofibrosis. Blood 2019;134(Supplement_1):558.

167. Krishnan A, Pagane M, Roshal M, et al. Evaluation of tagraxofusp (SL-401) alone and in combination with ruxolitinib for the treatment of myeloproliferative neo-plasms. Blood 2019;134(Supplement_1):2967.

168. Krishnan A, Li B, Pagane M, et al. Evaluation of combination tagraxofusp (SL-401) and hypomethylating agent (HMA) therapy for the treatment of chronic myelomonocytic leukemia (CMML). Blood 2018;132(Supplement 1):1809.

169. O'Sullivan JM, Harrison CN. Myelofibrosis: clinicopathologic features, prog-nosis, and management. Clin Adv Hematol Oncol 2018;16(2):121–31.

170. Rampal R, Al-Shahrour F, Abdel-Wahab O, et al. Integrated genomic analysis il-lustrates the central role of JAK-STAT pathway activation in myeloproliferative neoplasm pathogenesis. Blood 2014;123(22):e123–33.

171. Ciurea SO, Merchant D, Mahmud N, et al. Pivotal contributions of megakaryo-cytes to the biology of idiopathic myelofibrosis. Blood 2007;110(3):986–93.

172. Verstovsek S, Manshouri T, Pilling D, et al. Role of neoplastic monocyte-derived fibrocytes in primary myelofibrosis. J Exp Med 2016;213(9):1723–40.

173. Agarwal A, Morrone K, Bartenstein M, et al. Bone marrow fibrosis in primary myelofibrosis: pathogenic mechanisms and the role of TGF-beta. Stem Cell In-vestig 2016;3:5.

174. Verstovsek S, Hasserjian RP, Pozdnyakova O, et al. PRM-151 in myelofibrosis: efficacy and safety in an open label extension study. Blood 2018; 132(Supplement 1):686.

175. Verstovsek S, Mesa RA, Foltz LM, et al. PRM-151 in myelofibrosis: durable effi-cacy and safety at 72 weeks. Blood 2015;126(23):56.

176. Eliades A, Papadantonakis N, Bhupatiraju A, et al. Control of megakaryocyte expansion and bone marrow fibrosis by lysyl oxidase. J Biol Chem 2011; 286(31):27630–8.

177. Wen QJ, Yang Q, Goldenson B, et al. Targeting megakaryocytic-induced fibrosis in myeloproliferative neoplasms by AURKA inhibition. Nat Med 2015; 21(12):1473–80.

178. Psaila B, Wang G, Rodriguez-Meira A, et al. Single-Cell Analyses Reveal Megakaryocyte-Biased Hematopoiesis in Myelofibrosis and Identify Mutant Clone-Specific Targets. Mol Cell 2020;78(3):477–492 e478.

179. Sakaguchi S, Miyara M, Costantino CM, et al. FOXP3+ regulatory T cells in the human immune system. Nat Rev Immunol 2010;10(7):490–500.

180. Hasselbalch HC. Perspectives on chronic inflammation in essential thrombocy-themia, polycythemia vera, and myelofibrosis: is chronic inflammation a trigger and driver of clonal evolution and development of accelerated atherosclerosis and second cancer? Blood 2012;119(14):3219–25.

181. Keohane C, Kordasti S, Seidl T, et al. JAK inhibition induces silencing of T Help-er cytokine secretion and a profound reduction in T regulatory cells. Br J Hae-matol 2015;171(1):60–73.

182. Sharma MD, Hou DY, Baban B, et al. Reprogrammed foxp3(+) regulatory T cells provide essential help to support cross-presentation and CD8(+) T cell priming in naive mice. Immunity 2010;33(6):942–54.

183. Kadia TM, Ma H, Zeng K, et al. Phase I clinical trial of CK0801 (cord blood reg-ulatory T cells) in patients with bone marrow failure syndrome (BMF) including aplastic anemia, myelodysplasia and myelofibrosis. Blood 2019; 134(Supplement_1):1221.

184. Balkwill F, Mantovani A. Inflammation and cancer: back to Virchow? Lancet 2001;357(9255):539–45.
185. Hasselbalch HC, Bjorn ME. MPNs as inflammatory diseases: the evidence, consequences, and perspectives. Mediators Inflamm 2015;2015:102476.
186. Hermouet S, Hasselbalch HC, Cokic V. Mediators of inflammation in myeloproliferative neoplasms: state of the art. Mediators Inflamm 2015;2015:964613.

Advancing Effective Clinical Trial Designs for Myelofibrosis

Heidi E. Kosiorek, MS, Amylou C. Dueck, PhD*

KEYWORDS

- Clinical trials • Myelofibrosis • Adaptive designs • Biostatistics • Endpoints
- Symptoms • Quality of life • Phase I design

KEY POINTS

- Phase I and phase II adaptive designs may be useful for clinical trials of myelofibrosis.
- Clinical trial designs in myelofibrosis have shifted in recent years to accommodate new challenges in the post–JAK inhibitors approval era.
- Despite the availability of standardized response criteria, alternative measures of response in clinical trials evaluating newer agents may be warranted.
- Patient-reported symptoms remain a key outcome in myelofibrosis clinical trials, particularly in the phase III setting; a validated questionnaire is available for measurement of patient symptom burden.

INTRODUCTION

Myelofibrosis (MF) is a myeloproliferative neoplasm (MPN) associated with bone marrow fibrosis, cytopenias, constitutional symptoms, hepatosplenomegaly, and/or extramedullary hematopoiesis. Patients are at risk for premature death due to disease progression, leukemic transformation, thrombohemorrhagic complications, and infections. MF is a rare cancer and can be primary in nature or the result of post–polycythemia vera (PV) or post-essential thrombocythemia (ET) transformation, with a median age of onset of 67 years.[1] Median survival in MF from diagnosis ranges from 2.3 years to 15.9 years, depending on risk category, and thus MF can become chronic in nature for patients with low-risk disease.[2] A majority of patients have intermediate or high-risk disease and are eligible to receive JAK inhibitor treatment as first-line therapy.

Effectiveness of ruxolitinib, a JAK inhibitor, for reduction of splenomegaly and symptom relief in MF was demonstrated in both COMFORT-I and COMFORT-II phase III

Department of Health Sciences Research, Division of Biomedical Statistics and Informatics, Johnson Research Building, 13400 East Shea Boulevard, Scottsdale, AZ 85259, USA
* Corresponding author.
E-mail address: dueck.amylou@mayo.edu

Hematol Oncol Clin N Am 35 (2021) 431–444
https://doi.org/10.1016/j.hoc.2020.12.009
0889-8588/21/© 2020 Elsevier Inc. All rights reserved.

hemonc.theclinics.com

trials.[3,4] Fedratinib, also a JAK inhibitor, was effective for reducing splenomegaly and symptom burden in more than one-third of patients with MF in an international, double-blind, placebo-controlled trial.[5] Food and Drug Administration (FDA) approval of both JAK inhibitors as MF treatments has changed the treatment landscape for MF and thus increased complexity of clinical trial designs in MF. Many patients with MF have insufficient response, intolerance, or loss of initial response to ruxolitinib.[6] Thus, clinical trials likely will shift to focus on development of novel agents for patients who become resistant to or intolerant of either of these agents. Alternative approaches also may include testing of experimental agents in combination with an approved JAK inhibitor.

Evaluating efficacy and response in clinical trials is challenging because MF response criteria are multifaceted and incorporate hematologic parameters, bone marrow fibrosis, splenomegaly, transfusion dependency, and symptom measures along with molecular and cytogenetic changes. Considering alternative ways to measure response with newer agents may be warranted. This article focuses discussion on clinical trial designs as related to therapeutics for treatment of MF (primary, post-PV, or post-ET types). Nonpharmacologic interventions may represent promising therapeutic strategies and improve MF patient care.[7,8] Challenges in designing symptom management trials in cancer with complementary and alternative medicines are discussed by Buchanan and colleagues.[9]

PHASE I

Phase I trials are conducted to understand how well a drug/biologic can be tolerated in a small number of patients and may represent a first-in-human study. Phase I studies also can be used to evaluate standard-of-care treatment combined for the first time with another tested therapy or a new modality (eg, immunotherapy). Determining the maximum tolerated dose (MTD) for further testing is the goal of a phase I dose-escalation trial. Typically, the design starts with the lowest dose and escalates dosing levels until the MTD is reached based on dose-limiting toxicities (DLTs). Ethical considerations include minimizing both the number of patients treated at subtherapeutic doses as well as the number of patients treated at overly toxic dose levels. Phase I trials can be categorized generally as (1) rule based, (2) model based, and (3) model assisted (**Table 1**). Rule-based designs assign patients to dose levels according to prespecified rules based on actual DLT observations. Model-based designs assign patients to dose levels based on estimating the target toxicity level from a statistical model of the dose-toxicity relationship. Model-assisted designs are a newer class of designs that reside partway between rule-based and model-based designs, in which designs are based on underlying statistical models but decision rules can be prespecified.

Rule-Based Designs

The standard 3 + 3 design is considered a rule-based design and is the most commonly used phase I design, although other up-and-down phase I designs exist. More than 90% of published phase I trials used a 3 + 3 design due to ease of use and simplicity of prespecifying decisions in advance.[10] No prior assumptions about the dose-toxicity relationship are needed, other than assuming a nondecreasing dose-toxicity curve. In brief, 3 patients are treated per dose level to assess for DLT, usually over the first cycle of treatment. If no patients experience DLTs, the dose is escalated for the next cohort of 3 patients. If 1 patient has a DLT, an additional 3 patients are treated at this level with dose escalation only if none of these additional patients experiences DLTs. This process continues through the increasing dose levels

Table 1
Selected characteristics of phase I designs

Design Characteristics	Rule Based	Model Assisted	Model Based
Examples	3 + 3 Up/down	mTPI, mTPI-2 Keyboard BOIN	CRM EWOC BLRM
Predetermined dose escalation rules set up before study	Yes	Yes	No
Computationally intensive, repeated estimation of dose-toxicity curve	No	No	Yes
Targets any prespecified DLT rate	No	Yes	Yes
Number of patients treated at MTD can be >6	No	Yes	Yes
Rapid dose escalation	No	Yes	Yes
Good operating characteristics relative to sample size	No	Yes	Yes
Allocates a high percentage of patients to the MTD	No	Yes	Yes
Provides overdose control	Yes	Yes	Yes
Does not escalate the dose when the latest treated patient experiences toxicity and never deescalates the dose when the latest treated patient does not experience toxicity	No	Yes	Yes

Abbreviation: BLRM, Bayesian logistic regression model.

and if greater than or equal to 2 patients experience DLTs at a given dose level, the prior dose level is defined as the MTD. Therefore, the MTD is chosen as the highest dose level where 6 patients are treated with less than 2 experiencing DLTs. The 3 + 3 design assumes that the target probability for DLT takes values that are close to either 1/6 or 1/3. Disadvantages of the 3 + 3 design are that only 1/3 patients are treated at optimal doses,[11] and this design may start far from the target dose, representing a more conservative approach. This is especially problematic in rare tumor types where large numbers of patients may not be available for study and there are concerns for underdosing, and, therefore, subtherapeutic benefit of a significant number of patients might be realized. Despite these downfalls, the 3 + 3 continues to be used due to its ease of use, simplicity, and lack of software needed to implement the design. Furthermore, it is well received by institutional review boards and other regulatory agencies. Simple up-and-down, rolling 6, and accelerated titration designs also are considered rule based.

Model-Based Designs

Model-based designs have seen increasing development during the past decade with many variations. These include the continual reassessment method (CRM) and escalation with overdose control (EWOC) along with other adaptive designs. Model-based designs assume a parametric model for the relationship between dose and toxicity. The general approach starts with an initial estimate of the probability of DLT for the initial dose level and then observing the patient for occurrence of a DLT. After each patient, the probability estimate is revised and the next patient is assigned to the target dose level based on these updated estimates. These steps are repeated until the recommended dose level from the model does not change. The CRM approach does not depend on the starting dose level and the model can result in skipping dose levels (although restrictions often are implemented to moderate escalation in many studies). Benefits of the CRM approach are that fewer numbers of patients typically are needed to find the MTD than in the rule-based or model-assisted methods.[12] Disadvantages, however, include increased logistical burden and the requirement of ongoing data entry and monitoring after each patient. This can be difficult, especially for multicentered trials. Software is required to implement this approach and a strong collaboration with a biostatistician is needed.

The EWOC is an extension of the CRM method and is a Bayesian adaptive dose-finding design. Similar to the CRM, the estimated dose-toxicity curve is updated continuously. A feasibility bound parameter is prespecified in order to control concerns about overdosing, and dose escalation does not proceed if the probability of overdosing exceeds this prespecified value.[13] Unlike the CRM, the EWOC design produces consistent sequences of doses without dose skipping. Other modifications of the CRM include the Bayesian logistic regression model.[14] A time-to-event version (TITE-CRM) also is available.[15]

Model-Assisted Designs

Model-assisted designs represent a newer class of designs, with increasing use due in part to availability of software packages and online applications (R Shiny apps, Web sites, and so forth) for implementation. Model-assisted designs are based on underlying statistical models that represent a middle ground between the traditional rule-based and model-based designs with decisions that can be prespecified in advance for ease of use. An initial estimation (prior distribution) of the dose-toxicity curve is used and occurrence of toxicities in patients enrolled at each dose level provides an update to the statistical model, resulting in adjustment to this curve (posterior distribution). At the end of the trial, the posterior distribution is evaluated to identify the dose closest to the targeted toxicity level. Designs include the modified toxicity probability interval (mTPI), keyboard (which has been shown to be the same as the mTPI-2), Bayesian optimal interval design (BOIN), and others. These models have been shown to have good performance and superior operating characteristics compared with the 3 + 3 design in a variety of scenarios.[11] Another benefit is that the model-assisted designs can handle passive changes in the number of evaluable patients (such as when a patient becomes inevaluable after enrollment for the cohort closes) per dose level compared with the 3 + 3 design, which requires reopening in order to enroll additional patients to fill the required cohort of 3 patients when 1 or more of the patients become inevaluable.

The mTPI design specifies beforehand (a priori) 3 intervals corresponding to proper dosing, underdosing, and overdosing. A local beta-binomial probability model is used to describe the toxicities at the current dose level being studied. Dose-escalation decisions then are based on the unit probability mass (UPM) of the 3 intervals corresponding to the area under the posterior distribution curve. If the toxicity rate of the current dose level lies within the underdosing interval, then dose escalation is indicated. If the toxicity rate of the current dose level is within the proper dosing interval, remaining at the current dose level is indicated. If the toxicity rate of the current dose level is within the overdosing interval, then de-escalation is indicated. Dose-escalation decisions can be generated under a range of parameters (ie, do not have to assume toxicity of 1/3 or 1/6 like a 3 + 3 design). Recommended sample size for the mTPI design is $k \times (d + 1)$, where k is cohort size and d is the number of dose levels evaluated.[16] At the end of the study, toxicity data across all dose levels are combined to estimate the nondecreasing toxicity probabilities across the dose levels using a pool-adjacent-violators algorithm. The dose level with the toxicity probability closest to the target probability then is selected as the MTD. If no dose level has a toxicity probability within the target probability interval, the highest dose is considered the MTD or, if all doses have toxicity probability greater than the target probability, then no dose is selected. Overdosing is the biggest concern of the mTPI design due to the unequal width intervals of the UPM distribution. Therefore, extensions of the mTPI known as mTPI-2 and the keyboard designs were developed[17] and later shown to be identical.[18] These designs overcome the problem of overdosing by dividing the underdosing and overdosing intervals (also known as keys) into shorter subintervals. Thus, dose-escalation decisions are defined for the subintervals/keys to alleviate the concern of overdosing.

Risk of overdosing also is minimized by the BOIN design. Both mTPI and keyboard designs require calculating the posterior distribution (area under the curve) whereas the BOIN design relies on only comparison of the observed DLT rate at the current dose with fixed, prespecified escalation/de-escalation boundaries. An overdose control parameter is used to assure elimination of current and higher doses from the trial to prevent treating future patients if the DLT rate at the current dose level is greater than a prespecified threshold.[19] Similar to the mTPI design, once the prespecified sample size is exhausted, the MTD is computed based on isotonic regression. The BOIN design can be extended to use with combination of agents (BOIN-COMB) or late-onset toxicity (TITE-BOIN). A utility-based seamless phase I/II trial design (U-BOIN) for finding the optimal biological dose for targeted and immune therapies with the incorporation of a risk-benefit trade-off (between toxicity and efficacy) in order to reflect clinical practice more realistically.[20]

Phase I Designs of Combination Regimens

Dose escalation with drug combinations in a phase I setting can be examined in various ways. Depending on the mechanisms of action and potential for overlapping toxicities, consideration of the following approaches is warranted: alternating escalation of the agents in a series of sequential dose levels, simultaneous escalation of both agents, or escalation of 1 agent to the recommended dose for phase II trials while holding the other agent at a fixed (generally high or low) dose.[21] Bayesian models in this setting also are useful. The dose-toxicity probability curves are updated after each cohort of patients for both agents by using all toxicity data. Incorporating both toxicity and efficacy endpoints might be useful in the combination setting.[22,23] Synergism and interaction between agents should be considered carefully with pharmacokinetics.

PHASE II

Once the MTD has been established in phase I, a drug (or combination) may move to the phase II setting, in which the goal shifts to providing initial estimates of efficacy and ascertaining whether treatment warrants further development in future controlled trials (ie, phase III setting). Single-arm (nonrandomized) Simon 2-stage designs are some of the most popular phase II designs.[24] The hypothesis is tested in 2 (or more) stages in order to minimize the number of patients treated with a drug of low activity. The design is based on properties of the binomial distribution and requires specifying the largest success rate (typically, disease response rate) observed that would suggest a drug does not warrant further investigation. The design parameters are expressed in terms of the number of successes seen from n patients with a boundary (r) cutoff for determining whether to continue onto the second (or next) stage. The Simon optimal 2-

stage design has the minimum expected sample size overall and require fewer numbers of patients for the first stage whereas the minimax design requires the smallest total sample size overall.

Other phase II designs similar to the Simon 2-stage design include the Fleming version, which makes it possible to stop after the first stage if too few responses or too many responses are observed.[25] Single-arm (nonrandomized) 3-outcome phase II designs also exist in which the hypotheses tested also include the conclusion that the observed activity of the drug is borderline and the trial is inconclusive.[26]

A flexible, randomized, pick-the-winner design, in which patients are randomized to 1 of 2 or more experimental regimens may be used as a way to mimic clinical practice more closely, where there are many factors that determine a patient's choice of treatment including adverse events, cost, and treatment schedules.[27] In this case, the goal is to exclude a substantially inferior treatment for further study and select a substantially superior treatment for further study (continue on to phase III) when a superior treatment exists. If the observed difference in the success rate of the treatments (could include multiple arms) studied is larger than a prespecified difference, then the treatment with the highest success rate is selected. Otherwise, if the observed differences do not meet this requirement, other factors may be selected for the treatment of choice. This design is appropriate for selecting among experimental regimens (ie, selection design) and not versus a control (ie, screening design in which 1 of the randomized arms is a standard-of-care arm), because the selection design is not formally testing superiority (or more accurately, the null hypothesis that the success rates are equal). For a discussion of screening designs, see Rubinstein and colleagues.[28]

For small sample sizes and rare tumors, a design worth mentioning is the single-arm (nonrandomized) Gehan[29] design, which is a design with the minimum number of patients needed to conclude that a drug is worthy of further study or unlikely to be effective in a target number of patients. This design quickly screens out ineffective drugs in a timely manner. Based on the target effectiveness rate, the design calculates the chance of having a certain number of consecutive failures in a row (under the null hypothesis), and 1 or more successes observed in the required sample size are noteworthy for further study. For example, target effectiveness of 25% requires observing at least 1 success out of 9 patients to warrant further study of the drug.

In the phase II arena, several Bayesian trial designs exist. The Bayesian optimal phase II design is a flexible design that can include several interim analyses, can handle efficacy and toxicity endpoints together, and can apply to single-arm and 2-arm trials.[30] Similar to the designs detailed previously, it minimizes the expected sample size if the regimen has low activity and controls the type 1 error rate. A TITE version also is available for real-time interim decisions when patients' outcomes still may be pending, such as immunotherapy trials.[31]

Particularly in the era following ruxolitinib and fedratinib approval for MF, combination trials of novel agents combined with these standard-of-care drugs will become the norm. In addition, patients who are deemed refractory or resistant to JAK inhibitor therapies will be prime candidates for studying the effects of single-agent novel therapies. Designing studies that target these unique subpopulations of MF patients is crucial for trial conduct and conserving trial resources.

PHASE III

Phase III trials typically are designed to assess effectiveness of a new intervention versus standard of care, in a randomized setting. Designs can be specified as testing superiority, equivalence, or noninferiority (NI). There has been a recent interest in NI studies, in which the hypothesis of interest is that the difference between the experimental treatment and active control (ie, standard of care) lies within a difference margin of interest or that the new treatment is as good as the current treatment given. In 2005, fewer than 100 NI trials were published versus 600 NI trials published in 2015.[32] The NI difference margin chosen should be prespecified in advance of the study and can be estimated based on past performance of the active comparator arm in prior studies. In addition, FDA guidance exists as to how to select this margin.[33] The NI hypothesis is tested using a 1-sided test of the upper bound of the 97.5% CI, including the margin of interest. This may decrease the sample size needed compared with a superiority trial design if superiority of the experimental regimen is expected relative to standard of care.

Adhering to high standards of study conduct in NI trials is crucial because deviations (eg, treatment nonadherence, protocol violations, and attrition) typically create bias toward an NI result (ie, making the arms look more similar). Such biases typically are of lesser concern in superiority trials because they are in the direct of the null hypothesis (not to suggest that superiority trials can be carried out in a sloppy fashion!). In addition, NI trials should be analyzed using both intent-to-treat (ie, patients according to their randomized assignment) and per protocol (ie, patients according to their treatment received) approaches. Only reporting intent-to-treat analyses may bias results toward a false-positive conclusion of NI, because the difference obtained is narrower between treatments if substantial amounts of nonadherence, crossover, or loss to follow-up occur. Caution should be taken when interpreting studies that initially were designed with superiority in mind and then fail to show a difference; NI based on the absence of a significant treatment difference for a superiority study (ie, post hoc analysis is not appropriate) cannot be concluded. Trials can be designed to test NI first and then subsequently test for superiority difference after NI is established. **Fig. 1** shows the conclusions that can be made based on the upper bound of the CI for treatment differences of various scenarios. NI trials might be useful for comparing newer agents with standards of care in MF.

ADAPTIVE AND OTHER DESIGNS

Adaptive designs incorporate opportunities to change aspects of the study based on accumulating data and interim analyses. Changes typically are prespecified and detailed in advance. Changes made to the study can include fluctuating randomization probabilities to increase enrollment in treatment arm(s) that are doing well, sample size re-estimation, and interim methods for early stopping for efficacy and/or futility.[34] Hypotheses can be changed from NI to superiority, or eligibility criteria can be modified to enrich enrollment of subgroups that are deriving benefit (such as biomarker enrichment designs). Outcomes and analysis methods also can be modified based on accumulating data. Advantages of adaptive designs include increased flexibility and possible efficiency gains, but interim analyses rely on accurate data being quickly available for patients. Caution should be taken when interpreting treatment effects at the conclusion of the study because they are dependent on the adaptations made throughout the study.

Master trials using umbrella or basket designs have been incorporated into clinical trial design in order to accelerate drug development. Basket trials evaluate a targeted therapy in multiple diseases that have a common molecular alteration, whereas umbrella trials evaluate multiple targeted therapies for a single disease, stratified by subgroups based on molecular signatures. The Beat AML trial is an umbrella trial, sponsored by the Leukemia & Lymphoma Society, that is focused on testing novel targeted therapies and

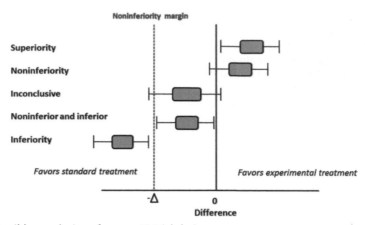

Fig. 1. Possible conclusions from an NI trial design.

combination studies in specific genomic subtypes for acute myeloid leukemia based on results of next-generation sequencing (NCT03013998).[35] As the landscape of MF treatment options and biomarkers evolves, the necessity for the basket/umbrella approach may be warranted.

ENDPOINTS IN MYELOFIBROSIS

As clinical trial designs evolve in MF, so must the endpoints used for evaluating treatment success. Typically, response in MF is assessed via International Working Group (IWG) consensus criteria.[36] Alternative response criteria are being examined, such as decreased bone marrow fibrosis in patients who have moderate or severe fibrosis, such as in the ongoing MPN-RC 118 clinical trial (NCT03895112). Overall survival has been shown to differ by risk, although this endpoint may not be feasible when median survival is expected to be long. Median survival for patients under 60 with primary MF ranged from 2.4 years to 13.4 years from diagnosis depending on International Prognostic Scoring System risk level.[37] These estimates were similar to those reported by Cervantes and colleagues.[2] A planned phase III trial (NCT04576156) of imetelstat versus best available therapy, however, recently was designed using overall survival as the primary endpoint. This trial of 320 patients (randomized 2:1) targets enrollment of patients with JAK inhibitor refractory MF and is designed to detect a 40% reduction in death (that is, a hazard ratio of 0.60 or improvement in median survival from 14 months in the best available therapy arm to 23 months in the imetelstat arm). The timely observation of deaths and strong hazard ratio both contribute to this design maintaining a feasible sample size. Overall survival as a primary endpoint likely is not feasible in a small to moderately sized trial in earlier stage disease where overall survival is expected to be much longer (eg, a combined analysis of the COMFORT-I/II trials reported a median survival of 5.3 years for the ruxolitinib arms and 2.3 years for the control arms[38]).

Splenomegaly and spleen size changes typically are evaluated in clinical trials based on imaging, such as computed tomography (CT) or magnetic resonance imaging (MRI). For example, the primary endpoint in the JAKARTA trial (NCT01437787) was the proportion of patients achieving greater than or equal to 35% reduction from baseline in spleen volume at the end of cycle 6 measured by MRI or CT, with a follow-up scan 4 weeks later. These endpoints, however, may limit trial enrollment to only patients with enlarged spleens, thus limiting generalizability to the larger MF patient population. In addition, clinical trial costs may be increased due to imaging costs outside standard of care.

To control overall type 1 error (ie, α) across endpoints in a clinical trial, sequential testing of endpoints can be performed in a hierarchical fashion. In this instance, the primary endpoint serves as the gatekeeper for secondary analysis, such that if the primary null hypothesis was rejected, then formal statistical testing can be undertaken for the subsequent secondary efficacy endpoints sequentially in a prespecified order. If the primary null hypothesis is not rejected, formal sequential testing of secondary endpoints is halted. In the phase III SIMPLIFY-1 trial (NCT01969838), formal sequential testing was stopped after the first secondary endpoint (total symptom score [TSS] response at week 24) and the subsequent secondary endpoints involving anemia response were not evaluated formally, although they would have supported benefit of the experimental therapy.[39] An alternative approach that avoids such a scenario is simultaneous testing, but usually at a cost of increased sample size, which is needed in order to split α across hypothesis tests.

Complex endpoints looking at both toxicity and efficacy combined may be useful, particularly in phase I and phase II trials. Development of better endpoints using pooled data and consortium-based work in MF is vital to evaluating newer agents and drug classes with differing mechanisms of action. For phase I/II trials, toxicity and efficacy of molecularly targeted agents may not follow traditional dose-toxicity relationships historically seen with cytotoxic therapies. As such, toxicity and efficacy may not be dose dependent in a monotonic fashion. An area of interest for future trials is the investigation of biomarkers that could provide more rapid efficacy signals rather than using typical response criteria that require several cycles or more of therapy before response assessment is known. This is an area of ongoing work and still early in development. For trials intended to support drug approval by a regulatory agency, careful discussion prior to protocol finalization with the regulatory agency (eg, the FDA in the United States) regarding study design, patient population, and primary/secondary endpoints is needed in order to support successful registration. Recommended endpoints may differ based on earlier stage disease versus the refractory setting and may involve coupling an endpoint demonstrating clinical activity (eg, spleen response), with an endpoint demonstrating patient benefit (eg, clinically meaningful improvement in patient-reported symptom burden).

PATIENT-REPORTED OUTCOMES

Clinical trials increasingly have been incorporating patient-reported outcomes (PROs). Symptom burden in patients with MPNs is assessed via the MPN Symptom Assessment Form (MPN-SAF) or the abbreviated TSS, which assesses the most clinically relevant symptoms—fatigue, concentration problems, early satiety, inactivity, night sweats, pruritus, bone pain, abdominal discomfort, weight loss, and fever.[40] Recently, to harmonize MF symptom burden questionnaires across academic and industry partners, the MF-SAF version 4.0 was developed and includes 7 items: fatigue, night sweats, pruritus, abdominal discomfort, pain, early satiety, and bone pain. The MF-SAF version 4.0 is recommended for use in MF trials and is available as a 7-day diary (24-hour recall) or 1-time (1-day recall) assessment.[41] Graphical display of TSS data appears in **Fig. 2** and follows recommendations for optimal visualization of PROs by Snyder and colleagues.[42] Statistical analysis should be conducted on the TSS as well as individual symptom items to ensure maximal use of data.

Symptom response for an individual patient in MF trials has historically been defined as a decrease (improvement) from baseline by 50%; however, this may not represent

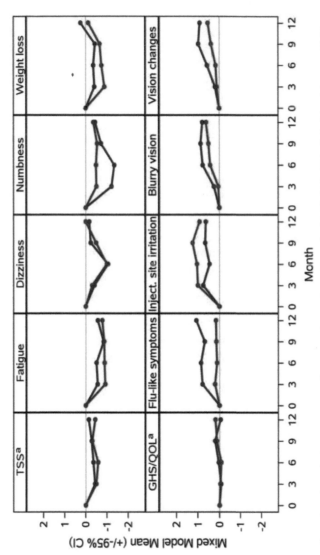

Fig. 2. Mean changes from baseline during treatment for PROs. [a]MPN-SAF TSS and EORTC QLQ-C30 global health status/QOL transformed to a 0–10 scale, where 10 represents the worst outcome for consistency with other displayed items. EORTC QLQ-C30, European Organisation for Research and Treatment of Cancer Quality of Life Questionnaire Core 30; GHS/QOL, global health status/quality of life. Inject. Injection.

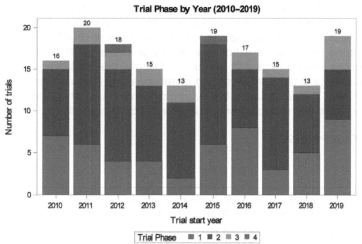

Trial Phase by Year (2010–2019)

Interventional trials with a start date from 2010–2019 were included.
Observational and behavioral studies were not included.

Fig. 3. Clinical trials conducted in myelofibrosis (2010–2019) by phase of study.

an attainable endpoint, particularly in patients with lower baseline symptom burden. Investigating other symptom response definitions is an ongoing area of investigation, with decreases smaller than 50% likely representing meaningful improvements.

In addition to assessment of MF symptom burden, other PROs should be used in clinical trials to assess important domains of health-related quality of life during a patient's treatment course. A possible approach is described by Kluetz and colleagues.[43]

MYELOFIBROSIS TRIALS DURING THE PAST DECADE

Frequency of clinical trials from 2010 to 2019 for MF treatment is presented in **Fig. 3**. Data were abstracted from ClinicalTrials.gov and reviewed for phase and trial design. A total of 165 treatment interventional studies, including MF patients (some with MF as the primary cohort and others including MF along with other MPN/myelodysplastic syndrome or hematologic malignancies related cohorts), were reviewed. A median of 16.5 (range 13–20) trials were initiated per year: 33% phase I, 56% phase II, 10% phase III, 1% phase IV, and 47% industry sponsored. For phase I trials with dose escalation (n = 41/54 [76%]), the majority proposed a standard 3 + 3 design (or other rule-based design) or did not specifically detail the dose escalation schema; fewer than 5 dose escalation trials were explicitly described as model-based or model-assisted. Approximately half of the phase I trials (23/54 [43%]) included combination treatment, with 17/23 (74%) using ruxolitinib or fedratinib. Median number of primary/secondary outcomes was 6.0 (range 1–28) across all studies. Primary and secondary endpoints were reviewed for patient-reported quality of life, symptoms, or other PROs. Overall, 63/165 (38%) studies included at least 1 PRO endpoint as a primary/secondary endpoint; 28% in phase I, 36% in phase II, and 82% in phase III. Median target enrollment for the phase III trials (n = 16) was 192 patients; only 2 phase III trials planned to enroll greater than 500 patients.

SUMMARY

Key design features of phase I, phase II, and phase III drug trials have been presented and discussed. For phase I trials in MF, incorporation of model-assisted and model-based approached are encouraged in order to maximize therapeutic benefits and include novel methods of dose escalation. Clinical trial designs in MF have shifted in recent years to accommodate new challenges in the post–JAK inhibitors approval era, and trials testing combination agents and/or employing NI or adaptive designs may become more prevalent in the future. Despite the availability of standardized response criteria, alternative measures of response with newer agents may be warranted. Finally, PROs, including MF symptom burden and other domains of health-related quality of life should be encouraged as endpoints in clinical trial designs.

CLINICS CARE POINTS

- A small number of phase I dose-escalation trials utilized a model-based or assisted design in MF clinical trials conducted from 2010 to 2019; 43% included combination treatment.
- Standard and adaptive phase I and phase II designs are appropriate in MF.
- Consideration of combination treatment clinical trial designs in the post–JAK inhibitor approval era with a small patient population is encouraged.
- Disease response by IWG criteria and patient-reported symptom burden assessed using MF-SAF version 4.0 are standard, but additional endpoints are needed in some settings.

CONFLICTS OF INTEREST DISCLOSURE(S)

Dr A.C. Dueck receives royalties from commercial licensing of the MPN-SAF. Data analysis and writing of this publication were supported by National Cancer Institute grants P01 CA108671 and P30 CA015083.

REFERENCES

1. Mesa RA, Silverstein MN, Jacobsen SJ, et al. Population-based incidence and survival figures in essential thrombocythemia and agnogenic myeloid metaplasia: an Olmsted County Study, 1976-1995. Am J Hematol 1999;61(1):10–5.
2. Cervantes F, Dupriez B, Pereira A, et al. New prognostic scoring system for primary myelofibrosis based on a study of the International Working Group for Myelofibrosis Research and Treatment. Blood 2009;113(13):2895–901.
3. Harrison C, Kiladjian JJ, Al-Ali HK, et al. JAK inhibition with ruxolitinib versus best available therapy for myelofibrosis. N Engl J Med 2012;366(9):787–98.
4. Verstovsek S, Mesa RA, Gotlib J, et al. A double-blind, placebo-controlled trial ofruxolitinib for myelofibrosis. N Engl J Med 2012;366(9):799–807.
5. Pardanani A, Harrison C, Cortes JE, et al. Safety and efficacy of fedratinib in patients with primary or secondary myelofibrosis: a randomized clinical trial. JAMA Oncol 2015;1(5):643–51.
6. Harrison CN, Schaap N, Mesa RA. Management of myelofibrosis after ruxolitinib failure. Ann Hematol 2020;99:1177–91.
7. Surapaneni P, Scherber RM. Integrative approaches to managing myeloproliferative neoplasms: the role of nutrition, exercise, and psychological interventions. Curr Hematol Malig Rep 2019;14:164–70.
8. Huberty J, Eckert R, Dueck A, et al. Online yoga in myeloproliferative neoplasm patients: results of a randomized pilot trial to inform future research. BMC Complement Altern Med 2019;19:121.

9. Buchanan DR, White JD, O'Mara AM, et al. Research-design issues in cancer-symptom–management trials using complementary and alternative medicine: Lessons from the National Cancer Institute Community Clinical Oncology Program Experience. J Clin Oncol 2005;23(27):6682–9.

10. Rogatko A, Schoeneck D, Jonas W, et al. Translation of innovative designs into phase I trials. J Clin Oncol 2007;25(31):4982-4986.

11. Zhou H, Yuan Y, Nie L. Accuracy, safety, and reliability of novel phase I trial designs. Clin Cancer Res 2018;24:4357–64.

12. O'Quigley J, Pepe M, Fisher L. Continual reassessment method: a practical design for phase I clinical trials in cancer. Biometrics 1990;46:33–48.

13. Babb J, Rogatko A, Zacks S. Cancer phase I clinical trials: efficient dose escalation with overdose control. Stat Med 1998;17:1103–20.

14. Neuenschwander B, Branson M, Gsponer T. Critical aspects of the Bayesian approach to phase I cancer trials. Stat Med 2008;27(13):2420-2439.

15. Yuan Y, Lin R, Li D, et al. Time-to-event Bayesian optimal interval design to accelerate phase I trials. Clin Cancer Res 2018;24(20):4921–30.

16. Ji Y, Wang SJ. Modified toxicity probability interval design: a safer and more reliable method than the 3+3 design for practical phase I trials. J Clin Oncol 2013; 31(14):1785–91.

17. Yan F, Mandrekar SJ, Yuan Y. Keyboard: a novel Bayesian toxicity probability interval design for phase I clinical trials. Clin Cancer Res 2017;23:3994–4003.

18. Zhou H, Murray TA, Pan H. Comparative review of novel model-assisted designs for phase I clinical trials. Stat Med 2018;37:2208–22.

19. Yuan Y, Hess KR, Hilsenbeck SG, et al. Bayesian optimal interval design: a simple and well-performing design for phase I oncology trials. Clin Cancer Res 2016; 22(17):4291–301.

20. Zhou Y, Lee JJ, Yuan Y. A utility-based Bayesian optimal interval (U-BOIN) phase I/II design to identify the optimal biological dose for targeted and immune therapies. Stat Med 2019;38(28):5299–316.

21. Le Tourneau C, Lee JJ, Siu LL. Dose escalation methods in phase I cancer clinical trials. J Natl Cancer Inst 2009;101(10):708-720.

22. Yin G, Li Y, Ji Y. Bayesian dose-finding in phase I/II clinical trials using toxicity and efficacy odds ratios. Biometrics 2006;62(3):777–87.

23. Zhang L, Yuan Y. A practical Bayesian design to identify the maximum tolerated dose contour for drug combination trials. Stat Med 2016;35(27):4924–36.

24. Simon R. Optimal two-stage designs for phase II clinical trials. Control Clin Trials 1989;10:1–10.

25. Fleming TR. One-sample multiple testing procedure for phase II clinical trials. Biometrics 1982;38:143–51.

26. Sargent DJ, Chan V, Goldberg RM. A three-outcome design for phase II clinical trials. Control Clin Trials 2001;22(2):117–25.

27. Sargent DJ, Goldberg RM. A flexible design for multiple armed screening trials. Stat Med 2001;20:1051–60.

28. Rubinstein LV, Korn EL, Freidlin B, et al. Design issues of randomized phase II trials and a proposal for phase II screening trials. J Clin Oncol 2005;23:7199–206.

29. Gehan E. Clincial trials in cancer research. Environ Health Perspect 1979;32: 31–48.

30. Zhou H, Lee JJ, Yuan Y. BOP2: Bayesian optimal design for phase II clinical trials with simple and complex endpoints. Stat Med 2017;36(21):3302–14.

31. Lin R, Coleman RL, Yuan Y. TOP: Time-to-event Bayesian optimal phase II trial design for cancer immunotherapy. J Natl Cancer Inst 2020;112(1):38–45.

32. Mauri L, D'Agostino RB. Challenges in the design and interpretation of noninferiority trials. N Engl J Med 2017;377:1357–67.
33. Non-inferiority clinical trials to establish effectiveness, guidance for industry. U.S. Department of Health and Human Services. FDA-2010-D-0075; 2016. Available at: https://www.fda.gov/regulatory-information/search-fda-guidance-documents/non-inferiority-clinical-trials.
34. Adaptive design clinical trials for drugs and biologics guidance for industry. U.S. Department of Health and Human Services. FDA-2018-D-3124; 2019. Available at: https://www.fda.gov/regulatory-information/search-fda-guidance-documents/adaptive-design-clinical-trials-drugs-and-biologics-guidance-industry.
35. Burd A, Schilsky RL, Byrd JC, et al. Challenges and approaches to implementing master/basket trials in oncology. Blood Adv 2019;3(14):2237–43.
36. Tefferi A, Cervantes F, Mesa R, et al. Revised response criteria for myelofibrosis: International Working Group-Myeloproliferative Neoplasms Research and Treatment (IWG-MRT) and European LeukemiaNet (ELN) consensus report. Blood 2013;122(8):1395–8.
37. Vaidya R, Siragusa S, Huang J, et al. Mature survival data for 176 patients younger than 60 years with primary myelofibrosis diagnosed between 1976 and 2005: evidence for survival gains in recent years. Mayo Clin Proc 2009; 84(12):1114–9.
38. Verstovsek S, Gotlib J, Mesa RA, et al. Long-term survival in patients treated with ruxolitinib for myelofibrosis: COMFORT-I and -II pooled analyses. J Hematol Oncol 2017;10(1):156.
39. Mesa RA, Kiladjian JJ, Catalano JV, et al. SIMPLIFY-1: A Phase III Randomized Trial of Momelotinib Versus Ruxolitinib in Janus Kinase Inhibitor-Naïve Patients With Myelofibrosis. J Clin Oncol 2017;35(34):3844–50.
40. Emanuel RM, Dueck AC, Geyer HL, et al. Myeloproliferative Neoplasm (MPN) Symptom Assessment Form total symptom score: prospective international assessment of an abbreviated symptom burden scoring system among patients with MPNs. J Clin Oncol 2012;30:4098–103.
41. Gwaltney C, Paty J, Kwitkowski VE, et al. Development of a harmonized patient-reported outcome questionnaire to assess myelofibrosis symptoms in clinical trials. Leuk Res 2017;59:26–31.
42. Snyder C, Smith K, Holzner B, et al. Making a picture worth a thousand numbers: recommendations for graphically displaying patient-reported outcomes data. Qual Life Res 2019;28(2):345–56.
43. Kluetz PG, Slagle A, Papadopoulos EJ, et al. Focusing on core patient-reported outcomes in cancer clinical trials: symptomatic adverse events, physical function, and disease-related symptoms. Clin Cancer Res 2016;22(7):1553–8.

Moving?

Make sure your subscription moves with you!

To notify us of your new address, find your **Clinics Account Number** (located on your mailing label above your name), and contact customer service at:

Email: journalscustomerservice-usa@elsevier.com

800-654-2452 (subscribers in the U.S. & Canada)
314-447-8871 (subscribers outside of the U.S. & Canada)

Fax number: 314-447-8029

Elsevier Health Sciences Division
Subscription Customer Service
3251 Riverport Lane
Maryland Heights, MO 63043

*To ensure uninterrupted delivery of your subscription, please notify us at least 4 weeks in advance of move.

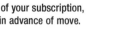